This book is t
or before t!

Species Differences in Thyroid, Kidney and Urinary Bladder Carcinogenesis

International Agency For Research On Cancer

The International Agency for Research on Cancer (IARC) was established in 1965 by the World Health Assembly, as an independently financed organization within the framework of the World Health Organization. The headquarters of the Agency are in Lyon, France.

The Agency conducts a programme of research concentrating particularly on the epidemiology of cancer and the study of potential carcinogens in the human environment. Its field studies are supplemented by biological and chemical research carried out in the Agency's laboratories in Lyon and, through collaborative research agreements, in national research institutions in many countries. The Agency also conducts a programme for the education and training of personnel for cancer research.

The publications of the Agency contribute to the dissemination of authoritative information on different aspects of cancer research. Information about IARC publications, and how to order them, is available via the Internet at: **http://www.iarc.fr**

Cover

Depiction of the ligand-binding cavities in α_{2u}-globulin (blue cloud) and mouse urinary protein (MUP) (red cloud) as determined by X-ray crystallography. For α_{2u}-globulin, the shape of the binding cavity is essentially spherical, resulting from the orientation of two phenylalanine residues which close off the back of the cavity. The two phenylalanine residues in α_{2u}-globulin are replaced by leucine and alanine, respectively in MUP, resulting in a binding cavity that is elongated and flattened (red cloud) relative to the binding pocket in α_{2u}-globulin. Although the binding cavities of the two proteins are similar in volume, the actual overlap in shape (the highlighted, pink region) is very small. The spherical binding cavity in α_{2u}-globulin is far less restrictive, thereby allowing for a broad spectrum of chemicals to bind to the protein.

Species Differences in Thyroid, Kidney and Urinary Bladder Carcinogenesis

Edited by :

C.C. Capen, E. Dybing, J.M. Rice and J.D. Wilbourn

IARC Scientific Publications No. 147

International Agency for Research on Cancer, Lyon

1999

Published by the International Agency for Research on Cancer,
150 cours Albert Thomas, F-69372 Lyon cedex 08, France

Distributed by Oxford University Press, Walton Street, Oxford OX2 6DP, UK (Fax: +44 1865 267782) and in
the USA by Oxford University Press, 2001 Evans Road, Carey, NC 27513, USA (Fax: +1 919 677 1303).
All IARC publications can also be ordered directly from IARC*Press*
(Fax: +33 4 72 73 83 02; E-mail: press@iarc.fr).

IARC Library Cataloguing in Publication Data

Species differences in thyroid, kidney and urinary
    bladder carcinogenesis / editors, C.C. Capen .... [et al.]

    (IARC Scientific publications ; 147)

1. Bladder Neoplasms 2. Kidney Neoplasms 3. Thyroid Neoplasms I. Capen, C.C.
    (Charles C.) II. Series

    ISBN 92 832 2147 8   (NLM Classification: W1)
    ISSN 0300–5085

Printed in France

Achevé d'imprimer sur rotative par l'imprimerie Darantiere à Dijon-Quetigny
Dépôt légal : 2ᵉ trimestre 1999 - N° d'impression : 99-0436

Foreword

In the absence of adequate human cancer data, it is biologically plausible and prudent to regard agents for which there is sufficient evidence of carcinogenicity in experimental animals as if they presented a carcinogenic risk to humans. However, the possibility that an agent causes cancer in animals through a mechanism that does not operate in humans must be taken into account. During recent years, evidence has developed that certain neoplasms commonly seen in bioassays for carcinogenicity in rodents can develop through such species-specific mechanisms. These include urinary bladder carcinomas associated with urolithiasis and with certain urinary precipitates; renal cortical neoplasms arising specifically in male rats in association with alpha-2 urinary (α_{2u}) globulin nephropathy, and thyroid follicular-cell tumours associated with imbalances in thyroid stimulating hormone levels. All of these conditions involve persistent hyperplasia in specific cell types from which neoplasms arise.

This publication originates from a Workshop held in Lyon during 3–7 November 1997, which was attended by invited experts from different countries, to consider how rodent tumours of urinary bladder, renal cortex, and thyroid gland should be treated within the *IARC Monographs on the Evaluation of Carcinogenic Risks to Humans*. The main product of the workshop was the Consensus Report, which is published in the first part of this volume, and was agreed by all participants. Each participant also prepared and presented an authored paper, which includes the views of the authors and also reflects the outcome of specialty group discussions held during the meeting.

The International Agency for Research on Cancer is grateful for financial support of this meeting by the U.S. National Institute of Environmental Health Sciences, the U.S. Environmental Protection Agency, and the European Commission.

P. Kleihues
Director, IARC

Species Differences in Thyroid, Kidney and Urinary Bladder Carcinogenesis
Lyon, 3–7 November 1997
List of participants

J.B. Beckwith
Loma Linda University
School of Medicine
Department of Pathology and
Human Anatomy
AH 327
Loma Linda, CA 92350, USA

A. Blair
Division of Cancer
Epidemiology and Genetics
National Cancer Institute
Executive Plaza North 418
6130 Executive Boulevard
Bethesda, MD 20892, USA

C.C. Capen
Department of Veterinary
Biosciences
College of Veterinary Medicine
Ohio State University
1925 Coffey Road
Columbus, OH 43210–1093
USA

S.M. Cohen
Department of Pathology and
Microbiology
University of Nebraska
Medical Center
600 South 42nd Street
Box 983135
Omaha NE 68198–3135, USA

W. Dekant*
Institut für Toxikologie und
Pharmakologie
Universität Würzburg
Versbacher Str. 9
97078 Würzburg, Germany

E. Dybing
Department of Environmental
Medicine
National Institute of Public
Health
PO Box 4404 Torshov
0403 Oslo
Norway

S. Franceschi
Epidemiology Unit
Aviano Cancer Centre
Via Pedemontana
Occidentale 12
33081 Aviano PN
Italy

S. Fukushima
Department of Pathology
Osaka City University
Medical School
1-4-54 Asahi-machi
Abeno-ku
Osaka 545, Japan

A. Fusco
Dipartimento di Biologia e
Patologia Cellulare e
Molecolare
Facoltà di Medicina e Chirurgia
Universita di Napoli
'Federico II'
via Pansini 5
80131 Naples
Italy

G.C. Hard
American Health Foundation
1 Dana Road
Valhalla, NY 10595, USA

J. Huff
Program of Environmental
Carcinogenesis
National Institute of
Environmental Health
Sciences
PO Box 12233
Research Triangle Park,
NC 27709, USA

C. La Vecchia
Istituto di Ricerche
Farmacologiche
'Mario Negri'
via Eritrea 62
20157 Milan
Italy

L. D. Lehman-McKeeman
Procter & Gamble Co.
Miami Valley Laboratories
PO Box 538707
Cincinnati, OH 45239-8707
USA

R.M. McClain
Department of Toxicology
and Pathology
Hoffmann-La Roche, Inc.
340 Kingsland St.
Nutley, NJ 07710 USA

A. Mellemgaard
Danish Cancer Society
Division of Cancer
Epidemiology
DK-2100 Copenhagen
Denmark

R.L. Melnick
National Institute of Environ-
mental Health Sciences
PO Box 12233
Research Triangle Park,
NC 27709, USA

R. Oyasu
Department of Pathology
Northwestern University
Medical School
Ward Memorial Building
303 East Chicago Avenue
Chicago, IL 60611-3008, USA

T. Sanner
Department for
Environmental and
Occupational Cancer
Norwegian Radium Hospital
Montebello
0310 Oslo, Norway

J.A. Swenberg
Environmental Sciences and
Engineering and Pathology
University of North Carolina
CP 7400
Rosenau Hall, Room 357
Chapel Hill, NC 27599, USA

B. Terracini
Unit of Tumour Epidemiology
Department of Biological
Science and Human
Oncology
University of Turin
Via Santena 7
10126 Turin, Italy

G.A. Thomas
Thyroid Carcinogenesis
Group
Strangeways Research
Laboratory
University of Cambridge
Wort's Causeway
Cambridge CB1 4RN
UK

D. Williams
Thyroid Carcinogenesis
Group
Strangeways Research
Laboratory
University of Cambridge
Wort's Causeway
Cambridge CB1 4RN, UK

Observers

**U.S. National Cancer
Institute**
D.G. Longfellow
Chemical and Physical
Carcinogenesis Branch
Division of Cancer Biology
National Cancer Institute
Suite 220 MSC 7055
6006 Executive Boulevard
Bethesda, MD 20892-7055
USA

European Union
J. Hart*
European Chemicals Bureau
Joint Research Centre
TP 641
I-21020 Ispra, Italy

**Japanese National Institute
of Health and Nutrition**
T. Yano
Division of Applied Food
Research
National Institute of Health
and Nutrition
1-23-1 Toyama
Shinjukui
Tokyo 162, Japan

IARC Secretariat
B. Ahn
M. Blettner
P. Boffetta
P. Brennan
K. Kjaerheim
V. Krutovskikh
N. Malats
D. McGregor
C. Partensky
J. Rice
H. Vainio
J. Wilbourn
H. Yamasaki

*Unable to attend

Contents

Species Differences in Thyroid, Kidney and Urinary Bladder Carcinogenesis
C. C. Capen, E. Dybing, J. M. Rice and J. D. Wilbourn, eds
IARC Scientific Publications No. 147
International Agency for Research on Cancer, Lyon, 1999

Consensus Report

Introduction

The *IARC Monographs* programme is an international consensus approach to the identification of chemicals and other agents that may present carcinogenic hazards to humans. The *Monographs* assess the strength of the published scientific evidence for such identifications, which are based primarily on epidemiological studies of cancer in humans and bioassays for carcinogenicity in mice and rats. Information that may be relevant to the mechanisms by which the putative carcinogen acts is also considered in making an overall evaluation of the strength of the total evidence for carcinogenicity to humans.

Following a meeting on mechanisms of carcinogenesis[1] held in 1992, a series of IARC publications have dealt with specific topics on generic mechanisms of carcinogenesis that are relevant to overall evaluations of carcinogenic hazards of certain groups of chemicals to humans. These include reports on *Peroxisome Proliferation and its Role in Carcinogenesis* in 1995[2] and *Mechanisms of Fibre Carcinogenesis* in 1996[3].

In the *IARC Monographs* programme, an agent with *sufficient evidence* of carcinogenicity in experimental animals and *inadequate evidence* of carcinogenicity in humans will ordinarily be placed in the category *Group 2B – the agent (or mixture) is possibly carcinogenic to humans*. When there is strong evidence that carcinogenesis in experimental animals is mediated by mechanisms that do operate in humans, the agent may be upgraded to *Group 2A – probably carcinogenic to humans*. However, the classification scheme allows for down-grading into *Group 3 – the agent (or mixture) is not classifiable as to its carcinogenicity to humans* if there is strong, consistent evidence that the mechanism of carcinogenicity in experimental animals does not operate in humans or is not predictive of carcinogenic risk to humans.

Numerous agents that are carcinogenic to the thyroid follicular epithelium, renal cortical epithelium or urinary bladder urothelium in experimental animals, humans or both have been evaluated in the *IARC Monographs* (see Appendix 1). A recurring theme is that both clearly genotoxic and some apparently non-genotoxic agents cause tumours in each of these tissues in experimental rodents. A second recurring theme is that, in bioassays for carcinogenicity in rodents, tumours in these tissues are often accompanied by tumours at other sites.

As a general rule, tumour morphology in rodents is similar for tumours at a given site, irrespective of the nature of the inducing agent. Thus, agents that may be acting by fundamentally different carcinogenic mechanisms may not be distinguishable by histopathology alone. However, in some cases, carcinogenic activity has been detected only in the thyroid follicular epithelium in rodents in association with a defined hormonal mechanism, in the male rat renal cortex in the presence of α_{2u}-globulin[4]-associated nephropathy or in the urinary bladder in rodents in the presence of urinary precipitates or calculi. The predictive value of tumours arising in any of these circumstances may be different from that of histologically similar neoplasms that arise in the same organs in rats or mice when these mechanisms or processes do not operate.

This IARC workshop was held in Lyon on 3–7 November 1997 to examine the scientific basis for possible species differences in mechanisms by which thyroid follicular-cell tumours in mice and

---

[1]Vainio, H., Magee, P.N., McGregor, D.B. & McMichael, A.J., eds (1992) *Mechanisms of Carcinogenesis in Risk Identification* (IARC Scientific Publications No. 116), Lyon, IARC

[2]IARC (1995) *Peroxisome Proliferation and its Role in Carcinogenesis. Views and Expert Opinions of an IARC Working Group* (IARC Technical Report No. 24), Lyon, IARC

[3]Kane, A.B., Boffetta, P., Saracci, R. & Wilbourn, J.D., eds (1996) *Mechanisms of Fibre Carcinogenesis* (IARC Scientific Publications No. 140), Lyon, IARC

[4]The protein is a urinary globulin and is properly designated α_{2u}-globulin (Roy, A.K. & Neuhaus, D.W. *Proc. Soc. Exp. Biol. Med.*, **121**, 894–899,1966). It is not a micro(μ)globulin, as the term $\alpha_{2\mu}$-globulin would suggest and this latter designation which has sometimes been used for the urinary globulin is to be avoided.

rats, renal tubule-cell tumours in male rats and urinary bladder tumours in rats may be produced. The workshop also addressed the predictive value of these tumours for the identification of carcinogenic hazards to humans when they occur alone and when they occur along with tumours in other organs. The workshop did not formally evaluate the carcinogenic hazard posed by any agent; such evaluations are undertaken in the context of the the *IARC Monographs* programme.

In the following sections, etiological risk factors in humans and experimental animals as well as the hypotheses underlying the proposed species-specific mechanisms for each of the above-mentioned tumour types are summarized. The applicability of the underlying mechanisms to humans is also discussed, and current gaps in knowledge are highlighted. Finally, for each tumour type, recommendations are presented on how the mechanistic data could be used in the overall evaluation of carcinogenicity to humans.

The Consensus Report uses the background scientific reviews that were prepared before the workshop by individual participants. These individual authored papers formed the basis for the discussions that were held and are included in the second part of this volume.

Follicular-cell neoplasms of the thyroid

Human thyroid follicular-cell tumours
Incidence, etiology and pathology of thyroid tumours in humans
Thyroid cancer represents about 0.5% of cancers recorded among men and about 2% of those recorded among women. In most countries, incidence rates are below 2 per 100 000 men and 4 per 100 000 women. Mortality rates are 5–10-fold lower than incidence rates, especially among women. There is evidence that in the last three decades mortality has been slowly decreasing, while the recorded incidence has been increasing in most developed countries (see Franceschi & Dal Maso, this volume).

Ionizing radiation is the only known human thyroid carcinogen; a history of adenoma and goitre are established risk factors for thyroid carcinoma. The evidence for other factors, including iodine deficiency and iodine excess, hormonal and reproductive factors, is less consistent. Wide

variations exist in the clinical behaviour of thyroid cancer, depending upon the histological type.

Benign thyroid tumours derived from follicular cells are relatively common in humans, while carcinomas are uncommon. Tumours derived from C cells (medullary carcinoma) are not included in this discussion. Carcinomas are subdivided into differentiated tumours, which retain both structural and functional follicular cell differentiation, and the undifferentiated tumours, which lack these features. Undifferentiated carcinomas are rare, rapidly progressive tumours. Differentiated carcinomas form up to 90% of clinically detected thyroid carcinomas and can be divided into two main groups: papillary carcinoma and follicular carcinoma. This classification was originally based on the dominant architectural pattern of the tumour, but it is now applied to describe tumours that are characterized by differing cytology, encapsulation, distribution of metastases and molecular biology; architectural pattern is of less importance in classification. Small papillary carcinomas, formerly called occult, are relatively frequent, but of little clinical significance. It seems likely that no more than a small proportion of microcarcinomas progress to clinically significant tumours. In the past, these microcarcinomas were usually found incidentally in surgical specimens or at autopsy. They are now increasingly found using ultrasound or other techniques.

The differing histological types occur at different frequencies in different countries, with Iceland and Hawaii showing the highest incidence of thyroid carcinomas, 80% of which are papillary carcinomas. These countries have a high dietary iodine intake, but it is not clear whether this plays a role in the high thyroid cancer incidence. Follicular carcinomas are proportionally more common in countries with low iodine intake, and the ratio of papillary to follicular carcinoma has changed in several countries after iodination of the diet. It is not certain, however, that the increasing incidence of papillary carcinoma is causally related to an increase in dietary iodine, as there has been a general trend for papillary carcinomas to increase for several decades. Incidence figures are influenced by several factors, including changing diagnostic techniques. In patients with congenital defects in thyroid hormone synthesis, with consequently elevated levels of thyroid-stimulating hormone (TSH), follicular adenomas are common and cancer, when it occurs, is almost always follicular in type. It therefore seems likely that high circulating levels of TSH in humans are associated with an increased incidence of tumours of the follicular type.

The role of other hormonal factors (see Franceschi & Dal Maso, this volume) has been suspected on the basis of the high female-to-male incidence ratio and the rapid rise in the incidence of thyroid cancer (largely papillary carcinoma) in females at puberty. Ten published case–control studies from the USA, Europe and Asia have studied the influence of reproductive and menstrual factors and use of exogenous female hormones on the incidence of thyroid cancer. A moderately increased risk was seen in parous women and in those who underwent an early menopause or who used oral contraceptives. The level of risk diminishes with time after these events or cessation of oral contraceptive use. Diagnostic ascertainment bias may play a role, since the majority of thyroid carcinomas in young women are detected as a consequence of medical examination for other reasons (e.g., oral contraceptive use, premenopausal complaints).

Mechanistic considerations in humans
Papillary carcinoma appears to arise directly from the follicular cell without any precursor lesion; it is the major type of thyroid cancer induced by radiation exposure and there is no evidence that it is causally linked to elevated TSH. Rearrangements of tyrosine kinase receptor genes (*ret* or *trk*) occur in a proportion of cases of papillary cancer and *ret* rearrangements have been identified in papillary microcarcinomas (see Thomas & Williams, this volume).

Follicular carcinoma appears to arise by progression from follicular adenoma. *Ras* mutations have been found in a proportion of follicular cancers, whereas tyrosine kinase receptor gene rearrangements have not been detected. The relationship between incidence of follicular carcinoma and iodine intake and the association of follicular but not papillary carcinoma with dyshormonogenesis suggest that prolonged TSH elevation may be associated with an increased risk of follicular carcinoma in humans. This effect does not appear to be large. The effect of TSH is mimicked in patients with Graves' disease with circulating autoantibodies

that bind to the TSH receptor; these patients are often treated with drugs such as methimazole, which may also cause a TSH increase. There is no evidence of a substantial increase in frequency of thyroid cancer in these patients, suggesting that short-term elevation of TSH in adults is not relevant to the incidence of human thyroid carcinoma.

In humans, ionizing radiation induces mostly papillary carcinomas. Children are much more sensitive to the thyroid carcinogenic effects of ionizing radiation than are adults.

Thyroid follicular-cell tumours in rodents
Incidence, etiology and pathology
Spontaneous thyroid tumours derived from the follicular cell occur in 1–3% of laboratory rats and mice (adenomas and carcinomas combined in a variety of strains of rats aged two or more years). In general, male rats show a higher incidence of follicular-cell tumours than female rats (see Thomas & Williams, this volume).

In rodents neoplasms derived from the thyroid follicular cell are not subdivided on the basis of pathological and molecular biological criteria into papillary and follicular types as in human patients. Thyroid tumours in rodents are usually follicular in architecture and do not possess the morphological or cytological features that are considered to be diagnostic for papillary thyroid carcinoma in humans. Most thyroid neoplasms in rodents that develop spontaneously or following exposure to xenobiotic chemicals are well demarcated lesions composed of variably sized colloid-containing follicles lined by hyperchromatic follicular cells. There often is evidence of progression of focal hyperplastic lesions to follicular cell adenomas and occasionally carcinomas. In contrast, the thyroid tumours that develop in mice transgenic for the human papillary carcinoma oncogene (*ret/PTC1*) do show morphological features seen in human papillary carcinomas (papillary infoldings, frequent nuclear grooves and intranuclear cytoplasmic inclusions). In comparison to the human tumours, little is known about the molecular biology of rodent thyroid tumours.

The thyroid follicular cell is one of the more common target sites for tumorigenesis in long-term toxicological studies in rats. Both genotoxic and non-genotoxic agents have been shown to induce thyroid follicular-cell tumours. Non-genotoxic agents can be divided into those which have effects directly on the thyroid (blocking uptake of iodine into the follicular cell, e.g., perchlorate; inhibiting thyroid peroxidase, e.g., thioureas, etc.; or inhibiting hormone release, e.g. lithium) and those which have effects on thyroid hormone catabolism and excretion (e.g., agents such as lupiditine which increase uptake into the hepatic cell or those such as phenobarbital which increase thyroid hormone loss from the liver through enzyme induction). The only known common pathway through which these agents act is the pituitary–thyroid feedback mechanism involving TSH. Among the genotoxic agents that cause thyroid tumours, some (e.g., certain dianilines) may also affect thyroid homeostasis.

A group of agents that induce thyroid follicular tumours by a non-genotoxic mechanism are also associated with the induction of liver tumours, although not necessarily in the same species (see McClain & Rice, this volume).

Radiation (exposure to either external radiation or to isotopes of iodine) has been shown to induce thyroid tumours in both rats and mice. At high doses, the mechanism of radiation thyroid carcinogenesis may involve not only genotoxic activity but also an effect through interference with thyroid hormone homeostasis leading to an increase in plasma TSH. Experimental evidence from rats shows a bell-shaped rather than a linear dose–response curve at high radiation levels, with the dose which gives the peak tumorigenic response in the rat thyroid lying within the range which demonstrably interferes with thyroid function (see Thomas & Williams, this volume).

Mechanistic considerations in rodents

The role of TSH-induced growth in the development of thyroid follicular tumours in rodents may be related to the increased chance of mutation that accompanies increased mitotic activity or to the increased chance of expansion of clones of cells bearing pre-existing mutations. The evidence that in rodents thyroid hormone imbalance alone leads to tumour formation is based on studies on the effect of iodine deficiency, partial thyroidectomy and transplantation of TSH-secreting tumours. Each of these regimes induced thyroid tumours in rodents without the use of any other agent. The frequency of tumour induction is higher if administration of a mutagen is followed

by goitrogen-induced sustained high TSH than if either the mutagen or the goitrogen is given separately. The importance of post-mutagenic growth is shown by the abolition of mutagen-induced carcinogenesis if all TSH-induced growth is suppressed. Additional evidence for the carcinogenic role of TSH-induced growth due to agents interfering with thyroid hormone homeostasis has been provided by experiments showing that return of the TSH level to normal using thyroid hormone abolishes the tumour-promoting effect of phenobarbital on the thyroid (see McClain & Rice, this volume).

Species differences relevant to thyroid carcinogenesis

Species differences in thyroid biochemistry and physiology

There are several species differences in thyroid physiology. Thyroxine-binding globulin (TBG) is the predominant plasma protein in humans and non-human primates that binds and transports thyroid hormone in the blood. This protein has binding affinities 3 and 5 orders of magnitude greater than the other two thyroxine-binding proteins, albumin and pre-albumin, respectively. The lack of TBG in the adult rat is an important difference.

Major differences are also present in the half-life of thyroxine, 12 h in the rat versus 5–9 days in humans, and in the serum level of TSH which is 25 or more times higher in the rodent than in humans. The rat also exhibits enhanced thyroid hormone elimination with less efficient enterohepatic recirculation than humans. The histology of the resting rodent thyroid is similar to that of the stimulated human gland, with small follicles lined by tall follicular cells. Thus, both the physiological parameters and the histological appearance indicate that the rodent thyroid gland is more active and operates at a higher level with respect to thyroid hormone turnover as compared to the human gland.

Species differences in goitrogenic effects

In general, the goitrogenic effects of chemicals do not operate via a species-specific mechanism. An exception is the goitrogenic effect of sulfonamides.

Some species, including rodents, are sensitive to sulfonamides, whereas no goitrogenic effects are observed at high dosages in monkeys or at therapeutic doses in humans. The biochemical basis for this species difference has been shown to be a marked species difference in the inhibition of thyroid gland peroxidase *in vitro* between rats and primates. The monkey is also less sensitive to the inhibition of thyroid peroxidase and the goitrogenic effects of propylthiouracil; however, this difference was not as great as with the sulfonamides.

Species differences in thyroid carcinogenesis

The weight of the evidence suggests that rodents are more sensitive than human subjects to thyroid tumour induction due to hormonal imbalances that cause elevated TSH levels.

Gaps in our knowledge

At the population level, it would be useful to obtain incidence and mortality data from areas of the world which have never been assessed but which are likely to have extreme variations with respect to iodine intake and other exposures (e.g., low-level radiation) potentially associated with thyroid cancer risk. Concurrent surveys on distribution by histological type should also be planned. The role of dietary habits, low-level radiation and cancer family history in different types of thyroid cancer should also be studied further by means of analytical epidemiology techniques.

Molecular studies of genes known to be involved in human thyroid tumours (e.g., *ret, ras, trk, p53*) should be expanded to link genetic changes to environmental factors where the latter are known (e.g. radiation). Other genes involved in thyroid carcinogenesis need to be identified, including germ-line mutations involved in familial thyroid tumours.

Similar molecular biological studies need to be carried out in animal thyroid tumours, both spontaneous and induced, so that any alterations can be linked to morphological changes and to the inducing agents used.

Renal-cell neoplasms of the kidney

Incidence, etiology and pathology of renal carcinomas in humans

Approximately three-fourths of human renal-cell carcinomas are conventional (clear-cell) carcinomas, the majority of which are associated with somatic alterations on chromosome 3 including the von Hippel-Lindau (*VHL*) gene. Other major renal-cell carcinoma subtypes are associated with distinctive cytogenetic features not involving the *VHL* gene. The most common of these are the papillary (chromophil) carcinomas associated with polysomies of chromosomes 7, 17 and other chromosomes and with deletion of the Y chromosome in tumours of males. Chromophobe carcinomas are another cytogenetically and morphologically distinct subgroup, characterized by hypodiploidy with loss of multiple chromosomes. It is important for future epidemiological and biological studies to consider these and other recently characterized tumour subgroups as potentially distinct entities involving different pathogenic mechanisms (see Beckwith, this volume).

The incidence rates of renal-cell carcinoma are highest in northern Europe, Australia and North America (6–8 per 100 000 in men, 3–4 per 100 000 in women), intermediate in southern Europe and Japan and low in the rest of Asia, Africa and South America. Incidence rates have been increasing in most populations, although the rate of increase seems to be slowing down in some countries and levelling off in a few others. The incidence in men is 2–3 times that in women (see Mellemgaard, this volume).

Two risk factors (cigarette smoking and obesity) have consistently been found to increase the risk of renal-cell carcinoma and together account for approximately 40% of cases in high-risk countries. Cigarette smoking increases the risk approximately two-fold and a dose–response effect as well as an effect of cessation have been demonstrated. Other tobacco products have not been associated with renal-cell carcinoma risk to the same extent.

Obesity (defined as a high body-mass index) increases risk in women and, to some extent, also in men. The increase in risk may be as high as 3–4-fold in very obese women. It is not known whether the diet, peripheral oestrogen synthesis or some other factors are responsible for the association.

Human exposure to gasoline and *d*-limonene is particularly interesting in the light of these agents' ability to induce α_{2u}-globulin nephropathy and renal tumours in male rats. Although some case–control studies have found an approximately 50% increase in risk among individuals exposed to gasoline after adjustment for other risk factors, other studies gave negative results and cohort studies of refinery workers and gasoline station attendants have yielded inconsistent findings. Furthermore, no studies have looked at leaded and unleaded gasoline separately. No epidemiological study has focused on d-limonene, but studies of diet and renal-cell carcinoma have not suggested an association with intake of fruit juice or citrus fruit which contain d-limonene.

The use of phenacetin increases the risk of urothelial cancer and, to a lesser extent, that of renal-cell carcinoma, but this drug is no longer available in most western countries. Other analgesics (e.g., aspirin and paracetamol) do not seem to influence the risk of renal-cell carcinoma.

Some studies have shown a moderate increase in risk of renal-cell carcinoma among users of diuretics or other antihypertensive drugs. It is unknown whether it is the medical condition, the drug itself or shared risk factors for renal-cell carcinoma and the medical condition that are responsible.

A possible role of diet and several occupational and environmental exposures (e.g., asbestos, cadmium, lead, pesticides, dry-cleaning processes, trichloroethylene, fungal toxins) in inducing human renal-cell carcinoma remains unresolved.

Mechanisms of renal-cell carcinogenicity in rodents

In the rodent kidney, several mechanisms of chemically induced carcinogenesis have been identified based on reasonably robust data-sets from the published literature. These mechanisms can be categorized as follows:

A. *Direct DNA reactivity*. Some model genotoxic carcinogens (or their metabolites), particularly certain N-nitroso compounds, are known to interact directly with DNA of renal tubule cells, causing genomic alterations.

B. *Indirect DNA damage mediated by oxidative stress*. At least two compounds (potassium bromate and ferric nitrilotriacetate) have been shown to generate reactive oxygen species in rodent kidneys, which in turn have the potential to cause genomic alterations.

C. *Sustained stimulation of cell proliferation*. A number of non-genotoxic chemicals appear to lead to the development of renal cell tumours through a process involving prolonged renal tubule cell injury coupled with regenerative cell proliferation. This mechanistic pathway can be further subcategorized as involving either

(i) a regenerative response to chemically induced cytotoxicity (chloroform has been suggested as an example of a chemical that directly affects proximal tubule cells causing cytotoxicity, cell death and compensatory cell proliferation); or

(ii) a regenerative response not dependent on direct chemical cytotoxicity but on cytotoxicity resulting from impairment of a physiological process; this is the proposed mechanism for α_{2u}-globulin nephropathy and the associated renal carcinogenesis.

Kidney tumours induced by chemicals in category C tend to occur in low incidence (usually less than 30%), even at high doses, with a long latency, and may exhibit sex-dependent differences and in some cases, species-specificity. This is in contrast to chemicals representing mechanistic categories A and B that can induce high (up to 100%) incidences of renal tumours which may have relatively short latent periods, and are not typified by sex-specificity.

α_{2u}-Globulin-associated nephropathy as a mechanism of renal tubule cell carcinogenesis in male rats

α_{2u}-Globulin nephropathy is a syndrome that occurs exclusively in male rat kidney. A diverse group of non-genotoxic chemicals have been shown to cause acute renal changes manifested as the accumulation of this urinary globulin in phagolysosomes of renal proximal tubule cells. The toxicity appears to be caused by the accumulation of a single, major male rat-specific protein, α_{2u}-globulin (see Swenberg & Lehman-McKeeman, this volume). The α_{2u}-globulin accumulating in the male kidney is synthesized in the liver, where its expression represents about 1%

of total hepatic mRNA. Hepatic synthesis of α_{2u}-globulin is regulated by complex hormonal interactions, particularly androgens, whereas in female rats, oestrogens repress hepatic synthesis. Lysosomal accumulation of α_{2u}-globulin leads to death of individual renal cells and compensatory cell proliferation which may result in atypical tubule hyperplasia and ultimately renal tubule tumours. Several agents that induce α_{2u}-globulin nephropathy have been shown to promote both spontaneously and chemically initiated tubule epithelial cells to preneoplastic and neoplastic lesions in male rat kidney. Furthermore, a quantitative relationship between sustained renal-cell proliferation and the promotion of preneoplastic and/or neoplastic lesions has been established, providing support for the conclusion that sustained renal cell proliferation is causally related to the development of renal tumours in male rats.

The contribution of α_{2u}-globulin to the species-specificity of the nephropathy has been shown in several ways. First, it has been determined that the NBR strain of rats that does not synthesize the hepatic form of α_{2u}-globulin, does not develop α_{2u}-globulin nephropathy and is not susceptible to renal tumour promotion by these agents. Additionally, it has been shown that, although mice are resistant to renal toxicity following exposure to agents that induce α_{2u}-globulin nephropathy, transgenic mice engineered to synthesize α_{2u}-globulin developed the nephropathy. Mechanistic studies have demonstrated that the requisite step in the development of the syndrome is the ability of a chemical (or metabolite(s)) to bind reversibly, and specifically, to α_{2u}-globulin. Binding of chemicals to α_{2u}-globulin appears to alter the lysosomal degradation of the protein, leading to its accumulation in phagolysosomes. Furthermore, a comprehensive survey of structurally-related proteins along with experimental analyses has provided evidence that, although other species, including humans, synthesize proteins that are similar to α_{2u}-globulin, differences in ligand-binding properties, physiological function and renal handling of these homologues preclude their involvement in this protein droplet nephropathy. For example, although mice synthesize mouse urinary protein (MUP), a protein that shares approximately 90% amino acid sequence identity with α_{2u}-globulin and which is considered the murine

homologue of α_{2u}-globulin, this protein does not contribute to a similar syndrome in mice.

An alternative hypothesis to the accumulation and impaired degradation of α_{2u}-globulin (see Melnick & Kohn, this volume) proposes that α_{2u}-globulin in male rats may serve to transport and concentrate the ligand within proximal tubule cells. Release of the ligand or subsequent metabolism of the ligand may produce cytotoxicity. However, one compound, 2,4,4-trimethyl-2-pentanol, has been tested and not found to be cytotoxic in primary cultures of renal tubule fragments. Although there are no data supporting this alternative hypothesis, it can be concluded that a process involving α_{2u}-globulin as a vector for chemically induced injury would remain exclusive to the male rat.

There are differences in opinion as to whether the hypothesis linking α_{2u}-globulin nephropathy to the induction of kidney tumours is consistent with the available data on chemicals or mixtures proposed to act through this mechanism. Such differences have been attributed to a lack of compliance with the criteria that must be fulfilled in order to state that the mechanism by which chemicals induce renal tubule cell tumours is exclusively through an accumulation of the rat male-specific α_{2u}-globulin. The Working Group therefore formulated the following criteria (all of which must be met) for concluding that an agent causes kidney tumours through an α_{2u}-globulin-associated response (Table 1).

Numerous chemicals have been shown to induce hyaline droplets in the kidneys of male rats. However, for many of these there is a lack of sufficient data and/or adherence to previous developed criteria, that characterize a chemical causing kidney tumours solely through an α_{2u}-globulin-associated response. Swenberg and Lehman-McKeeman (see this volume) have judged that only seven of 40 chemicals and mixtures which induce hyaline droplets in male rat kidney have fully met the criteria in Table 1 for an α_{2u}-globulin-associated response. All of the remaining chemicals need additional data in order to determine whether they meet these criteria. Some chemicals which induce hyaline droplets in the kidney in male rats are excluded by these criteria (see Swenberg & Lehman-McKeeman, this volume).

Table 1. Criteria for an agent causing kidney tumours through an α_{2u}-globulin-associated response in male rats

- Lack of genotoxic activity (agent and/or metabolite) based on an overall evaluation of in-vitro and in-vivo data
- Male rat specificity for nephropathy and renal tumorigenicity
- Induction of the characteristic sequence of histopathological changes in shorter-term studies, of which protein droplet accumulation is obligatory
- Identification of the protein accumulating in tubule cells as α_{2u}-globulin
- Reversible binding of the chemical or metabolite to α_{2u}-globulin
- Induction of sustained increased cell proliferation in the renal cortex
- Similarities in dose–response relationship of the tumour outcome with the histopathological end-points (protein droplets, α_{2u}-globulin accumulation, cell proliferation).

Do similar mechanisms occur in humans?

A requisite step in the development of α_{2u}-globulin nephropathy is the binding of a chemical (or metabolite) to α_{2u}-globulin. α_{2u}-Globulin is a member of a superfamily of proteins that bind and transport a variety of ligands. Many of these proteins are synthesized in mammalian species, including humans. Therefore, the question of a similar mechanism occurring in humans can be addressed by determining whether these structurally homologous proteins can function in humans in a manner analogous to α_{2u}-globulin. This question can be answered both qualitatively and quantitatively.

The protein content of human urine is very different from that of rat urine, as humans excrete very little protein (about 1% of the concentration in male rats). Human urinary protein is also predominantly a species of high molecular weight, and there is no protein in human plasma or urine identical to α_{2u}-globulin.

With respect to the α_{2u}-globulin superfamily, it has been shown that MUP, the protein most similar to α_{2u}-globulin, does not contribute to a similar syndrome in mice, and the lack of a response in female rats, which synthesize many other proteins of this superfamily, demonstrates that these proteins are unlikely to contribute to the renal toxicity.

Saturable binding of 2,4,4-trimethyl-2-pentanol and d-limonene-1,2-oxide to α_{2u}-globulin can be shown in vitro, but these chemicals do not bind to other members of the α_{2u}-globulin superfamily. Furthermore, it has been shown that 2,4,4-trimethyl-2-pentanol does not bind specifically to any low molecular weight protein isolated from male human kidney, indicating that there are no proteins constitutively present in human kidney that are similar to α_{2u}-globulin. The X-ray-derived crystal structure of α_{2u}-globulin further supports the unique binding property of this protein. Other superfamily proteins are characterized by flattened, elongated binding pockets, whereas the ligand-binding site in α_{2u}-globulin is distinguished by its spherical, non-restrictive shape.

From a quantitative perspective, adult male rat kidneys reabsorb about 35 mg of α_{2u}-globulin per day. Female rats synthesize less than 1% of the amount of α_{2u}-globulin reabsorbed by male rats, but no α_{2u}-globulin is detected in the female rat kidney and female rats do not develop the nephropathy. The most abundant α_{2u}-globulin superfamily protein in human kidney and plasma is α_1-acid glycoprotein, and this protein does not bind to agents that induce α_{2u}-globulin nephropathy in rats.

Taken together, there is no evidence that a mechanism similar to α_{2u}-globulin nephropathy occurs in humans.

Gaps in knowledge

For many chemicals that induce hyaline droplets in male rat kidney, there is insufficient information to evaluate whether this response is associated with an α_{2u}-globulin-related mechanism. The most important data gaps are therefore those required to establish whether such chemicals fulfil the criteria for an α_{2u}-globulin-associated response.

Because d-limonene is currently being evaluated as a cancer chemopreventive agent, it should be possible to establish in humans whether this agent produces nephrotoxicity at the high doses used in those clinical trials.

There is also a need for further epidemiological studies of gasoline exposure, preferably with quantitative exposure assessment and sufficient data on other risk factors to allow adjustment for potential confounding factors.

There is a need for further evaluation of quantitative relationships between the various intermediate steps in order to improve prediction of the carcinogenic response of chemicals operating through the α_{2u}-globulin-associated mechanism.

Information on effects of chemicals on lysosomal function relative to their abilities to cause α_{2u}-globulin accumulation is needed.

Kinetic models linking α_{2u}-globulin accumulation and ligand dosimetry after multiple dosing are needed.

Clarification of whether an endogenous ligand exists for α_{2u}-globulin would help in understanding the physiological function of this protein and might further delineate the mechanisms underlying α_{2u}-globulin-associated pathology in the kidneys of male rats. Mechanisms of cell death should be investigated.

A hypothesis has been put forward that α_{2u}-globulin serves to concentrate nephrotoxic ligands and that the renal pathology is related to a release of such bound ligands. Additional experiments designed to examine this hypothesis are warranted.

Urinary bladder neoplasms

Incidence, etiology and pathology of urinary bladder tumours in humans

Incidence and mortality rates for bladder cancer tend to be higher in developed countries than in developing countries. Between 1973 and 1994, bladder cancer incidence in the United States showed moderate increases in both sexes and various races, whereas mortality tended to decline, particularly in men. In the early 1990's, most age-adjusted mortality rates for men within Europe fell within the range of 5–8 per 100 000. Rates for women were between 1 and 3 per 100 000 in most countries and showed no appreciable changes over time. In most of western Europe, mortality has declined in generations born since 1940.

Transitional-cell carcinoma of the bladder accounts for about 95% of bladder cancer, although squamous-cell carcinomas are more common in certain regions, such as the Middle East (see La Vecchia & Airoldi, this volume).

Cigarette smoking is recognized as the main cause of bladder carcinoma and accounts for about 50% of cases in most developed countries. A high risk of bladder carcinoma has been observed in workers exposed to some aromatic amines. Based on these and other occupational risks (e.g., among leather workers, truck drivers and aluminium production workers), it has been estimated that 5–10% of bladder carcinomas in industrialized countries were due to exposures of occupational origin.

A number of other factors have been evaluated as possible human bladder carcinogens. Several studies have investigated the association between coffee consumption and bladder cancer risk. Although excess risks have been reported in some studies, the lack of dose– or duration–risk relationships leaves this issue open to discussion. There is also no convincing evidence of any appreciable risk of bladder cancer from personal use of hair dyes.

Two cancer chemotherapeutic drugs, cyclophosphamide and chlornaphazine, and treatment with ionizing radiation have been shown to cause bladder cancer in humans. Heavy consumption of phenacetin-containing analgesics was strongly associated with lower urinary tract carcinomas including bladder carcinomas in several studies, but paracetamol-containing analgesics have not been shown to have such effects.

Infectious agents and other diseases of the urinary tract, which may cause chronic inflammation, have a major influence on bladder cancer risks in northern Africa and the Middle East and other areas where *Schistosoma haematobium* infestation is endemic. In these regions, there is a consistent relationship between carcinomas (especially squamous-cell carcinomas) of the bladder and urinary schistosomiasis.

The role of urinary tract infections other than those associated with schistosomiasis on bladder carcinogenesis is more difficult to assess. Most findings, however, are consistent with a 2-3-fold elevated risk. The association appears to be stronger for squamous-cell carcinomas and may be stronger in women.

With reference to urinary tract stones, four case–control studies published between the 1960s and the 1980s found relative risks between 1.0 and 2.5. At least three more recent case–control studies and one record-linkage cohort study gave a relative risk between 1.2 and 1.4 for a history of urinary tract stones. An interesting feature of these investigations was that the association was stronger in women, with statistically significant relative risks higher than 2. Although there exists a potential for recall bias in the case–control studies and uncontrolled confounding in the cohort study, these findings suggest that the presence of urinary tract stones is associated with bladder carcinoma in humans.

No epidemiological study has addressed the issue of a possible role of persistent crystalluria as a risk factor for urothelial carcinoma in humans. Likewise, quantitative studies on cellular proliferation and possible precursors of bladder carcinoma in relation to the presence of bladder stones and/or urinary infections in humans are lacking.

Overall, epidemiological data do not indicate that saccharin and other artificial sweeteners are related to human bladder cancer, although studies in children are scanty. Occasional observations of increased or decreased risks in some subgroups are to be regarded as fluctuations within a series of multiple comparisons.

Calculi-, amorphous precipitate- and microcrystalluria-associated irritation, cell proliferation and urinary bladder carcinogenesis in mice and rats

Many non-genotoxic chemicals have been shown to induce formation of microcrystals, amorphous precipitates and/or calculi in the urine of mice and rats (see Fukushima & Murai, this volume). Such chemicals include uric acid, calcium oxalate, uracil, thymine, melamine and others. The proliferative and tumorigenic effects produced in the bladder of these rodents require the concentration of the chemical in the urine to be sufficiently high to lead to precipitate formation and ultimately to calculi.

The ability of chemicals to produce calculi varies with species, strain and sex, as do the proliferative and tumorigenic responses. Calculus formation is also dependent on specific chemical and physical conditions of the urine (e.g., pH, volume), which have not been completely delineated. Marked increased urothelial cell proliferation (e.g., papillomatosis in rats) is caused by the presence of a calculus. The same response is observed when chemically inert materials (e.g., glass beads, paraffin wax and cholesterol pellets) are surgically implanted into the bladder of rodents, or when physiological conditions are altered leading to calculus formation (e.g., uric acid metabolism following portacaval shunt). The extent of the proliferation is dependent on the abrasiveness of the surface of the implanted pellet or the number and size of calculi.

These proliferative effects of calculi are commonly sustained in rodents since these species are normally horizontally positioned allowing the object to remain within the lumen of the urinary bladder, with less chance of elimination. If the calculus is removed before a neoplasm is produced, the proliferative changes are rapidly reversed. Bacterial urinary tract infections can enhance the formation of calculi. If the calculus remains in the urinary bladder for an extended period of time, it may lead to cancer formation.

Microcrystalluria is associated with irritation and cell proliferation but its association with bladder carcinomas is less clear.

Are calculi associated with irritation and cell proliferation in humans and do the mechanisms of carcinogenesis mediated by such effects in rodents operate in humans?

Urinary bladder calculi, irrespective of composition, cause irritation and cell proliferation in humans (see Fukushima & Murai, this volume). There is some epidemiological evidence that urinary tract cancer in humans is associated with a history of calculi in the bladder (see La Vecchia & Airoldi, this volume). The risk in humans may not be as great as that in rodents because the calculi are usually voided spontaneously or removed by surgical procedures. Thus, although there are quantitative differences in the carcinogenic response to calculi between species, the effect is not species-specific. However, calculus formation is dependent on attainment in the urine of critically high concentrations of the constituent chemicals which form the calculus. The carcinogenic effects are also dependent on reaching a threshold concentration for calculus formation.

Urinary bladder carcinogenesis produced by chemicals causing calcium phosphate containing precipitates in the urine of rats

High doses of several sodium salts of moderate to strong organic acids (see Cohen, this volume) produce a calcium phosphate-containing precipitate in the urine of rats and increased urothelial proliferation. Increased bladder tumour incidences are seen when these sodium salts are administered after treatment with bladder carcinogens such as N-[4-(5-nitro-2-furyl)-2-thiazolyl]formamide (FANFT) or N-butyl-N-(4-hydroxybutyl)nitrosamine (BBN). One exception is sodium hippurate, which reduces the pH of the urine to below 6.5, so that precipitate does not form.

Other sodium salts such as sodium *ortho*-phenylphenate and trisodium nitrilotriacetate which do not cause formation of calcium phosphate-containing precipitates in the urine of rats have other biological properties which are associated with their carcinogenic effects in the urinary bladder of rats.

In the 1970s, sodium saccharin was fed to rats at high doses in the diet in a two-generation protocol (before conception, throughout gestation, lactation and post-weaning, for the lifetime of the animal) and found to be carcinogenic to the urinary bladder. Subsequent studies have demonstrated that if administration begins at birth, tumour response is similar to that observed when exposure began before conception. The male rat is considerably more susceptible than the female rat. Administration beginning before five weeks of age also produced an increased incidence of tumours, although less than when administration began at birth or earlier. Administration of sodium saccharin to rats beginning at six to eight weeks of age, as in a standard two-year bioassay, did not produce a tumorigenic response. Monkeys treated with 25 mg/kg bw/day sodium saccharin starting at birth, and mice, hamsters and guinea-pigs treated with high doses of sodium saccharin in the diet starting at an adult age (doses of the same order of magnitude as those given to rats) did not show proliferation or neoplastic effects in the urinary bladder.

In relation to other sodium salts of moderate to strong organic acids (the most extensively studied being sodium ascorbate), an effect on the urothelium has been identified mainly in male rats using either short-term studies evaluating cell proliferation in the bladder epithelium or in studies in which high doses of the sodium salt were administered after an initial period of treatment with a bladder carcinogen, such as FANFT or BBN. However, two-generation studies have not been reported for any of these other sodium salts. Only a few of these sodium salts have been studied in mice and no proliferative effect on urothelium has been observed. None of the other sodium salts has been studied in other species

Saccharin, ascorbate and the other chemicals being discussed are sodium salts of moderate to strong acids. They are nearly completely ionized at physiological pH, and as anionic structures do not interact with DNA. Genotoxicity assays *in vivo* have been nearly entirely negative. Also, the evidence does not support a role of contaminants of these chemicals as the cause of the urinary tract effects in rats. The carcinogenic action of these sodium salts involves the formation of a calcium phosphate-containing precipitate in the urine of the rats fed high dietary doses. This causes cell death of superficial layers of the urothelium, leading to regenerative hyperplasia and ultimately to tumours. Quantitative aspects of the cell proliferation help to explain the necessity for administration beginning at weaning or earlier. The formation of this precipitate requires a urinary pH above 6.5. Administration of the corresponding acids of the sodium salts does not produce a proliferative effect on the rat bladder epithelium. In addition, any treatment which produces acidification of the urine inhibits both formation of the calcium phosphate-containing precipitate and the neoplastic effects of these sodium salts on urothelium. Acidification can be accomplished by co-administration of the sodium salt with ammonium chloride or administration in semi-synthetic diets, such as AIN-76A, which produce markedly acidic urine.

Formation of this precipitate appears to require high urinary concentrations of protein, as found in rats. Male rats are more susceptible than female rats, presumably because of the higher concentration of protein in their urine, secondary to excretion of large amounts of α_{2u}-globulin. Administration of sodium saccharin or sodium ascorbate to NBR male rats, which do not excrete high concentrations of α_{2u}-globulin, results in little to no hyperplastic response in the urinary bladder.

Even in male rats, which are the most sensitive animals, high doses are required for formation of the precipitate, induction of the cytotoxicity and induction of proliferative responses in the urothelium. In general, at a level of 1% of the diet, there was no statistically significant effect for either sodium saccharin or sodium ascorbate, and only slight effects were seen at doses of 2.5–3.0% of the diet. Most of the other sodium salts have been evaluated at doses equimolar to 5% sodium saccharin or as 5% of the diet.

Mice are resistant to the proliferative effects of sodium saccharin and the other sodium salts which have been studied, despite also having appropriate urinary pH, high urinary protein concentrations, and high osmolality like the rat. However, urinary concentrations of calcium and phosphate are considerably lower in the mouse than in the rat, and this greatly reduces the potential for formation of a calcium phosphate precipitate.

Studies in monkeys, including one investigation in which sodium saccharin was administered at a dose of 25 mg/kg bw per day for 18–23 years beginning immediately after birth, showed no evidence of formation of the precipitate or cytotoxic or proliferative changes in the urinary tract. These findings may be due to the lower doses of sodium saccharin as well as the much lower concentrations of protein and lower osmolality in the urine of non-human primates than in mice and rats.

Do the mechanisms of carcinogenesis involving calcium phosphate-containing precipitate formation, cell death and cell proliferation, operate in humans?

Extensive epidemiological studies in humans have failed to show an increased risk of urinary bladder cancer secondary from use of artificial sweeteners. Healthy humans have very low concentrations of urinary protein and much lower urinary osmolalities than rodents, two of the critical parameters required for the formation of cytotoxic calcium phosphate-containing precipitate. In individuals with nephrotic syndrome, there is proteinuria that can attain protein concentrations nearly as high as those found in rats. However, the osmolality does not increase above normal levels in humans (50–500 mosmol/kg). The highest osmolalities that could be attained in humans have been estimated theoretically at approximately 1200 mosmol/kg,

compared with 1400–2000 mosmol/kg in saccharin-treated rats. Thus the epidemiological, experimental animal and mechanistic data suggest that the tumorigenic response in the urinary bladder of rats generated by these sodium salts is a species- and dose-specific phenomenon that does not occur in humans.

Since epidemiological reports on high dietary intakes of sodium, calcium and vitamin C related to bladder cancer are scattered and the results are inconclusive, no inference on mechanisms of carcinogenesis can be drawn.

Gaps in mechanistic knowledge

Few data are available on mechanistic pathways which occur subsequent to calculus formation in the urinary bladder of rodents or humans. *p53* and *H-ras* mutations are not found in urinary bladder tumours in rats treated with calculus-inducing agents. However, the molecular and genetic events involved in cell cytotoxicity, regenerative hyperplasia and tumour formation are unknown. Amorphous precipitates may vary widely in composition and no generalization can be drawn that is universally applicable to all such precipitates. There is little information regarding the reasons for quantitative differences in carcinogenic response to different agents between species and sexes.

Urinary precipitate produced by certain sodium salts consists mainly of calcium phosphate and this precipitate is cytotoxic to the urothelium. Mechanisms leading to urothelial cell death are not known. Critical factors essential for the formation of the urinary precipitate have not been fully identified and the physical and chemical mechanisms for the formation (or the lack of formation) of the precipitate need to be more clearly defined.

Conclusions

The overall conclusions of the Working Group were formulated by providing answers to questions concerning how the mechanistic data reviewed in the previous sections can be used in making overall evaluations of carcinogenicity to humans.

How can mechanistic data on thyroid-stimulating hormone (TSH)-associated follicular-cell neoplasms in rodents be used in making overall evaluations of carcinogenicity to humans?

Agents that lead to the development of thyroid neoplasia through an adaptive physiological mechanism belong to a different category from those that lead to neoplasia through genotoxic mechanisms or through mechanisms involving pathological responses with necrosis and repair.

Agents causing thyroid follicular-cell neoplasia in rodents solely through hormonal imbalance can be identified using the following criteria.

- There is a lack of genotoxic activity (agent and/or metabolite) based on an overall evaluation of in-vitro and in-vivo data
- The presence of hormone imbalance has been demonstrated under the conditions of the carcinogenicity assay.
- The mechanism whereby the agent leads to hormone imbalance has been defined.

When tumours are observed both in the thyroid and at other sites, they should be evaluated separately on the basis of the modes of action of the agent.

Agents that induce thyroid follicular tumours in rodents through interference with thyroid hormone homeostasis can, with few exceptions, also interfere with thyroid hormone homeostasis in humans if given at a sufficient dose for a sufficient time. These agents can be assumed not to be carcinogenic in humans at exposure levels which do not lead to alterations in thyroid hormone homeostasis.

How can mechanistic data on α_{2u}-globulin-associated renal-cell neoplasms in male rats be used in making overall evaluations of carcinogenicity to humans?

In making overall evaluations of carcinogenicity to humans, it can be concluded that production of renal-cell tumours in male rats by agents that fulfil all of the following criteria for an α_{2u}-globulin-associated response is not predictive of carcinogenic hazard to humans:

- Lack of genotoxic activity (agent and/or metabolites) based on an overall evaluation of in-vitro and in-vivo data
- Male rat specificity for nephropathy and renal tumorigenicity
- Induction of the characteristic sequence of histopathological changes in shorter-term studies, of which protein droplet accumulation is obligatory

- Identification of the protein accumulating in tubule cells as α_{2u}-globulin
- Reversible binding of the chemical or metabolite to α_{2u}-globulin
- Induction of sustained increased cell proliferation in renal cortex
- Similarities in dose–response relationship of the tumour outcome with the histopathological end-points (protein droplets, α_{2u}-globulin accumulation, cell proliferation)

In situations where an agent induces tumours at other sites in the male rat or tumours in other laboratory animals, the evidence regarding these other tumour responses should be used independently of the α_{2u}-globulin-associated tumorigenicity in making the overall evaluation of carcinogenicity to humans.

How can mechanistic data on calculi- and micro-crystalluria-associated urinary bladder neoplasms in mice and rats contribute to making overall evaluations of carcinogenicity to humans?

For chemicals producing bladder neoplasms in rats and mice as a result of calculus formation in the urinary bladder, the response cannot be considered to be species-specific; thus, the tumour response is relevant to an evaluation of carcinogenicity to humans. There are quantitative differences in response between species and sexes. Calculus formation is dependent on the attainment in the urine of critical concentrations of constituent chemicals which form the calculus; therefore, the biological effects are dependent on reaching threshold concentrations for calculus formation. Microcrystalluria is often associated with calculus formation, but its relevance to species-specific mechanisms cannot be assessed.

How can mechanistic data on urinary calcium phosphate-containing precipitate-associated bladder neoplasms in rats contribute to making overall evaluations of carcinogenicity to humans?

Calcium phosphate-containing precipitates in the urine of rats, such as those produced by the administration of high doses of some sodium salts, including sodium saccharin and sodium ascorbate, can result in the production of urinary bladder tumours. This sequence can be considered to be species- and dose-specific and is not known to occur in humans.

In making overall evaluations of carcinogenicity to humans, it can be concluded that the production of bladder cancer in rats via a mechanism involving calcium phosphate-containing precipitates is not predictive of carcinogenic hazard to humans, provided that the following criteria are met:

- the formation of the calcium phosphate-containing precipitate occurs under the conditions of the carcinogenicity bioassay which is positive for cancer induction;
- prevention of the formation of the urinary precipitate results in prevention of the bladder proliferative effect;
- the agent (and/or metabolites) shows a lack of genotoxic activity, based on an overall evaluation of in-vitro and in-vivo data;

- the agent being evaluated does not produce tumours at any other site in experimental animals;
- there is evidence from studies in humans that precipitate formation or cancer does not occur in exposed populations.

In situations where an agent induces tumours at other sites in rats or tumours in other laboratory animals, the evidence regarding these other tumour responses should be used independently of information on tumours associated with calcium phosphate-containing precipitates in making the overall evaluation of carcinogenicity to humans.

Species Differences in Thyroid, Kidney and Urinary Bladder Carcinogenesis
C.C. Capen, E. Dybing, J.M. Rice and J.D. Wilbourn, eds
IARC Scientific Publications No. 147
International Agency for Research on Cancer, Lyon, 1999

Species differences in chemical carcinogenesis of the thyroid gland, kidney and urinary bladder

E. Dybing and T. Sanner

Introduction

It is well known that carcinogens show quantitative differences in activity between species (Gold *et al.*, 1984, 1986, 1987, 1990, 1993a, 1995). A classic example is 2-naphthylamine, which appears to be much more potent in humans and dogs than in rats (Kriek, 1969; Radomski, 1979; Gold *et al.*, 1984). Rats, on the other hand, are much more susceptible towards the hepatocarcinogenicity of 2-acetylaminofluorene than mice or hamsters, while guinea-pigs and monkeys appear to be resistant (Miller *et al.*, 1964; Dyer *et al.*, 1966; Miller, 1970; Gold *et al.*, 1984). Aflatoxin B_1 is a very potent liver carcinogen in rats but is less potent in monkeys and hamsters and essentially noncarcinogenic in feeding experiments in mice (Herrold, 1969; Wogan, 1973; Gold *et al.*, 1984; Thorgeirsson *et al.*, 1994). Many of these quantitative species differences in carcinogenic activity may be attributed to differences in carcinogen metabolism (Dybing & Huitfeldt, 1992). In general, however, the quantitative differences in carcinogenic activity between animals are not large. Differences in potency between rats and mice are within a factor of 10 for 74% and within a factor of 100 for 98% of known carcinogens, respectively (Gaylor & Chen, 1986; Gold *et al.*, 1989).

All chemicals for which there is sufficient evidence of carcinogenicity in humans and that have been studied adequately in experimental animals have shown carcinogenic activity in at least one animal species (Wilbourn *et al.*, 1986; Tomatis *et al.*, 1989). Such an association makes it plausible that chemicals which have shown carcinogenic activity in experimental animals also have carcinogenic potential in humans (US Environmental Protection Agency, 1996; IARC, 1998).

Furthermore, animal bioassays have revealed carcinogens that were subsequently found to cause cancer in humans (Wilbourn *et al.*, 1986; Tomatis *et al.*, 1989; Huff, 1992; Tomatis *et al.*, 1997). However, recent evidence indicates that some experimental carcinogens may act through species-specific mechanisms, so that the assumption that all experimental carcinogens are potential human carcinogens may not always be valid (Swenberg *et al.*, 1992; Hard *et al.*, 1993; Cohen & Lawson, 1995).

The present overview considers tumour development in the thyroid gland, kidney and urinary bladder in the context of species-specificity in chemical carcinogenesis. In order to illustrate this, some examples are presented of carcinogens which show species differences in activity at these target sites (Tables 1–3). Such differences may, in principle, be of a quantitative as well as a qualitative nature. In the following presentation and quantitative comparisons, extensive use is made of the data in the Carcinogenic Potency Database (CPDB) of Gold *et al.* (1984, 1986, 1987, 1990, 1993a, 1995). It must be recognized that categorization of carcinogenesis and noncarcinogenicity in the CPDB is based on the evaluation by the authors of the studies included in the database. Thus, there may be discrepancies between the classification of chemicals in this database and that following the more comprehensive evaluation performed by the International Agency for Research on Cancer (IARC).

General mechanisms of carcinogens

Chemical carcinogenesis is a multistep process involving genetic and epigenetic alterations whereby normal cells are converted into malignant ones (Weinstein, 1988; Boyd & Barrett, 1990;

Table 1. Mutagenicity of chemicals which have been evaluated in the carcinogenic potency database as carcinogenic in the thyroid gland in rats and/or mice[a]

Mutagenicity in *Salmonella*	Rat	Mouse
Mutagenic	*ortho*-Anisidine.HCl**	3-Amino-4-ethoxyacetanilide*
	2,4-Diaminoanisole sulfate**	HC Blue No.1**
	1-Ethyl-1-nitrosourea	2,4-Diaminoanisole sulfate**
	Ethylene thiourea**	Ethylene thiourea**
	Glycidol**	4,4'-Methylenedianiline. 2HCl**
	Iodinated glycerol**	1,5-Naphthalenediamine**
	4,4'-Methylenebis(*N,N*-dimethyl)-	4,4'-Oxydianiline**
	benzenamine**	CI pigment red 2**
	4,4'-Methylenedianiline.2HCl**	4,4'-Thiodianiline**
	4,4'-Oxydianiline**	
	para-Rosaniline.HCl**	
	4,4'-Thiodianiline**	
	Zinc dimethyldithiocarbamate*	
Nonmutagenic	3-Aminotriazole**	Chlorinated paraffins (C_{12}, 60% chlorine)**
	Chlorinated paraffins (C_{12}, 60% chlorine)**	Diethylstilboestrol**
	N,N '-Diethylthiourea*	Ethionamide*
	Malonaldehyde, sodium salt**	Sulfamethazine
	Methimazole	2,3,7,8-Tetrachlorodibenzo-*para*-dioxin**
	2,3,7,8-Tetrachlorodibenzo-*para*-dioxin**	
	Trimethylthiourea*	
	Vinyl acetate	
No evaluation	Bemitradine	Oxazepam
	1-Ethylnitroso-3-(2-oxopropyl)urea	
	Mirex, photo-	
	N-Nitrosobis(2-oxopropyl)amine	
	Propylthiouracil**	
	Thiouracil**	

[a] From Gold & Zeiger, 1997

* Tested in both species but positive at some site only in one species

**Tested in both species and positive at some site in both species

Harris, 1992; Barrett, 1993, 1995). The starting point of the carcinogenic process involves a mutational, irreversible cellular change, either induced by a chemical agent or occurring spontaneously. Thereafter, the initiated cell is clonally expanded by epigenetic factors which selectively influence cellular proliferation. Subsequently, multiple genetic changes must occur before the clonally expanded, preneoplastic cells develop into a malignant tumour. These sequential steps have been termed initiation, promotion and progression, respectively, and can be characterized morphologically and biochemically (Bird, 1995; Dragan *et*

al., 1995; Mehta, 1995). Specific changes in gatekeeper genes, predisposing genes or modifying genes may selectively affect rates of tumour initiation or tumour progression (Kinzler & Vogelstein, 1996).

Barrett (1993) has described three basic mechanisms by which a substance can influence the multistep carcinogenic process: (1) by inducing a heritable mutation in a critical gene; (2) by inducing a heritable, epigenetic change in a critical gene; or (3) by increasing clonal expansion of a cell with a heritable alteration in a critical gene, allowing an increased probability of additional

Table 2. Mutagenicity of chemicals which have been evaluated in the carcinogenic potency database as carcinogenic in the kidney in rats and/or mice[a]

Mutagenicity in Salmonella	Rat	Mouse
Mutagenic	Aflatoxin B$_1$* 1-Amino-2-methylanthraquinone** 2-Amino-4-nitrophenol * 2-Amino-5-nitrothiazole* ortho-Anisidine.HCl** Azoxymethane Bromate, potassium* Bromodichloromethane** Coumarin** Formic acid 2-[(5-nitro-2-furyl)-2-thiazolyl]hydrazide** 1-(2-Hydroxyethyl)-1-nitrosourea** 8-Methoxypsoralen N-{[3-(5-Nitro-2-furyl)-1,2,4-oxadiazol-5-yl]-methyl}-acetamide N-[5-(5-Nitro-2-furyl)-1,3,4-thiadiazol-2-yl]acetamide** ortho-Nitroanisole** 1-[(5-Nitrofurfurylidene)amino]hydantoin** N-Nitrosodiethanolamine N-Nitrosodimethylamine** Cl Acid Orange 3* Phenacetin** Quercetin* Streptozotocin** 1,2,3-Trichloropropane** Vinyl chloride**	Bromodichloromethane** 1,3-Butadiene** 2,4-Diaminophenol.2HCl* N-Hydroxy-2-acetylamino-fluorene** Phenacetin** Cl Pigment Red 3** Streptozotocin** Tris(2,3-dibromopropyl)-phosphate** Vinylidene chloride *
Nonmutagenic	Benzofuran** Caffeic acid** Captafol** Chlorinated paraffins (C$_{12}$, 60% chlorine)** Chloroform** 3-(p-Chlorophenyl)-1,1-dimethylurea * Chlorothalonil* Cinnamyl anthranilate** Citrinin 1,4-Dichlorobenzene** 3,4-Dihydrocoumarin** Dimethyl methylphosphonate* Hexachlorobutadiene Hexachloroethane** Hydroquinone** Isophorone* Lead acetate* d-Limonene* α-Methylbenzyl alcohol*	ortho-Benzyl-para-chlorophenol* Caffeic acid** Chloroform** Daminozide** Hydroquinone** Mercurymethylchloride Nitrilotriacetic acid** Ochratoxin A**

17

Table 2 (contd)		
Mutagenicity in *Salmonella*	**Rat**	**Mouse**
Nonmutagenic	Mirex**	
	Nitrilotriacetic acid**	
	Nitrilotriacetic acid, trisodium salt, monohydrate*	
	Ochratoxin A**	
	Phenazone	
	Phenylbutazone**	
	ortho-Phenylphenate, sodium*	
	Tetrachloroethylene**	
	Tris(2-chloroethyl)phosphate*	
No evaluation	2-Amino-5-(5-nitro-2-furyl)1,3,4-oxadiazole	1,2-Di-*n*-butylhydrazine.HCl
	2-Amino-5-(5-nitro-2-furyl)1,3,4-thiadiazole	Dichloroacetylene**
	Barbital sodium	3-Hydroxy-*para*-butyrophenetidine
	Dichloroacetylene**	Lead acetate, basic**
	Diethylacetamide	
	Dimethoxane	
	4,6-Dimethyl-2-(5-nitro-2-furyl)pyrimidine	
	N-4-(4'-Fluorobiphenyl)acetamide	
	Hexamethylmelamine	
	2-Hydrazino-4-(5-nitro-2-furyl)thiazole**	
	Lead acetate, basic**	
	2-Methoxy-3-aminodibenzofuran	
	Z-Methyl-O,N,N-azoxyethane	
	N-(N-Methyl-*N*-nitrosocarbamoyl)-1-ornithine	
	L-5-Morpholinomethyl-3-[(5-nitrofurfurylidene)-amino]-2-oxazolidinone.HCl	
	3-(5-Nitro-2-furyl)imidazo(1,2-α)pyridine**	
	1-Nitroso-1-hydroxyethyl-3-chloroethylurea	
	N-Oxydiethylene thiocarbamyl-*N*-oxydiethylene sulfenamide	

[a] From Gold & Zeiger, 1997

*Tested in both species but positive at some site only in one species

**Tested in both species and positive at some site in both species

Table 3. Mutagenicity of chemicals which have been evaluated in the carcinogenic potency database as carcinogenic in the urinary bladder[a]

Mutagenicity in Salmonella	Rat	Mouse
Mutagenic	Allyl isothiocyanate* 2-Amino-4-(5-nitro-2-furyl)thiazole** 4-Amino-2-nitrophenol* ortho-Anisidine.HCl** N-Butyl-N-(4-hydroxybutyl)nitrosamine 4-Chloro-ortho-phenylenediamine** meta-Cresidine** para-Cresidine** Cyclophosphamide** CI Disperse Blue 1* IQ.HCl 2-Naphthylamine** N-[4-(5-Nitro-2-furyl)-2-thiazolyl]formamide** ortho-Nitroanisole** N-Nitroso-N-methyl-N-dodecylamine N-Nitrosodibutylamine** N-Nitrosodiethylamine N-Nitrosopyrrolidine Phenacetin** Quercetin* para-Quinone dioxime* ortho-Toluidine.HCl** Trp-P-2 acetate**	2-Acetylaminofluorene** 4-Aminodiphenyl ortho-Anisidine.HCl** para-Cresidine** N-Hydroxy-2-acetylaminofluorene** N-[4-(5-Nitro-2-furyl)-2-thiazolyl]formamide** Phenacetin** Telone II**
Nonmutagenic	Acetaminophen** 11-Aminoundecanoic acid* Diethylene glycol Melamine* Nitrilotriacetic acid** Nitrilotriacetic acid, trisodium salt, monohydrate* N-Nitrosodiphenylamine* Phenazone ortho-Phenylphenate sodium* ortho-Phenylphenol* Saccharin, sodium* ortho-Toluenesulfonamide Uracil**	Uracil**
No evaluation	Fosetyl Al 2-Methoxy-3-aminodibenzofuran N-Nitroso-N-methyl-N-tetradecylamine N-Nitroso-N-methyldecylamine N-Nitrosobis(2-oxopropyl)amine ortho-Nitrosotoluene N-Oxydiethylene thiocarbamyl-N-oxydiethylene sulfenamide	2-Aminodiphenylene oxide 4-Chloro-4'-aminodiphenylether** 4-Ethylsulfonylnaphthalene-1-sulfonamide

[a] From Gold & Zeiger, 1997
*Tested in both species but positive at some site only in one species
**Tested in both species and positive at some site in both species

events. Theoretically, chemical carcinogenesis could thus be induced by compounds which act through any one of these mechanisms. Other substances may induce tumours by two or even all three mechanisms. There is ample evidence that mutagens may cause cancer. Most, but not all, human carcinogens are active in a variety of genetic toxicology tests (Bartsch & Malaveille, 1990; Shelby & Zeiger, 1990). However, there are a number of experimental carcinogens which are not mutagens: only about 50% of the experimental carcinogens identified by the US National Toxicology Program are mutagens (Tennant et al., 1987; Zeiger et al., 1990; Ashby & Tennant, 1991). In this review, carcinogenic activity will be related to mutagenicity in the Salmonella test (Ames et al., 1975), as reported in the CPDB, although it must be recognized that some carcinogens found to be negative in the Salmonella test show clear evidence of genotoxicity in other test systems, such as ochratoxin (Dirheimer, 1996; see Table 2) and hydroquinone (Chen et al., 1994; see Table 2).

There has been much debate about whether nonmutagenic carcinogens can act through stimulation of cell proliferation (Ames & Gold, 1990; Cohen & Ellwein, 1990; Preston-Martin et al., 1990; Weinstein, 1991; Cohen & Ellwein, 1992; Huff, 1992; Melnick et al., 1993). It is proposed that such agents can fix DNA damage occurring spontaneously during cellular replication or that which is induced by other mutagenic agents. In addition, nonmutagenic carcinogens may enhance the probability of additional genetic events during clonal expansion of initiated cells. Mitogenesis is certainly crucial to the carcinogenic process (Ames & Gold, 1990; Preston-Martin et al., 1990; Weinstein, 1991; Barrett, 1993). Mitosis may be induced through cellular signals resulting from the interaction of external agents with cellular receptors. An increase in cell numbers may also be achieved by inhibition of apoptosis (Schulte-Hermann et al., 1993; Goldsworthy et al., 1996). In addition, replicative cell proliferation may be initiated as a secondary event to tissue damage induced after generally high exposures to cytotoxic agents.

A schematic categorization of chemical carcinogens is depicted in Figure 1 (modified from Cohen & Ellwein, 1992). It must be recognized that such a scheme may be excessively simplistic, since several mechanisms may operate in concert (Barrett, 1993, 1995).

Cancer of the thyroid gland

There are a number of important species differences in thyroid gland physiology which are important for the development of thyroid tumours (Dohler et al., 1979; Capen, 1994; McClain, 1995). The half-life of thyroxine is much shorter in rats (12–24 h) than in humans (5–9 days) and the serum levels of thyroid-stimulating hormone (TSH) are 25 times higher in rodents than in man (Dohler et al., 1979). Further, rats require about a 10-fold higher production of thyroxine than do humans (Dohler et al., 1979). In addition, the human plasma high-affinity thyroxine-binding globulin is absent in rodents, cats and rabbits (Dohler et al., 1979). This absence results in the blood transport of more free thyroxine in these species compared to humans, and predisposes the former to higher levels of metabolism and excretion. Iodine deficiency readily induces thyroid gland neoplasia in rodents (Axelrad & Leblond, 1955), whereas a clear etiological role for endemic goitre in humans has not been established (Pendergast et al., 1961; Doniach, 1970), although an excess risk of thyroid cancer has, in some studies, been associated with goitre (Ron et al., 1987; Salabè, 1994; D'Avanzo et al., 1995) (see also Franceschi & Dal Maso, this volume).

Thyroid gland neoplasia may be induced both directly by mutagenic carcinogens and indirectly through hormone imbalance (Furth, 1959; Capen, 1994; McClain, 1995). Treatment of rodents with a number of antithyroid substances induces a high incidence of thyroid tumours (Napalkov, 1990). Such hormonal imbalance may occur either through inhibition of thyroid hormone production, secretion or peripheral conversion, or through alteration of metabolism resulting in increased biliary excretion of conjugates. All of these mechanisms lead to a compensatory sustained increase in the synthesis and secretion of TSH through negative feedback on the pituitary gland. Antithyroid agents, such as thiourea, propylthiouracil and methimazole, and sulfonamides, such as sulfadiazine and sulfamethazine, are effective inhibitors of thyroid hormone synthesis in rats, whereas they are much less potent in monkeys (Takayama *et al.*, 1986). The marked difference in inhibition of thyroid peroxidase between rats and monkeys appears to constitute the biochemical basis for this species difference (Takayama *et al.*, 1986; Swenberg *et al.*, 1992). Among rodents, the rat is more sensitive towards the thyroid neoplastic effect of sulfamethazine than the mouse (Littlefield *et al.*, 1989, 1990).

Many chemicals can, at high doses, alter thyroid function in rodents via enzyme induction leading to increased disposition of thyroxine (Hill *et al.*, 1989; McClain, 1989). In such cir-

cumstances, a compensatory increase in TSH will, if the chemical exposure is prolonged, lead to thyroid gland neoplasia (McClain, 1989). The classical inducer phenobarbital has been shown to act as a thyroid gland tumour promoter in rats (McClain *et al.*, 1988). The promoting effect of enzyme inducers on thyroid gland tumorigenesis is usually greater in rats than in mice, with males generally more sensitive than females (Capen, 1994).

The thyroid gland is a target site for 6% of 354 rat carcinogens and 3% of 299 mouse carcinogens

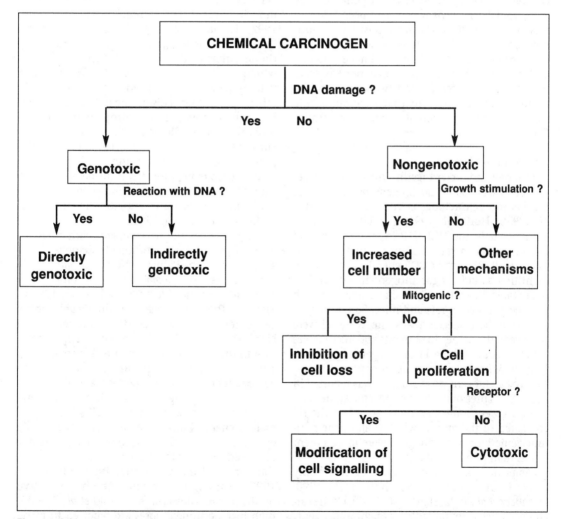

Figure 1. Schematic categorization of chemical carcinogens (modified after Cohen & Ellwein, 1992)

in the CPDB (Gold *et al.*, 1993b). Similar figures were reported for 379 National Cancer Institute/National Toxicology Program (NCI/NTP) long-term studies (Huff *et al.*, 1991). In all, 34 of the CPDB chemicals have been identified as thyroid gland carcinogens in rats and/or mice (Table 1). Additional studies have been added to the CPDB since Gold *et al.* (1993b) calculated the frequencies of tumours at different target sites, the number of substances inducing tumours at a particular site in Tables 1–3 may be higher than those which can be calculated from the percentages given by Gold *et al.* (1993b). Of the 25 thyroid carcinogens which have been tested in rats and mice, 20 (80%) were positive in both species at any site, but only seven were positive in the thyroid gland in both rats and mice (Tables 1 and 4). Five of these seven carcinogens were mutagenic in *Salmonella* and two were not. The thyroid gland carcinogens that were mutagenic were all much more potent in rats than in mice (Table 4).

Cancer of the kidney

The kidney and ureter together constitute a target site for 13% of 354 rat carcinogens, but only 4% of the 299 mouse carcinogens in the CPDB (Gold *et al.*, 1993b). Huff *et al.* (1991) found that 7% of the carcinogens in the NCI/NTP experiments caused kidney cancer in rats and approximately 1% in mice. In all, 81 of the CPDB chemicals have been identified as kidney carcinogens in rats and/or mice (Table 2). Of the 57 renal carcinogens which have been tested in rats and mice, 38 (68%) were positive in both species at any site, while 11 were positive in the kidney in both rats and mice (Tables 2 and 4). Four of these 11 carcinogens were mutagenic in *Salmonella*, five were nonmutagenic and for two carcinogens no evaluation was reported in the CPDB. Three of the four mutagenic kidney carcinogens were somewhat more potent in the rat compared to the mouse, whereas all of the nonmutagenic kidney carcinogens were more potent in rats than in mice (Table 4).

Some nongenotoxic renal carcinogens are only active in the male rat (Borghoff *et al.*, 1990; Swenberg *et al.*, 1992; Hard *et al.*, 1993). Of the carcinogens listed in Table 2, 1,4-dichlorobenzene, dimethyl methylphosphonate, hexachloroethane, isophorone, *d*-limonene and tetrachloroethylene

cause hyaline droplet nephropathy which leads to replicative tubule cell proliferation via a reversible interaction with the male rat-specific urinary protein α_{2u}-globulin. Unleaded gasoline and its constituent 2,2,4-trimethylpentane, which also cause hyaline droplet nephropathy, renal cell proliferation and renal tumours (Short *et al.*, 1987, 1989), as well as *d*-limonene, act as tumour promoters in the kidney (Short *et al.*, 1989; Dietrich & Swenberg, 1991a; Hard *et al.*, 1993). No other member of the lipocalin protein superfamily (Flower, 1996), to which the α_{2u}-globulin protein belongs, binds hyaline droplet nephropathy-inducing agents (Lehman-McKeeman & Caudill, 1992). The uniqueness of the mechanism for this type of renal carcinogen is further substantiated by the fact that in the NCI-Black-Reiter rat strain, which lacks hepatic mRNA for α_{2u}-globulin (Chatterjee *et al.*, 1989), no hyaline droplets or other aspects of renal disease are induced by chemicals which induce hyaline droplets in males of other rat strains (Dietrich & Swenberg, 1991a,b). Further strengthening the association between the presence of α_{2u}-globulin and development of hyaline droplet nephropathy is the demonstration that *d*-limonene induces nephropathy in transgenic mice expressing α_{2u}-globulin (Lehman-McKeeman & Caudill, 1994).

The kidney is unusual compared with other target sites, in that the proportion of carcinogens that are positive in the kidney is greater for *Salmonella*-negative than for *Salmonella*-positive compounds, as recorded in the CPDB file (Gold *et al.*, 1993b). Many of the nonmutagenic kidney carcinogens cause renal tubule necrosis at higher doses. Nitrilotriacetic acid is a more potent nephrotoxicant in the rat than in the mouse (Anderson *et al.*, 1985), which corresponds with its relative tumorigenic potency in the two species (Table 4).

Long-term gavage studies with hydroquinone have shown increases in tubule cell adenomas of male Fischer 344 rats accompanied by renal tubule epithelial degeneration, but these effects were not observed in female rats or B6C3F$_1$ mice (US National Toxicology Program, 1989; Hard *et al.*, 1997). Although hydroquinone gives negative results in the *Salmonella* test (Gold *et al.*, 1993b), high intraperitoneal doses are reported to cause clastogenic effects in mouse bone marrow cells (Chen *et al.*, 1994). In cell proliferation studies

Target site	Carcinogen	Mutagenicity in Salmonella	TD$_{50}$ rats mg/kg bw/d	TD$_{50}$ mice mg/kg bw/d
Thyroid gland	2,4-Diaminoanisole sulfate	Mutagenic	162	1060
	Ethylene thiourea		7.42	82
	4,4'-Methylenedianiline. 2HCl		27.2	128
	4,4'-Oxydianiline		14.3	598
	4,4'-Thiodianiline		5.59	88.4
	Chlorinated paraffins (C$_{12}$, 60% chlorine)	Nonmutagenic	736	372
	2,3,7,8-Tetrachlorodibenzo-para-dioxin		0.10[b]	1.59[b]
Kidney	Bromodichloromethane	Mutagenic	152	137
	Phenacetin		547	1100
	Streptozotocin		0.78	2.44
	Tris(2,3-dibromopropyl)-phosphate		1.57	2.56
	Caffeic acid	Nonmutagenic	3930	4700
	Chloroform		119	153
	Hydroquinone		349	5320
	Nitrilotriacetic acid		2530	13800
	Ochratoxin A		0.058	358
	Dichloroacetylene	No evaluation	3.34	0.47
	Lead acetate, basic		107	986
Urinary bladder	ortho-Anisidine.HCl	Mutagenic	31.9	935
	para-Cresidine		88.4	44.7
	N-[4-(5-Nitro-2-furyl)-2-thiazolyl]-formamide		1.31	30.5
	Phenacetin		11700	37000
	Uracil	Nonmutagenic	ND[c]	ND[c]
	None	No evaluation	–	–

Table 4. Carcinogenic potency (TD$_{50}$) values for carcinogens positive at target site in both rats and mice[a]

[a] From Gold & Zeiger, 1997
[b] μg/kg bw/d
[c] No data found

with hydroquinone in Fischer 344 rats, bromo-deoxyuridine incorporation was increased in the kidney tubules of males but not females (English *et al.*, 1994). The underlying mechanism of hydro-quinone-induced nephrotoxicity remains to be fully elucidated (Whysner *et al.*, 1995). However, it has been suggested that the tumour response in rats linked to the rodent-specific chronic progressive nephropathy may have little relevance to humans (Hard *et al.*, 1997).

Long-term administration of chlorothalonil to rats leads to the development of renal tumours, a phenomenon associated with nephrotoxicity induced by a reactive thiol metabolite generated by the action of cysteine β-lyase (IPCS, 1996). Chlorothalonil is much less nephrotoxic in mice and dogs than in rats and much less nephrocarcinogenic in mice compared to rats (IPCS, 1996; Wilkinson & Killeen, 1996). The rat has much higher renal levels of γ-glutamyl transpeptidase and β-lyase, enzymes involved in chlorothalonil bioactivation, than other species, including humans (Wilkinson & Killeen, 1996).

However, there does not always appear to be such a good correlation between nephrotoxicity and nephrocarcinogenicity. Chloroform administered to B6C3F$_1$ mice by gavage did not cause kidney tumours (US National Cancer Institute, 1976), although shorter-term administration of chloroform induced degeneration and necrosis with subsequent cell proliferation in this strain of mice (Larson et al., 1994). In contrast, kidney tumours were seen after chloroform administration either by inhalation in male BDF$_1$ mice or in an aqueous-miscible toothpaste vehicle in male ICI mice (Roe et al., 1979). Chloroform also causes cytotoxicity and cell proliferation in renal tubules of Fischer 344 rats (Larson et al., 1994), although no renal tumour response was detected in a carcinogenicity bioassay in this strain (Matsushima, 1994). On the other hand, treatment of male Osborne–Mendel rats with chloroform by gavage results in the development of kidney tumours (US National Cancer Institute, 1976). There is a lack of intermediate end-points that may be linked to renal cancer development in this strain of rat.

There may also be sex and species differences for mutagenic nephrotoxic carcinogens. Vinylidene chloride, for example, causes renal necrosis and tumours only in male mice, but not in female mice or rats (WHO, 1990), a phenomenon which has been correlated with specific expression of cytochrome P450 2E1 in the kidney of male mice (Speerschneider & Dekant, 1995). These authors did not find evidence of P450 2E1 catalysis in human kidney microsomes, suggesting that vinylidene chloride-induced renal tumorigenesis may be sex- and species-specific.

Cancer of the urinary bladder

A number of chemicals have been shown to induce urinary bladder tumours associated with formation of urinary calculi after long-term administration of high doses to rodents (Wolkowski-Tyl et al., 1982; Clayson et al., 1995; Cohen, 1995a,b; Cohen & Lawson, 1995). In general, calculi form more readily in rats than in mice or the formation is similar in the two species. However, calculi–induced proliferation appears to be considerably greater in rats than in mice. This difference is partly due to a primarily papillomatous reaction in rats, whereas in mice it is predominantly a nodular response involving a smaller number of cells (Cohen & Lawson, 1995). The presence of calculi leads to erosion of the bladder surface with subsequent extensive regenerative hyperplasia that ultimately results in tumour formation. In general, these bladder carcinogens form calculi in the urine more readily in rats than in mice or at least to similar extents, whereas the proliferative response appears to be considerably greater in rats than in mice (Cohen & Lawson, 1995). There is also a sex difference, male rodents frequently being affected to a greater extent than females. The process involved in urothelial carcinogenesis related to calculus formation may be influenced by factors such as volume, osmolality, cationic and anionic concentration and quantitative and qualitative differences in the presence of urinary protein (Clayson et al., 1995; Cohen, 1995b).

Epidemiological studies have suggested that calculus formation in humans may be a risk factor, but the association is weak (Matanoski & Elliott, 1981; Burin et al., 1995). However, there are obvious differences in calculus residence time between rodents and humans related to the horizontal versus vertical status, which may make humans less sensitive than rodents towards tumour development caused by calculi-forming agents (DeSesso, 1995). Another factor affecting calculus residence time is the fact that the associated pain motivates humans to seek medical attention. Microcrystalluria produced by silicates also causes severe erosion of the urothelium, regenerative hyperplasia and tumour formation (Okamura et al., 1992). Amorphous calcium phosphate precipitates of a number of sodium salts, including sodium saccharin, ascorbate, glutamate, bicarbonate and chloride, are cytotoxic to the rat urothelium and generate a mild regenerative hyperplasia which is associated with the generation of bladder tumours (see Cohen, this volume). These effects are greater in male than in female rats and appear not to occur in mice, hamsters or monkeys (Ellwein & Cohen, 1990; Cohen & Lawson, 1995). There are clear cationic differences in the responses to saccharin, in that sodium saccharin produces both proliferative and tumorigenic effects, while potassium saccharin has less proliferative effect and calcium saccharin only a marginal effect (Cohen, 1995b). An involvement of the male-rat-specific α_{2u}-globulin in the carcinogenic effects of sodium salts in the urinary bladder is indicated by the lack of induction of epithelial cell proliferation by sodium saccharin or sodium L-ascorbate in male NCI-Black-Reiter rats (Uwagawa et al., 1994).

Tributyl phosphate induces urinary bladder hyperplasia and tumours in long-term experiments in rats (Weiner et al., 1997), but not in mice (Kotkoskie et al., 1997). This compound is an example of a nongenotoxic bladder carcinogen which causes urothelial cytotoxicity with marked regenerative hyperplasia, but without accompanying crystalluria, urinary precipitate or calculi (Arnold et al., 1997).

The urinary bladder and urethra are together a target site for 10% of the 354 rat carcinogens and 4% of the mouse carcinogens in the CPDB (Gold et al., 1993b). In contrast, the urinary bladder was reported to be the target organ for only 4% of the carcinogens in the 379 NCI/NTP studies examined by Huff et al. (1991). Cancer of the urinary bladder occurred in less than 1% of the NCI/NTP experiments in the mouse. In all, 50 of the CPDB chemicals have been identified as

urinary bladder carcinogens in rats and/or mice (Table 3). Of the 32 bladder carcinogens which have been tested in rats and mice, 20 (63%) were positive in both species at any site, whereas only five were positive in the urinary bladder in both rats and mice (Tables 3 and 4). Four of these five carcinogens were mutagenic in *Salmonella* and one was not. Three of the four mutagenic urinary bladder carcinogens were more potent in the rat than in the mouse (Table 4).

Discussion

Species differences in chemical carcinogenesis may in principle be either qualitative in nature when there are interspecies differences in pathogenetic mechanisms, or be due to quantitative differences in action (Table 5). For carcinogenic mechanisms that can operate across various species, there may be quantitative differences, either due to variation in carcinogen delivery leading to differences in target dose (kinetic differences) or due to dynamic factors resulting from differences in target sensitivity. A number of such dynamic factors may influence the outcome of the carcinogenic process, including variation in receptor levels and affinities, rates and degrees of cell proliferation or apoptosis, as well as in rates and degrees of DNA repair.

Overall concordance in neoplastic response between rats and mice exposed to a given chemical is in the order of 75% (Haseman & Huff, 1987; Gold et al., 1989; Huff et al., 1991). Among rat carcinogens, 76% are positive in the mouse, while 70% of mouse carcinogens are positive in the rat

---

Table 5. Principal types of species differences in chemical carcinogenesis

I. Qualitative differences

Species-specific differences in pathogenetic mechanisms

II. Quantitative differences

    A. Differences in kinetic factors

    Differences in carcinogen delivery leading to differences in target dose

    B. Differences in dynamic factors

    Differences in target sensitivity related to, e.g., receptor level and affinity, cell proliferation, apoptosis, DNA repair

---

(Gold *et al.*, 1989). Somewhat lower concordance has been found for the limited number of compounds that have been tested in hamsters as well as rats and mice. For these, 64% (21/33) of rat carcinogens are positive in hamsters and 61% (17/28) of mouse carcinogens are positive in hamsters (Gold *et al.*, 1991). There may be lower concordance between rodents and humans than between rodent species. Site-specific prediction between rats and mice is less accurate than overall prediction of positivity, since the likelihood is at most 52% that if a chemical induces tumours at a given site in one species, it will also do so at the same site in the other species (Gold *et al.*, 1991). With respect to mutagenicity, mutagens are more likely than nonmutagens to be carcinogenic, more likely to induce tumours at multiple target sites and more likely to be carcinogenic in two species (Gold *et al.*, 1993b; Tennant, 1993, Gray *et al.*, 1995).

Allen *et al.* (1988) attempted to compare potency estimates from epidemiological data with those from animal carcinogenesis bioassays. For the 23 chemicals that were selected, the bioassay data gave potency estimates that were highly correlated with potencies estimated from human studies. However, sufficient evidence of carcinogenicity according to the IARC criteria was available for only 11 of the 23 chemicals studied (IARC, 1987).

A number of nongenotoxic rodent thyroid carcinogens act through an indirect mechanism involving a sustained increase in TSH levels. Given the marked differences between humans and rodents in thyroid gland physiology, it seems probable that such chemicals will be quantitatively much less active in humans. In order to operate through this type of mechanism in humans, the exposures would need to be so high as to induce evidence of thyroid hormone imbalance before development of neoplasia. In addition to such indirectly acting thyroid carcinogens, a number of genotoxic rodent thyroid carcinogens have been identified. These genotoxic thyroid carcinogens are approximately an order of magnitude more potent in rats than in mice. Such thyroid carcinogens may be considered potential human carcinogens, but no information is available indicating what their tumorigenic potency in humans would be.

Rodent kidney carcinogens act through several different mechanisms. On the one hand, there are many kidney carcinogens that express mutagenic activity. Some of these, such as vinylidene chloride (WHO, 1990) and tris(2,3-dibromopropyl)phosphate (Söderlund *et al.*, 1980) also cause tubule necrosis, so that, in addition to having initiator potential, these carcinogens may elicit a strong promoting effect. Quantitative differences in tumorigenic potency between rats and mice for these compounds may in many instances be related to metabolic factors.

Chemicals inducing renal tumours in male rats through interaction with α_{2u}-globulin do so through a mechanism which does not operate in female rats or other species. This mechanism of carcinogenesis is thus in the true sense species-specific and qualitatively different from other mechanisms. However, it must be remembered that chemicals causing tumours in male rats through this mechanism may act as carcinogens in other organs and species through alternative mechanisms. Examples of such kidney carcinogens are unleaded gasoline (IARC, 1989) and 1,4-dichlorobenzene (US National Toxicology Program, 1987), both of which also induce hepatic tumours in mice.

Nongenotoxic rodent renal carcinogens are generally more potent in rats than mice, or are active only in rats. Several such carcinogens cause renal necrosis, resulting in subsequent replicative proliferation. Metabolic differences are often responsible for the observed species differences in necrogenic potency, and may also be of importance for species differences in tumorigenicity. In principle, this type of renal carcinogen could be active in humans provided that exposures are comparable in terms of relative tumorigenic potency.

Many nonmutagenic rodent urinary bladder carcinogens appear to act through an indirect mechanism involving formation of calculi and microcrystalluria, resulting in urothelial lesions with accompanying regenerative hyperplasia. Urinary bladder tumours associated with calcium phosphate-containing precipitates produced by some sodium salts are unique to the rat. On the other hand, there are also a number of rodent bladder carcinogens which are mutagenic. Rats appear generally to be more sensitive than mice towards both mutagenic and nonmutagenic bladder carcinogens. Both of these types of carcinogen could be active in humans. However, at least with respect to bladder carcinogens acting secondarily through calculus formation, humans appear to be less sensitive than rats.

It is important to recognize that most chemicals which are carcinogenic for the thyroid gland, kidney or urinary bladder are also carcinogenic at some other site (Table 6). It appears that more non-mutagens than mutagens show site-specificity for these target organs; however, only for the urinary bladder is the difference statistically different ($p = 0.02$). For the sites discusssed, only uracil is exclusively carcinogenic at the same site (urinary bladder) in both rats and mice.

Conclusions

1. There are many examples of quantitative differences in carcinogenic activity between rats and mice, whereas the database for quantitative comparisons between rodents and humans is small.

2. Mutagenic thyroid carcinogens are more potent in rats than in mice. Chemicals causing thyroid tumours through an indirect mechanism via sustained elevation of TSH levels are presumably much more potent in rats than in humans due to the large differences in thyroid physiology between these two species.

3. There is strong evidence that chemicals causing renal tumours in male rats via interaction with α_{2u}-globulin and accompanying hyaline droplet nephropathy act through a sex- and species-specific mechanism which does not occur in female rats or other species.

4. Renal toxicity and replicative proliferation is of importance for the activity of many mutagenic as well as nonmutagenic renal carcinogens. Sex and species differences in renal tumorigenesis may often be related to differences in the generation of toxic metabolites in the kidney.

5. The rat is generally more sensitive than the

Table 6. Site-specificity of chemicals which have been tested in both rats and mice and evaluated in the Carcinogenic Potency Database as carcinogenic in the thyroid gland, kidney or urinary bladder in either or both species[a]

Site	Mutagenic	Nonmutagenic
Thyroid gland	13% (2/15)[b] [Zinc dimethyldithiocarbamate {R}, 3-amino-4-ethoxyacetanilide {M}][c]	38% (3/8) [*N,N*-Diethylthiourea {R}, trimethylthiourea {R}, ethionamide {M}]
Kidney	8% (2/26) [CI Acid Orange 3 {R}, 2,4-diaminophenol.2HCl {M}]	26% (7/27) [Chlorothalonil {R}, dimethyl methylphosphonate {R}, lead acetate {R}, *d*-limonene {R}, α-methylbenzyl alcohol {R}, tris(2-chloroethyl)phosphate {R}, *ortho*-benzyl-*para*-chlorophenol {M}]
Urinary bladder	19% (4/21) [Allyl isothiocyanate {R}, 4-amino-2-nitrophenol {R}, *meta*-cresidine {R}, CI Disperse Blue {R}]	50% (5/10) [Melamine {R}, *N*-nitrosodiphenylamine {R}, *ortho*-phenylphenol, saccharin sodium {R}, uracil {R, M}]

[a] From Gold & Zeiger, 1997
[b] Number of chemicals carcinogenic only for given site versus number of chemicals carcinogenic for given site plus other sites
[c] R, rats; M, mice

mouse towards urinary bladder carcinogenesis. The rat is especially sensitive towards chemicals which cause urothelial toxicity and accompanying regenerative hyperplasia associated with calculus, microcrystalluria or precipitate formation.

7. Most of the carcinogens which are active in the thyroid gland, kidney or urinary bladder in both rats and mice are also active at another site.

References

Allen, B.C., Crump, K.S. & Shipp, A.M. (1988) Correlation between carcinogenic potency of chemicals in animals and humans. *Risk Anal.*, 8, 531–544

Ames, B.N. & Gold, L.S. (1990) Too many rodent carcinogens: mitogenesis increases mutagenesis. *Science*, 249, 970–971

Ames, B.N., McCann, J. & Yamasaki, E. (1975) Methods for detecting carcinogens and mutagens with the *Salmonella*/mammalian microsome mutagenicity test. *Mutat. Res.*, 31, 347–364

Anderson, R.L., Bishop, W.E. & Campbell, R.L. (1985) A review of the environmental and mammalian toxicology of nitrilotriacetic acid. *Crit. Rev. Toxicol.*, 15, 1–102

Arnold, L.L., Christenson, W.R., Cano, M., St. John, M.K., Wahle, B.S. & Cohen, S.M. (1997) Tributyl phosphate effects on urine and bladder epithelium in male Sprague-Dawley rats. *Fundam. Appl. Toxicol.*, 40, 247–255

Ashby, J. & Tennant, R.W. (1991) Definitive relationships among chemical structure, carcinogenicity and mutagenicity for 301 chemicals tested by the US NTP. *Mutat. Res.*, 257, 229–306

Axelrad, A.A. & Leblond, C.P. (1955) Induction of thyroid tumors in rats by a low iodine diet. *Cancer*, 8, 339–367

Barrett, J.C. (1993) Mechanisms of multistep carcinogenesis and carcinogen risk assessment. *Environ. Health Perspect.*, 100, 9–20

Barrett, J.C. (1995) Mechanisms for species differences in receptor-mediated carcinogenesis. *Mutat. Res.*, 333, 189–202

Bartsch, H. & Malaveille, C. (1990) Screening assays for carcinogenic agents and mixtures: an appraisal based on data in the IARC Monograph series. In: Vainio, H., Sorsa, M. & McMichael, A.J., eds, *Complex Mixtures and Cancer Risks* (IARC Scientific Publications No. 104), Lyon, IARC, pp. 65–74

Bird, R.P. (1995) Role of aberrant crypt foci in understanding the pathogenesis of colon cancer. *Cancer Lett.*, 93, 55–71

Borghoff, S.J., Short, B.G. & Swenberg, J.A. (1990) Biochemical mechanisms and pathobiology of α_{2u}-globulin nephropathy. *Ann. Rev. Pharmacol. Toxicol.*, 30, 349–367

Boyd, J.A. & Barrett, J.C. (1990) Genetic and cellular basis of multistep carcinogenesis. *Pharmacol. Ther.*, 46, 469–486

Burin, G.J., Gibb, H.J. & Hill, R.N. (1995) Human bladder cancer: descriptive statistics and evidence for a potential irritation-induced mechanism. *Food Chem. Toxicol.*, 33, 785–795

Capen, C.C. (1994) Mechanisms of chemical injury of thyroid gland. *Prog. Clin. Biol. Res.*, 387, 173–191

Chatterjee, B., Demyan, W.F., Song, C.S., Gary, B.D. & Roy, A.K. (1989) Loss of androgenic induction of α_{2u}-globulin gene family in the liver of NIH black rats. *Endocrinology*, 125, 1385–1388

Chen, H.W., Tomar, R. & Eastmond, D.A. (1994) Detection of hydroquinone-induced nonrandom breakage in the centromeric heterochromatin of mouse bone marrow cells using multicolor fluorescence in situ hybridization with the mouse major and minor satellite probes. *Mutagenesis*, 9, 563–569

Clayson, D.B., Fishbein, L. & Cohen, S.M. (1995) Effects of stones and other physical factors on the induction of rodent bladder cancer. *Food Chem. Toxicol.*, 33, 771–784

Cohen, S.M. (1995a) Cell proliferation in the bladder and implications for cancer risk assessment. *Toxicology*, 102, 149–159

Cohen, S.M. (1995b) Role of urinary physiology and chemistry in bladder carcinogenesis. *Food Chem.Toxicol.*, 33, 715–730

Cohen, S.M. & Ellwein, L.B. (1990) Cell proliferation in carcinogenesis. *Science*, 249, 1007–1011

Cohen, S.M. & Ellwein, L.B. (1992) Risk assessment based on high-dose animal exposure experiments. *Chem. Res. Toxicol.*, 5, 742–748

Cohen, S.M. & Lawson, T.A. (1995) Rodent bladder tumors do not always predict for humans. *Cancer Lett.*, 93, 9–16

D'Avanzo, B., La Vecchia, C., Franceschi, S., Negri, E. & Talamini, R. (1995) History of thyroid diseases and subsequent thyroid cancer risk. *Cancer Epidemiol. Biomarkers Prev.*, 4, 193–199

DeSesso, J.M. (1995) Anatomical relationships of urinary bladders compared: their potential role in the development of bladder tumors in humans and rats. *Food Chem. Toxicol.*, 33, 705–714

Dietrich, D.R. & Swenberg, J.A. (1991a) The presence of alpha$_{2u}$-globulin is necessary for d-limonene promotion of male rat kidney tumors. *Cancer Res.*, 51, 3512–3521

Dietrich, D.R. & Swenberg, J.A. (1991b) NCI-Black-Reiter (NBR) male rats fail to develop renal disease following exposure to agents that induce α_{2u}-globulin (α_{2u}) nephropathy. *Fundam. Appl. Toxicol.*, **16**, 749–762

Dirheimer, G. (1996) Mechanistic approaches to ochratoxin toxicity. *Food. Add. Contam.*, **13** (Suppl.), 45–48

Dohler, K.D., Wong, C.C. & von zur Muhlen, A. (1979) The rat as a model for the study of drug effects on thyroid function: consideration of methological problems. *Pharmacol. Ther.*, **5**, 305–318

Doniach, I. (1970) Aetiological consideration of thyroid carcinoma. In: Smithers, D., ed., *Neoplastic Diseases at Various Sites. Tumours of the Thyroid Gland*, Vol. 6, Edinburgh, E. & S. Livingston, pp. 55–72

Dragan, Y., Teeguarden, J., Campbell, H., Hsia, S. & Pitot, H. (1995) The quantitation of altered hepatic foci during multistage hepatocarcinogenesis in the rat: transforming growth factor α expression as a marker for the stage of progression. *Cancer Lett.*, **93**, 73–83

Dybing, E. & Huitfeldt, H.S. (1992) Species differences in carcinogen metabolism and interspecies extrapolation. In: Vainio, H., Magee, P.N., McGregor, D.B. & McMichael, A.J., eds, *Mechanisms of Carcinogenesis in Risk Identification* (IARC Scientific Publications No. 116), Lyon, IARC, pp. 501–522

Dyer, H.M., Kelly, M.G. & O'Gara, R.W. (1966) Lack of carcinogenic activity and metabolic fate of fluorenylacetamides in monkeys. *J. Natl Cancer Inst.*, **36**, 305–322

Ellwein, L.B. & Cohen, S.M. (1990) The health risks of saccharin revisited. *Crit. Rev. Toxicol.*, **20**, 311–326

English, J.C., Perry, L.G., Vlaovic, M., Moyer, C. & O'Donoghue, J.L. (1994) Measurement of cell proliferation in the kidneys of Fischer 344 and Sprague-Dawley rats after gavage administration of hydroquinone. *Fundam. Appl. Toxicol.*, **23**, 397–406

Flower, D.R. (1996) The lipocalin protein family: structure and function. *Biochem. J.*, **318**, 1–14

Furth, J. (1959) A meeting of ways in cancer research: thoughts on the evolution and nature of neoplasms. *Cancer Res.*, **19**, 241–258

Gaylor, D.W. & Chen, J.J. (1986) Relative potency of chemical carcinogens in rodents. *Risk Anal.*, **6**, 283–290

Gold, L.S. & Zeiger, E., eds, (1997) *Handbook of Carcinogenic Potency and Genotoxicity Databases*, Boca Raton, CRC Press

Gold, L.S, Sawyer, C.B., Magaw, R., Backman, G.M., de Veciana, M., Levinson, R., Hooper, N.K., Havender, W.R., Bernstein, L., Peto, R., Pike, M.C. & Ames, B.N. (1984) A carcinogenic potency database of the standardized results of animal bioassays. *Environ. Health Perspect.*, **58**, 9–319

Gold, L.S., de Veciana, M., Backman, G.M., Magaw, R., Lopipero, P. Smith, M., Blumenthal, M., Levinson, R., Bernstein, L. & Ames, B.N. (1986) Chronological supplement to the carcinogenic potency database: standardized results of animal bioassays published through December 1982. *Environ. Health Perspect.*, **67**, 161–200

Gold, L.S., Slone, T.H., Backman, G.M., Magaw, R., Da Costa, M., Lopipero, P., Blumenthal, M. & Ames, B.N. (1987) Second chronological supplement to the carcinogenic potency database: standardized results of animal bioassays published through December 1984 and by the National Toxicology Program through May 1986. *Environ. Health Perspect.*, **74**, 237–329

Gold, L.S., Bernstein, L., Magaw, R. & Slone, T.H. (1989) Interspecies extrapolation in carcinogenesis: prediction between rats and mice. *Environ. Health Perspect.*, **81**, 211–219

Gold, L.S., Slone, T.H., Backman, G.M., Eisenberg, S., Da Costa, M., Wong, M., Manley, N.B., Rohrbach, L. & Ames, B.N. (1990) Third chronological supplement to the carcinogenic potency database: standardized results of animal bioassays published through December 1986 and by the National Toxicology Program through June 1987. *Environ. Health Perspect.*, **84**, 215–285

Gold, L.S., Slone, T.H., Manley, N.B. & Bernstein, L. (1991) Target organs in chronic bioassays of 533 chemical carcinogens. *Environ. Health Perspect.*, **93**, 233–246

Gold, L.S., Manley, N.B., Slone, T.H., Garfinkel, G.B., Rohrbach, L. & Ames, B.N. (1993a) The fifth plot of the carcinogenic potency database: results of animal bioassays published in the general literature through 1988 and by the National Toxicology Program through 1989. *Environ. Health Perspect.*, **100**, 65–168

Gold, L.S., Slone, T.H., Stern, B.R. & Bernstein, L. (1993b) Comparison of target organs of carcinogenicity for mutagenic and non-mutagenic chemicals. *Mutat. Res.*, **286**, 75–100

Gold, L.S., Manley, N.B., Slone, T.H., Garfinkel, G.B., Ames, B.N., Rohrbach, L., Stern, B.R. & Chow, K. (1995) Sixth plot of the carcinogenic potency database: results of animal bioassays published in the general literature 1989 to 1990 and by the National Toxicology Program 1990 to 1993. *Environ. Health Perspect.*, **103** (Suppl 8), 3–122

Goldsworthy, T.L., Conolly, R.B. & Fransson-Steen, R. (1996) Apoptosis and cancer risk assessment. *Mutat. Res.*, **365**, 71–90

Gray, G.M., Li, P., Shlyakhter, I. & Wilson, R. (1995) An empirical examination of factors influencing prediction of carcinogenic hazard across species. *Reg. Toxicol. Pharmacol.*, **22**, 283–291

Hard, G.C., Rodgers, I.S., Baetcke, K.P., Richards, W.L., McGaughy, R.E. & Valcovic, L.R. (1993) Hazard evaluation of chemicals that cause accumulation of α_{2u}-globulin, hyaline droplet nephropathy, and tubule neoplasia in the kidneys of male rats. *Environ. Health Perspect.*, **99**, 313–349

Hard, G.C., Whysner, J., English, J.C., Zang, E. & Williams, G.M. (1997) Relationship of hydroquinone-associated rat renal tumors with spontaneous chronic progressive nephropathy. *Toxicol. Pathol.*, **25**, 132–143

Harris, C.C. (1992) Tumour suppressor genes, multistage carcinogenesis and molecular epidemiology. In: Vainio, H., Magee, P.N., McGregor, D.B. & McMichael, A.J., eds, *Mechanisms of Carcinogenesis in Risk Identification* (IARC Scientific Publications No. 116), Lyon, IARC, pp. 67–85

Haseman, J.K. & Huff, J.E. (1987) Species correlation in long-term carcinogenicity studies. *Cancer Lett.*, **37**, 125–132

Herrold, K.M. (1969) Aflatoxin induced lesions in Syrian hamsters. *Br. J. Cancer*, **23**, 655–660

Hill, R.N., Erdreich, L.S., Paynter, O.E., Roberts, P.A., Rosenthal, S.L. & Wilkinson, C.F. (1989) Thyroid follicular cell carcinogenesis. *Fundam. Appl. Toxicol.*, **12**, 629–697

Huff, J.E. (1992) Chemical toxicity and chemical carcinogenesis. Is there a causal connection? A comparative morphological evaluation of 1500 experiments. In: Vainio, H., Magee, P.N., McGregor, D.B. & McMichael, A.J., eds, *Mechanisms of Carcinogenesis in Risk Identification* (IARC Scientific Publications No. 116), Lyon, IARC, pp. 437–475

Huff, J., Cirvello, J., Haseman, J. & Bucher, J. (1991) Chemicals associated with site-specific neoplasia in 1394 long-term carcinogenesis experiments in laboratory rodents. *Environ. Health Perspect.*, **93**, 247–270

IARC (1987) *IARC Monographs on the Evaluation of Carcinogenic Risks to Humans*, Suppl. 7, *Overall Evaluations of Carcinogenicity: An Updating of* IARC Monographs Volumes 1 to 42, Lyon

IARC (1989) *IARC Monographs on the Evaluation of Carcinogenic Risks to Humans*, Vol. 46, *Diesel and Gasoline Engine Exhausts and Some Nitroarenes*, Lyon

IARC (1998) *IARC Monographs on the Evaluation of Carcinogenic Risks to Humans*, Preamble, Lyon

IPCS (1996) *Chlorothalonil* (Environmental Health Criteria 183), World Health Organization, International Programme on Chemical Safety, Geneva

Kinzler, K.W. & Vogelstein, B. (1996) Lessons from hereditary colorectal cancer. *Cell*, **87**, 159–170

Kotkoskie, L.A., Richter, W.R. & Auletta, C.S. (1997) A

dietary oncogenicity study of tributyl phosphate in the mouse. *The Toxicologist. Fundam. Appl. Toxicol.*, **36** (Suppl. 1), Abstract No. 833

Kriek, E. (1969) On the mechanism of action of carcinogenic aromatic amines. I. Binding of 2-acetylaminofluorene and N-hydroxy-2-acetylaminofluorene to rat liver nucleic acids in vivo. *Chem.-Biol. Interactions*, **1**, 3–17

Larson, J.L, Wolf, D.C. & Butterworth, B.E. (1994) Induced cytolethality and regenerative cell proliferation in the livers and kidneys of male B6C3F$_1$ mice given chloroform by gavage. *Fundam. Appl. Toxicol.*, **23**, 537–543

Larson, J.L., Wolf, D.C., Méry, S., Morgan, K.T. & Butterworth, B.E. (1995) Toxicity and cell proliferation in the liver, kidneys and nasal passages of female F-344 rats, induced by chloroform administration by gavage. *Food Chem. Toxicol.*, **33**, 443–456

Lehman-McKeeman, L.D. & Caudill, D. (1992) α_{2u}-Globulin is the only member of the lipocalin protein superfamily that binds to hyaline droplet inducing agents. *Toxicol. Appl. Pharmacol.*, **116**, 170–176

Lehman-McKeeman, L.D. & Caudill, D. (1994) *d*-Limonene induced hyaline droplet nephropathy in α_{2u}-globulin transgenic mice. *Fundam. Appl. Toxicol.*, **23**, 562–568

Littlefield, N.A., Gaylor, D.W., Blackwell, B.N. & Allen, R.R. (1989) Chronic toxicity/carcinogenicity studies of sulphamethazine in B6C3F$_1$ mice. *Food Chem. Toxicol.*, **27**, 455–463

Littlefield, N.A., Sheldon, W.G., Allen, R. & Gaylor, D.W. (1990) Chronic toxicity/carcinogenicity studies of sulphamethazine in Fischer 344/N rats: two-generation exposure. *Food Chem. Toxicol.*, **28**, 157–167

Matanoski, G.M. & Elliott, E.A. (1981) Bladder cancer epidemiology. *Epidemiol. Rev.*, **3**, 203–229

Matsushima,T. (1994) Carcinogenesis study of chloroform (inhalation). Japan Industrial Safety and Health Association. (Written correspondence to Byron Butterworth, Chemical Industries Institute of Toxicology, Research Triangle Park, NC, USA, August 9, 1994)

McClain, R.M. (1989) The significance of hepatic microsomal enzyme induction and altered thyroid function in rats: implications for thyroid gland neoplasia. *Toxicol. Pathol.*, **17**, 294–306

McClain, R.M. (1995) Mechanistic considerations for the relevance of animal data on thyroid neoplasia to human risk assessment. *Mutat. Res.*, **333**, 131–142

McClain, R.M., Posch, R.C., Bosakowski, T. & Armstrong, J.M. (1988) Studies on the mode of action for thyroid gland tumor promotion in rats by phenobarbital. *Toxicol. Appl. Pharmacol.*, **94**, 254–265

Mehta, R. (1995) The potential for the use of cell proliferation and oncogene expression as intermediate markers during liver carcinogenesis. *Cancer Lett.*, **93**, 85–102

Melnick, R.L., Huff, J.E., Barrett, J.C., Maronpot, R.R., Lucier, G. & Portier, C.J. (1993) Cell proliferation and chemical carcinogenesis: symposium overview. *Environ. Health Perspect.*, **101** (Suppl. 5), 3–7

Miller, J.A. (1970) Carcinogenesis by chemicals: an overview – G.H.A. Clowes memorial Lecture. *Cancer Res.*, **30**, 559–576

Miller, E.C., Miller, J.A. & Enomoto, M. (1964) The comparative carcinogenicities of 2-acetylaminofluorene and its N-hydroxy metabolite in mice, hamsters, and guinea pigs. *Cancer Res.*, **24**, 2018–2031

Napalkov, N.P. (1990) Tumours of the thyroid gland. In: Turusov, V.S. & Mohr, U., eds, *Pathology of Tumours in Laboratory Animals, Vol. 1, Tumours of the Rat*, 2nd edition (IARC Scientific Publications No. 99), Lyon, IARC, pp. 539–572

Okamura, T., Garland, E.M., Johnson, L.S., Cano, M., Johansson, S.L. & Cohen, S.M. (1992) Acute urinary tract toxicity of tetraethylorthosilicate in rats. *Fundam. Appl. Toxicol.*, **18**, 425–441

Pendergast, W.J., Milmore, B.K. & Marcus, S.C. (1961) Thyroid cancer and thyrotoxicosis in the United States. Their relationship to endemic goiter. *J. Chronic Dis.*, **13**, 22–38

Preston-Martin, S., Pike, M.C., Ross, R.K., Jones, P.A. & Henderson, B.E. (1990) Increased cell division as a cause of human cancer. *Cancer Res.*, **50**, 7415–7421

Radomski, J.L. (1979) The primary aromatic amines: their biological properties and structure–activity relationships. *Ann. Rev. Pharmacol. Toxicol*, **19**, 129–157

Roe, F.J.C., Palmer, A.K., Worden, A.N. & Van Abbe, N.J. (1979) Safety evaluation of toothpaste containing chloroform. I. Long-term studies in mice. *J. Environ. Pathol. Toxicol.*, **2**, 799–819

Ron, E., Kleinerman, R.A., Boice, J.D., Jr, LiVolsi, V.A., Flannery, J.T. & Fraumeni, J.F., Jr (1987) A population-based case–control study of thyroid cancer. *J. Natl Cancer Inst.*, **79**, 1–12

Salabè, G.B. (1994) Aetiology of thyroid cancer: an epidemiological overview. *Thyroidology*, **6**, 11–19

Schulte-Hermann, R., Bursch, W., Kraupp-Grasl, B., Oberhammer, F., Wagner, A. & Jirtle, R. (1993) Cell proliferation and apoptosis in normal liver and preneoplastic foci. *Environ. Health Perspect.*, **101** (Suppl. 5), 87–90

Shelby, M.D. & Zeiger, E. (1990) Activity of human carcinogens in the Salmonella and rodent bone-marrow cytogenetics tests. *Mutat. Res.*, **234**, 257–261

Short, B.G., Burnett, V.L., Cox, M.G., Bus, J.S. & Swenberg, J.A. (1987) Site-specific renal cytotoxicity and cell proliferation in male rats exposed to petroleum hydrocarbons. *Lab. Invest.*, **57**, 564–577

Short, B.G., Steinhage, W.H. & Swenberg, J.A. (1989) Promoting effects of unleaded gasoline and 2,2,4-trimethylpentane on the development of atypical cell foci and renal tubular cell tumors in rats exposed to N-ethyl-N-hydroxyethylnitrosamine. *Cancer Res.*, **49**, 6369–6378

Söderlund, E., Dybing, E. & Nelson, S.D. (1980) Nephrotoxicity and hepatotoxicity of tris(2,3-dibromopropyl)phosphate in the rat. *Toxicol. Appl. Pharmacol.*, **56**, 171–181

Speerschneider, P. & Dekant, W. (1995) Renal tumorigenicity of 1,1-dichloroethene in mice: the role of male-specific expression of cytochrome P450 2E1 in the renal bioactivation of 1,1-dichloroethene. *Toxicol. Appl. Pharmacol.*, **130**, 48–56

Swenberg, J.A., Dietrich, D.R., McClain, R.M. & Cohen, S.M. (1992) Species-specific mechanisms of carcinogenesis. In: Vainio, H., Magee, P.N., McGregor, D.B. & McMichael, A.J., eds, *Mechanisms of Carcinogenesis in Risk Identification* (IARC Scientific Publications No. 116), IARC, Lyon, pp. 477–500

Takayama, S., Aihara, K., Onodera, T. & Akimoto, T. (1986) Antithyroid effects of propylthiouracil and sulfamonomethoxine in rats and monkeys. *Toxicol. Appl. Pharmacol.*, **82**, 191–199

Tennant, R.W. (1993) Stratification of rodent carcinogenicity bioassay results to reflect relative human hazard. *Mutat. Res.*, **286**, 111–118

Tennant, R.W., Margolin, B.H., Shelby, M.D., Zeiger, E., Haseman, J.K, Spalding, J., Caspary, W., Resnick, M., Stasiewicz, S., Anderson, B. & Minor, R. (1987) Prediction of chemical carcinogenicity in rodents from in vitro genetic toxicity assays. *Science*, **236**, 933–941

Thorgeirsson, U.P., Dalgard, D.W., Reeves, J. & Adamson, R.H. (1994) Tumor incidence in a chemical carcinogenesis study of nonhuman primates. *Reg. Toxicol. Pharmacol.*, **19**, 130–151

Tomatis, L., Aitio, A., Wilbourn, J. & Shuker, L. (1989) Human carcinogens so far identified. *Jpn. J. Cancer Res.*, **80**, 795–807

Tomatis, L., Huff, J., Hertz-Picciotto, I., Sandler, D.P., Bucher, J., Boffetta, P., Axelson, O., Blair, A., Taylor, J., Stayner, L. & Barrett, J.C. (1997) Avoided and avoidable risks of cancer. *Carcinogenesis*, **18**, 97–105

US Environmental Protection Agency (1996) Proposed Guidelines for Carcinogen Risk Assessment (EPA/600/P-92/003C), Office of Research and Development, Washington DC

US National Cancer Institute (1976) Carcinogenesis Bioassay of Chloroform (National Technical Information Service No. PB264018/AS), Bethesda, MD

US National Toxicology Program (1987) Carcinogenesis Studies of 1,4-Dichlorobenzene in F344/N Rats and B6C3F1 Mice (NTP Technical Report Series No. 319), Research Triangle Park, NC

US National Toxicology Program (1989) *Toxicology and Carcinogenesis Studies of Hydroquinone* (NIH Publication No. 90-2821), US Department of Health and Human Services, Washington DC

Uwagawa, S., Saito, K., Okuno, Y., Kawasaki, H., Yoshitake, A., Yamada, H. & Fukushima, S. (1994) Lack of induction of epithelial cell proliferation by sodium saccharin and sodium L-ascorbate in the urinary bladder of NCI-Black-Reiter (NBR) male rats. *Toxicol. Appl. Pharmacol.*, **127**, 182–186

Weiner, M.L., Auletta, C.S. & Richter, W.R. (1997) A dietary oncogenicity study of tributyl phosphate in the rat. *The Toxicologist. Fundam. Appl. Toxicol.*, **36** (Suppl. 1), Abstract No. 884

Weinstein, I.B. (1988) The origins of human cancer: molecular mechanisms of carcinogenesis and their implications for cancer prevention and treatment – twenty-seventh G.H.A. Clowes memorial award lecture. *Cancer Res.*, **48**, 4135–4143

Weinstein, I.B. (1991) Mitogenesis is only one factor in carcinogenesis. *Science*, **251**, 387–388

WHO (1990) Vinylidene Chloride (Environmental Health Criteria 100), World Health Organization, Geneva

Whysner, J., Verna, L., English, J.C. & Williams, G.M. (1995) Analysis of studies related to tumorigenicity induced by hydroquinone. *Regul. Toxicol. Pharmacol.*, **21**, 158–176

Wilbourn, J., Haroun, L., Heseltine, E., Kaldor, J., Partensky, C. & Vainio, H. (1986) Response of experimental animals to human carcinogens: an analysis based upon the IARC Monographs programme. *Carcinogenesis*, **7**, 1853–1863

Wilkinson, C.F. & Killeen, J.C. (1996) A mechanistic interpretation of the oncogenicity of chlorothalonil in rodents and an assessment of human relevance. *Regul. Toxicol. Pharmacol.*, **24**, 69–84

Wogan, G.N. (1973) Aflatoxin carcinogenesis. *Meth. Cancer Res.*, **7**, 309–344

Wolkowski-Tyl, R., Chin, T.Y., Popp, J.A. & Heck, H.D. (1982) Chemically induced urolithiasis in weanling rats. *Am. J. Pathol.*, **107**, 419–421

Zeiger, E., Haseman, J.K., Shelby, M.D., Margolin, B.H. & Tennant, R.W. (1990) Evaluation of four in vitro genetic toxicity tests for predicting rodent carcinogenicity: confirmation of earlier results with 41 additional chemicals. *Environ. Mol. Mutag.*, **16** (Suppl. 18), 1–14

Corresponding author

E. Dybing
Department of Environmental Medicine, National Institute of Public Health,
Oslo, Norway; and Laboratory of Occupational and Environmental Cancer,
Institute of Cancer Research, Oslo, Norway

Species Differences in Thyroid, Kidney and Urinary Bladder Carcinogenesis
C.C. Capen, E. Dybing, J.M. Rice and J.D. Wilbourn, eds
IARC Scientific Publications No. 147
International Agency for Research on Cancer, Lyon, 1999

Hormonal imbalances and thyroid cancers in humans

S. Franceschi and L. Dal Maso

Introduction

In humans, the normal thyroid contains two lobes joined by an isthmus. Fibrous septa divide the gland into pseudolobules which, in turn, are composed of vesicles called follicles or acini. Follicle walls are composed of cuboidal epithelium. The lumen of follicles is filled with a proteinaceous colloid, which contains a protein, thyroglobulin, within the peptide sequence of which L-thyroxine (T_4) and 3,5,3-triiodo-L-thyronine (T_3) are synthesized and stored. T_4 and T_3, the active thyroid hormones, influence a diversity of metabolic processes: the growth and maturation of tissues, cell respiration, total energy expenditure, and the turnover of essentially all substrates, vitamins and hormones, including the thyroid hormones themselves (Wartofski, 1994). Thyroid function is regulated by pituitary (thyroid-stimulating hormone, TSH) and hypothalamic (thyrotropin-releasing hormone, TRH) mediators and by the glandular organic iodine content.

In humans, the great majority of thyroid cancers arise from the epithelial elements of the gland, mostly from the follicular cells (Robbins et al., 1984). Such carcinomas fall into two broad groups: differentiated and undifferentiated (anaplastic). The former group is subdivided into two types, papillary and follicular. Medullary carcinoma derives from parafollicular cells (i.e., calcitonin-producing cells) and accounts for 5–15% of most series of thyroid carcinomas (Franceschi et al., 1993). It has quite a separate aetiology from other thyroid carcinomas, inheritance being an important determinant (Ron, 1996) and it is not considered further in the present review.

Radiation is the only well defined risk factor for thyroid carcinoma. A pooled analysis of five cohort studies and two case–control investigations, cumulating over 3 000 000 person–years of follow-up and 700 thyroid cancers, showed that, for persons exposed to radiation before the age of 15 years, the dose–response relationship was best described by a linear equation, even down to very low doses (0.10 Gy) (Ron et al., 1995). In contrast, risk was not appreciably elevated for exposure to external radiation in adults and no clear excess following diagnostic or therapeutic iodine-131 exposure was detected (Ron, 1996).

The thyroid gland is not obviously related to female sex hormones in the way the breast, ovary and uterus are. However, most thyroid disorders, except endemic iodine-deficient goitre, are several-fold more prevalent in women than men. Overall, thyroid cancer shows a 2–3-fold higher incidence in females than in males in most populations (Franceschi et al., 1993). However, female-to-male ratios vary substantially by histological type, being about 3 for papillary carcinoma, 2 for follicular carcinoma and 1 for medullary and undifferentiated carcinoma. This points to the possibility that events related to reproductive and menstrual history may be determinants of the risk of developing the most frequent tumours at this site (i.e., papillary and follicular carcinomas).

Puberty, pregnancy and oral contraceptives are associated with enlargement of the thyroid gland and with increases in serum levels of total T_4 and T_3 caused partly by a rise in the concentration of thyroxine-binding globulin (TBG) (Surks et al., 1990). One possible mechanism for explaining the hormonal influence in the pathogenesis of thyroid cancer is that increased levels of female hormones may cause elevation of TSH levels, leading in turn to thyroid hyperplasia and finally to cancer. Experimentally, increased TSH secretion induces thyroid tumours in rodents (Williams, 1979). Some authors (Pacchiarotti et al., 1986) reported small but significant increases of TSH levels in the second and third trimesters of pregnancy, perhaps as a compensatory mechanism to meet the increased demand for thyroid hormones in this period. Furthermore, estrogen receptors have been found in thyroid cancers (Miki et al., 1990).

The main focus of the present review is on epidemiological data regarding the relationship between menstrual and reproductive factors and risk of cancer of the thyroid in women. The role of elevated TSH levels will also be considered briefly, on the basis of circumstances (e.g., benign thyroid disease or residence in areas endemic for goitre) or exposures (e.g., food intake) which may cause and/or indicate enhanced TSH secretion.

Female sex hormones and thyroid cancers

Of at least ten case–control studies which have provided data on female thyroid cancer and reproductive and menstrual factors, four were conducted in the United States of America: one each in Washington State (McTiernan et al., 1984a; 185 cases and 393 controls, below age 80 years), Los Angeles, California (Preston-Martin et al., 1987; 292 cases and 292 controls below age 55 years), Connecticut (Ron et al., 1987; 109 cases and 208 controls below age 80), and Hawaii (Kolonel et al., 1990; Goodman et al., 1992; 140 cases and 328 controls, no age limit).

Five studies were carried out in Europe, including one each in Italy (Franceschi et al., 1990; D'Avanzo et al., 1995; 291 cases and 427 controls, below age 75) and Switzerland (Levi et al., 1993; 100 cases and 318 controls below age 75). Three studies were performed in Sweden (southern Sweden, Wingren et al., 1993; 149 cases and 187 controls, below age 60; northern Sweden, Hallquist et al., 1993, 1994; 123 cases and 240 controls, below age 70; and Uppsala, Galanti et al., 1995a, 1997; 133 cases and 203 controls, below age 72). One further study was conducted in Shanghai, China (Preston-Martin et al., 1993; 207 cases and 207 controls).

Of 1729 cancer cases examined, 80% had papillary carcinoma and 14% follicular carcinoma. Undifferentiated and medullary carcinomas accounted for only 10 and 32 cases, respectively. Four per cent of the cases had other or unspecified types. Thus the present results apply almost exclusively to differentiated thyroid carcinomas, chiefly papillary ones.

In order to evaluate the association of thyroid cancer risk with hormone-related events and exposures, odds ratios (ORs) and corresponding 95% confidence intervals (CI) are presented. Multiple logistic regression equations conditioned on age and including a term for history of radiation therapy (the best known risk factor for thyroid cancer; Ron et al., 1995) were fitted to the original data. Adjustment for other potential confounding factors was also made, where possible.

Menstrual factors

Information on age at menarche in relation to thyroid cancer risk can be derived from 10 case–control studies (Table 1). In those of Kolonel et al. (1990), Franceschi et al. (1990) and Galanti et al. (1995a), late age at menarche was associated with non–significantly increased ORs around 1.6 for menarche at age 15 or above compared with age 12 or below. In most investigations, however, the distribution of cases and controls with respect to age at menarche was similar.

Some consistent findings emerged with respect to the influence of menopause (Table 2). In all investigations except one (Ron et al., 1987), a higher proportion of cases compared to controls had undergone menopause, although the age distributions of cases and controls were similar and age was allowed for. Significantly increased risk (over two-fold) was found by McTiernan et al. (1987), Kolonel et al. (1990) and Levi et al. (1993). ORs tended to be somewhat higher for artificial than natural menopause, but the association with early menopause persisted after allowance for type of menopause. Late age at menopause was, thus, associated with reduced thyroid cancer risk, ORs for menopause at age 53 or above compared to below 45 years being 0.34 (95% CI, 0.10–1.21) in Kolonel et al. (1990) and 0.50 (95% CI, 0.14–1.74) in Levi et al. (1993).

In addition to age at menarche and menopause, some investigations included information on menstrual irregularities. Although in those of Franceschi et al. (1990) and Levi et al. (1993), women who reported irregularities were at slightly increased risk, most studies did not find any clear association with this characteristic.

Reproductive factors

In all ten published investigations, women with

Table 1. Odds ratios and corresponding 95% confidence intervals[a] of thyroid cancer by age at menarche

Study and location	Age at menarche (years)		
	< 13	13, 14	>14
McTiernan et al. (1987) Western Washington, USA	1	1.19 (0.79–1.78)	1.35 (0.76–2.38)
Preston-Martin et al. (1987) Los Angeles, USA	1	0.94 (0.61–1.46)	0.91 (0.43–1.93)
Ron et al. (1987) Connecticut, USA	1	1.35 (0.80–2.25)	1.03 (0.48–2.20)
Kolonel et al. (1990) Hawaii, USA	1	1.03 (0.65–1.63)	1.71 (0.98–2.96)
Franceschi et al. (1990) Northern Italy	1	1.08 (0.78–1.50)	1.54 (0.94–2.51)
Levi et al. (1993) Vaud, Switzerland	1	1.42 (0.83–2.44)	1.14 (0.59–2.21)
Wingren et al. (1993) Southeastern Sweden	1	0.83 (0.48–1.44)	0.71 (0.36–1.42)
Hallquist et al. (1994) Northern Sweden	1	1.48 (0.85–2.57)	1.01 (0.51–1.99)
Galanti et al. (1995a) Uppsala, Sweden	1	0.82 (0.47–1.44)	1.67 (0.83–3.36)
Preston-Martin et al. (1993) Shanghai, China	1	0.67 (0.22–2.10)	0.59 (0.19–1.82)

[a] Estimates from multiple logistic regression equations conditioned on age and adjusted for radiation history and age.

children seemed to be at somewhat increased risk of thyroid cancer compared with nulliparae (Table 3). However, no clear trend of increasing risk with increasing number of births (Table 3) or pregnancies was generally seen and, in several investigations (Ron et al., 1987; Preston-Martin et al., 1993), ORs tended to peak in women with one or two births.

Incomplete pregnancies showed a pattern similar to that for full-term pregnancies. However, in a few studies (Ron et al., 1987; Kolonel et al., 1990; Levi et al., 1993; Preston-Martin et al., 1993), personal history of miscarriages, especially at first pregnancy attempt, and difficulties in conception (Kolonel et al., 1990) seemed directly associated with thyroid cancer risk.

In a cohort study of all women and men who were born in Norway between 1935 and 1974 (about 2.6 million individuals), number of children was significantly related to thyroid cancer risk in women (ORs, 1.3, 1.4, 1.5 and 1.7 for 1, 2, 3 and 4 or more children, compared with none), but not in men (Glattre & Kravdal, 1994). However, even childless women had a thyroid cancer risk well above that of all men.

Although this aspect has received far less attention than parity, a tendency for thyroid cancer risk to increase slightly with increasing age at first pregnancy emerged from several studies (Table 4). Compared with women who bore their first child below 20 years of age, those who bore their first child at age 30 or later showed ORs above one in virtually all investigations, although in none was the risk significant.

Use of exogenous female hormones

Results on the relationship between oral contraceptive (OC) use and thyroid cancer risk are shown in Table 5, after allowance for other risk covariates (i.e., radiation history, education, parity, and type of menopause). In four investigations (Preston-Martin et al., 1987, 1993; Levi et al., 1993;

Table 2. Odds ratios and corresponding 95% confidence intervals[a] of thyroid cancer by menopausal status

	Pre	Post	
		Natural	Artificial
McTiernan et al. (1987) Western Washington, USA	1	2.17 (0.94–5.01)	2.67 (1.30–5.48)
Preston-Martin et al. (1987) Los Angeles, USA	1	0.26 (0.04–1.50)	1.63 (0.64–4.15)
Ron et al. (1987) Connecticut, USA	1	0.90 (0.33–2.46)	0.80 (0.38–1.86)
Kolonel et al. (1990) Hawaii, USA	1	1.90 (0.78–4.61)	2.03 (0.88–4.66)
Franceschi et al. (1990) Northern Italy	1	1.34 (0.66–2.72)	1.91 (0.92–3.99)
Levi et al. (1993) Vaud, Switzerland	1	1.75 (0.46–6.59)	5.61 (1.68–18.74)
Galanti et al. (1995a) Uppsala, Sweden	1	1.37 (0.30–6.32)	2.37 (0.60–9.45)
Preston-Martin et al. (1993) Shanghai, China	1	2.97 (1.08–8.20)	8.36 (0.79–88.48)

The top of the menopausal status columns is labelled "Menopausal status" spanning Pre/Post.

[a] Estimates from multiple logistic regression equations conditioned on age, and adjusted for radiation history, hormonal replacement therapy and age.

Wingren et al., 1993), women who had ever used OCs were at somewhat elevated risk, but the association never attained statistical significance. No clear trend was seen with the number of years of OC use.

Two studies, from Connecticut (Ron et al., 1987) and Italy (Franceschi et al., 1990), showed elevated thyroid cancer risk in OC users for younger women (ORs, 1.8 and 1.4 respectively), but no relationship in middle–aged users. The most interesting findings, however, concern recency of OC use, since, in all these studies, risk was specifically increased for current OC use and declined with increasing time since stopping. ORs above 1.5 in current OC users were found by Preston-Martin et al. (1987), Ron et al. (1987) and Levi et al. (1993).

Data are scantier with reference to menopausal hormone replacement treatment. The ORs associated with ever having had such treatment were 1.4 in the Washington study (McTiernan et al., 1984a), 0.5 in the Connecticut study (Ron et al., 1987), 0.9 in the Hawaii study (Kolonel et al., 1990) and 1.1 in one Swedish study (Hallquist et al., 1994), in the absence, however, of any consistent relationship with duration of use or any other time-related variable.

Thyroid–stimulating hormone (TSH) and growth factors

By analogy with animal models, situations which cause (e.g., iodine deficiency) and/or indicate (goitre, nodules) enhanced TSH secretion have been associated with increased risk in humans (Williams, 1979). The evidence is not, however, totally consistent.

Since Wegelin (1928) reported a 10-fold higher prevalence of thyroid cancer at autopsy in Bern, an endemic goitre area, than in Berlin, an area non-endemic for goitre, goitre and/or iodine deficiency have been considered as probable risk factors for thyroid cancer. Some of highest incidence (Parkin et al., 1992) and mortality (Levi et al., 1994) rates (Table 6) for thyroid cancer worldwide have indeed been found in endemic goitre areas close to the Andes (Colombia, Cali; Ecuador, Quito) and the

Table 3. Odds ratios and corresponding 95% confidence intervals[a] of thyroid cancer by number of births

		Number of births			
	0	1	2	3	≥ 4
McTiernan et al. (1987) Western Washington, USA	1	1.54 (0.81–2.95)	1.10 (0.58–2.07)	1.54 (0.76–3.12)	1.55 (0.74–3.25)
Preston-Martin et al. (1987) Los Angeles, USA	1	1.23 (0.62–2.44)	1.14 (0.57–2.28)	1.30 (0.52–3.31)	1.15 (0.41–3.20)
Ron et al. (1987) Connecticut, USA	1	1.95 (0.88–4.32)	2.06 (0.96–4.43)	1.10 (0.44–2.76)	1.30 (0.52–3.24)
Kolonel et al. (1990) Hawaii, USA	1	0.79 (0.38–1.63)	0.75 (0.39–1.45)	0.52 (0.24–1.09)	1.64 (0.85–3.14)
Franceschi et al. (1990) Northern Italy	1	1.13 (0.68–1.89)	1.28 (0.78–2.09)	1.30 (0.71–2.37)	1.18 (0.62–2.24)
Levi et al. (1993) Vaud, Switzerland	1	1.06 (0.50–2.24)	1.14 (0.58–2.23)	1.59 (0.70–3.61)	0.93 (0.30–2.86)
Galanti et al. (1995a) Uppsala, Sweden	1	1.38 (0.64–3.01)	0.81 (0.39–1.68)	0.80 (0.34–1.90)	2.02 (0.57–7.17)
Preston-Martin et al. (1993) Shanghai, China	1	1.98 (1.04–3.75)	1.66 (0.60–4.58)	0.50 (0.15–1.61)	0.80 (0.25–2.63)

[a] Estimates from multiple logistic regression equations conditioned on age, and adjusted for radiation history, oral contraceptive use and age.

Alps (Switzerland, and Austria). Iceland and Hawaii, however, have outstandingly high rates of thyroid cancer, despite high levels of iodine intake (Goodman et al., 1988). Correction of iodine deficiency through the introduction of iodized salt (Wynder, 1952) or changed farming practices (Phillips, 1997) has proved successful as far as goitre elimination is concerned. With respect to thyroid cancer, clear declines in mortality have been reported in Switzerland (Wynder, 1952), but not in the United States (Ron, 1996).

Separate consideration of various histological types led to the suggestion that follicular and anaplastic carcinomas may be more frequent in endemic goitre areas, while papillary carcinomas may be enhanced by iodine excess (Williams, 1977; Williams et al., 1977). In Sweden, iodination of the food supply was started in 1936 and enhanced in 1966. Regional patterns of thyroid cancer incidence in the period 1958–81 in relation to the presence of former goitre endemicity have been reported (Pettersson et al., 1996). Incidence rates for all thyroid cancers combined were slightly lower in formerly iodine-deficient areas than in iodine-sufficient ones. The incidence of papillary cancer was higher in iodine-sufficient areas and higher in urban than in rural areas. Conversely, the incidence of follicular and anaplastic carcinoma was slightly elevated in iodine-deficient areas. However, upward trends in incidence rates of papillary carcinoma were similar in iodine-sufficient and iodine-deficient areas. Conversely, the decreases in incidence rates of anaplastic carcinoma were more marked in areas formerly affected by goitre endemicity.

Only two case–control studies have provided data on risk of thyroid cancer by residence in endemic goitre areas (Table 7). In the Italian study, the RR for having resided in endemic goitre areas was 1.3 for < 20 years of residence and 1.6 for 20 or more years (D'Avanzo et al., 1995). Residence before the age of 25 years seemed more influential (Franceschi et al., 1989). In the study in Sweden, a trend towards an association was found with duration of residence in endemic goitre areas (Galanti et al., 1995b). In neither study was any

Table 4. Odds ratios and 95% confidence intervals[a] of thyroid cancer by age at first birth

	Nulliparae	< 20	Age at first birth (years) 20–24	25–29	≥ 30
McTiernan et al. (1987) Western Washington, USA	0.70 (0.31–1.60)	1	0.85 (0.47–1.54)	0.70 (0.34–1.44)	1.45 (0.60–3.51)
Preston-Martin et al. (1987) Los Angeles, USA	6.22 (0.35–112.15)	1	1.73 (0.22–13.38)	46.00 (0.72–2908.75)	2.09(0.10–42.86)
Ron et al. (1987) Connecticut, USA	0.47 (0.13–1.62)	1	1.00 (0.40–2.50)	0.74 (0.26–2.05)	1.42(0.42–4.80)
Kolonel et al. (1990) Hawaii, USA	2.95 (1.09–8.01)	1	0.71 (0.36–1.42)	1.09 (0.52–2.28)	2.01(0.76–5.32)
Franceschi et al. (1990) Northern Italy	1.05 (0.46–2.39)	1	0.87 (0.45–1.69)	1.47 (0.74–2.94)	1.73(0.77–3.89)
Levi et al. (1993) Vaud, Switzerland	1.59 (0.39–6.39)	1	2.15 (0.64–7.19)	1.97 (0.56–6.88)	2.18(0.54–8.88)
Galanti et al. (1995a) Uppsala, Sweden	0.70 (0.21–2.29)	1	0.57 (0.25–1.28)	0.66 (0.28–1.55)	1.20(0.37–3.93)
Preston-Martin et al. (1993) Shanghai, China	0.51 (0.14–1.92)	1	1.20 (0.50–2.88)	1.33 (0.49–3.57)	1.34(0.39–4.66)

[a] Estimates from multiple logistic regression equations conditioned on age, and adjusted for radiation history, parity and age.

clear difference detected between papillary carcinomas and follicular carcinomas with respect to residence history.

Results are far more consistent with respect to the influence of previous benign thyroid diseases. Thyroid nodules (adenomas), when analysed separately, were usually associated with higher relative risks than goitre (Table 8). The possibility that ascertainment and/or recall bias somewhat exaggerated RR estimates must be borne in mind. In case–control studies, lower RRs (approximately equal to 6) associated with a positive history of goitre were reported, whereas no significant elevation of risk was seen for a history of hyperthyroidism or hypothyroidism (McTiernan et al., 1984b; Preston-Martin et al., 1987; Franceschi et al., 1989; Kolonel et al., 1990; Levi et al., 1991).

Regarding Graves' disease and its role in thyroid carcinogenesis, the first report was that of a 2.5% prevalence of thyroid cancer in 2114 hyperplastic thyroid glands (Olen and Klinck, 1966), 50% of which were papillary in type. However, no significant excess of thyroid cancer was reported among patients with Graves' disease in Olmsted County, Minnesota, USA (Munoz et al., 1978), nor among those with thyrotoxicosis in the US

Cooperative Thyrotoxicosis study (Dobyns et al., 1974).

In a retrospective follow-up study of 7338 women with either nontoxic nodular goitre, thyroid adenoma, hyperthyroidism, hypothyroidism, Hashimoto's thyroiditis, or no thyroid disease, treated between 1925 and 1974 at the Massachusetts General Hospital, a significant increase in thyroid cancer risk was observed only in women with thyroid adenoma (Goldman et al., 1990).

Finally, with respect to dietary influences, some foods (notably fish) contain large amounts of iodine, while others (e.g., milk, meat, eggs, etc.) can be important sources of iodine depending upon farming practices (Phillips, 1997). Some vegetables, most notably cruciferous vegetables, and certain staple foods, especially cassava and maize, contain goitrogenous substances. The few case–control studies in which dietary information was collected, however, discarded the possibility of any vegetables having an adverse effect on thyroid cancer risk, at least in affluent countries (Franceschi et al., 1993; Galanti et al., 1997). With respect to fish, they suggested that the association may be different according to the local iodine

Table 5. Odds ratios and corresponding 95% confidence intervals[a] of thyroid cancer by oral contraceptive use

	Oral contraceptive use	
	Never	Ever
McTiernan et al. (1987) Western Washington, USA	1	1.00 (0.60–1.68)
Preston-Martin et al. (1987) Los Angeles, USA	1	1.45 (0.81–2.59)
Ron et al. (1987) Connecticut, USA	1	1.13 (0.61–2.11)
Kolonel et al. (1990) Hawaii, USA	1	0.64 (0.39–1.07)
Franceschi et al. (1990) Northern Italy	1	0.95 (0.61–1.49)
Levi et al. (1993) Vaud, Switzerland	1	1.26 (0.70–2.29)
Wingren et al. (1993) Southeastern Sweden	1	1.22 (0.73–2.03)
Hallquist et al. (1994) Northern Sweden	1	0.82 (0.47–1.42)
Galanti et al. (1995a) Uppsala, Sweden	1	0.93 (0.51–1.69)
Preston-Martin et al. (1993) Shanghai, China	1	1.57 (0.87–2.84)

[a] Estimates from multiple logistic regression equations conditioned on age, and adjusted for radiation history, education, parity, type of menopause, and age.

Table 6. Highest incidence and mortality rates of thyroid cancer in females (world-standardized) and female to male (F to M) ratios

Country, area	Rate	F to M Ratio
	Incidence [a]	
Colombia, Cali	6.6	3.7
Ecuador, Quito	6.3	2.2
US, Los Angeles, Japanese	6.9	4.9
Filipino	7.9	1.7
US, Hawaii, White	8.7	3.2
Japanese	6.3	1.5
Hawaiian	9.6	1.8
Filipino	24.2	3.7
Chinese	11.3	1.4
Philippines, Manila	8.6	2.5
Iceland	8.3	1.3
	Mortality [b]	
Iceland	0.9	1.0
Hungary	0.9	1.5
Malta	0.8	1.6
Austria	0.8	1.3
Singapore	0.8	1.0
Switzerland	0.7	1.2
Italy	0.7	1.4
Germany, FRG	0.7	1.2
Germany, GDR	0.7	1.4
Finland	0.7	1.4
Czechoslovakia	0.7	1.4
Israel	0.7	1.2

[a] From Parkin et al. (1992)
[b] From Levi et al. (1994)

availability (i.e., there may be a positive association in the presence of iodine excess, but a negative one with iodine deficiency) (Franceschi et al., 1993; Glattre et al., 1993).

Discussion

Several menstrual and reproductive factors have been related to thyroid cancer risk, but often subsequent studies have failed to confirm the findings. This is not surprising since investigations on these topics have not included more than a few hundred women and the available data indicate that these factors are only weakly related to thyroid cancer risk, if at all. Even the few consistent findings (i.e., associations with early menopause, late age at first birth, and recent OC use) may well have been missed in smaller data–sets. Indeed, the associations

observed are often of similar magnitude (e.g., age at first birth), though not always in the same direction (e.g., age at menopause), as those reported for breast cancer (Lipworth, 1995), which required studies of several thousand cases to be adequately assessed (Collaborative Group on Hormonal Factors in Breast Cancer, 1996; Talamini et al., 1996). Thus, these data suggest that menstrual and reproductive factors are weak correlates of subsequent thyroid cancer risk. The apparently stronger effect of most menstrual and reproductive factors on neoplasms occurring at younger age (Franceschi et al., 1993) suggests that hormonal factors have a late–stage (promotional) effect on

Duration of	Sex		Age (years)		Type		All
residence (years)	Male	Female	< 50	> 50	Papillary	Follicular	
Italy[a]							
Never	1	1	1	1	1	1	1
< 20	0.9	1.6	1.3	1.1	1.3	1.9	1.3
> 20	1.1	2.2[b]	2.5[b]	1.1	1.7	1.9	1.6
Age at 1st residence							
≤ 25	0.7	1.1	–	–	–	–	1.0
< 25	1.4	2.7[b]	–	–	–	–	2.4[b]
Sweden[c]							
Never	–	–	1	1	1	1	1
≤ 10	–	–	1.3	0.8	0.9	1.8	1.1
11–20	–	–	0.7	0.9	0.9	0.3	0.8
21–40	–	–	0.8	2.3	1.1	1.9	1.3
> 41	–	–	2.0	1.7	1.5	1.2	1.5
Age at 1st residence							
< 1	1.2	1.1	–	–	0.9	1.8	1.1
1–10	0.9	1.0	–	–	0.9	0.3	0.8
11–20	0.5	2.1	–	–	1.1	1.9	1.3
> 21	0.9	0.9	–	–	1.5	1.2	1.5

Table 7. Relative risk of thyroid cancer by residence in endemic goitre areas. Italy, 1986–92 and Sweden 1980–92

[a] Franceschi et al. (1989) and D'Avanzo et al. (1995).
[b] Statistically significant (95% confidence interval does not include unity).
[c] Galanti et al. (1995b).

thyroid cancer, as on several other hormone-related neoplasms, and their influence seems to level off soon after exposure ceases (Day, 1983; Bruzzi et al., 1988).

Some of the associations observed, including the association with early or artificial menopause, may well be due to diagnostic or ascertainment bias since, for instance, women undergoing surgical menopause may be more carefully surveyed for any hormonal — including thyroid — imbalance (Franceschi et al., 1993). Likewise, some excess of cancer risk in current OC users could be due to increased surveillance for thyroid masses among OC users. The majority of thyroid carcinomas in young women, in fact, are detected in the absence of symptoms or signs, as a consequence of examination for other reasons (Franceschi et al., 1993). However, these findings may reflect a real association restricted to current or recent use. Again, this pattern of risk is similar to that described for breast cancer, for which the association with OC use seems also to be exclusive to current or recent users (Collaborative Group on Hormonal Factors in Breast Cancer, 1996; La Vecchia et al., 1996). A better quantification of the roles of reproductive and menstrual factors and, of greater public health importance, OCs and hormone replacement therapy will emerge from a pooled analysis of individual data from 14 studies, partly unpublished, including about 2300 female cases of thyroid cancer and 3700 control women.

With respect to the role of elevated TSH levels, epidemiological findings on thyroid cancer excess in iodine-rich areas as well as in iodine-deficient areas seem contradictory. Both iodine deficiency and iodine excess may lead to enhanced TSH secretion. Endemic goiter due to iodine excess has been demonstrated in Japanese and Norwegian

Table 8. Relative risk of thyroid cancer in females by history of benign nodules and goitre

Reference	Type of case-control study	Benign nodules	Goitre
McTiernan et al. (1987)	Population-based	10.5[a]	
Preston-Martin et al. (1987)	Population-based	12.0	6.6
Ron et al. (1987)	Population-based	33.3	5.6
Franceschi et al. (1989)	Hospital-based	Infinity[b]	9.6
Preston-Martin et al. (1993)	Hospital-based	16.0	7.0
Goldman et al. (1990)	Historical follow-up	11.7	2.6
Levi et al. (1991)	Hospital-based	18.3	3.8

[a] Benign nodules and/or goitre
[b] No control subjects reported the disease.

fishermen who eat large quantities of iodine-rich seaweed (Suzuki et al., 1965; Okamura et al., 1987), and in locations in China where iodine concentration in drinking water is very high (Li et al., 1987), and iodine-rich salt or pickled vegetables (Zhu et al., 1984) are ingested in large quantities. Direct epidemiological evidence is, however, very scanty. Only one study provided information on TSH levels in the preclinical phase of thyroid cancer (Thoresen et al., 1988), in which 43 patients with thyroid cancer were compared with 128 healthy controls, for whom sera had been collected on average four years earlier, in a large Norwegian serum bank. No difference in TSH level was found, whereas levels of TBG were increased among thyroid cancer patients compared with controls. The increased TBG levels were interpreted as either a secretory product from a slowly growing subclinical tumour or a leakage phenomenon from normal follicles (Thoresen et al., 1988).

Although the importance of accurate histological typing in the study of thyroid cancer cannot be overemphasized, the possibility that correction of iodine deficiency can induce an increase in papillary carcinomas (the so–called papillarization hypothesis) (Rolon, 1986) remains difficult to confirm, but seems unlikely (Pettersson et al., 1996). The elimination of iodine deficiency has been accompanied in affluent countries by elevation of diagnostic standards (e.g., use of thyroid scintigraphy, ultrasound, and fine-needle biopsy). Such improvements account in large part for the increased incidence, since a 'pool' of individuals with clinically silent papillary carcinomas is probably present in most populations, as shown by the high prevalence of such lesions (up to over 30%) in autopsy series (Franceschi et al., 1993; Ron, 1996).

Acknowledgements
The authors wish to thank Mrs Anna Redivo for editorial assistance and the investigators who provided original data.

References
Bruzzi, P., Negri, E., La Vecchia, C., Decarli, A., Palli, D., Parazzini, F. & Del Turco, M.R. (1988) Short term increase in risk of breast cancer after full term pregnancy. Br. Med. J., 297, 1096–1098

Collaborative Group on Hormonal Factors in Breast Cancer (1996) Breast cancer and hormonal contraceptives: collaborative reanalysis of individual data on 53 297 women with breast cancer and 100 239 women without breast cancer from 54 epidemiological studies. Lancet, 347, 1713–1727

D'Avanzo, B., La Vecchia, C., Franceschi, S., Negri, E. & Talamini, R. (1995) History of thyroid diseases and subsequent thyroid cancer risk. Cancer Epidemiol. Biomarkers Prev., 4, 193–199

Day, N.E. (1983) Time as a determinant of risk in cancer epidemiology: the role of multistage models. Cancer Surv., 2, 577–593

Dobyns, B.M., Sheline, G.E., Workman, J.B., Tompkins, E.A., McConahey, W.M. & Becker, D.V. (1974) Malignant and benign neoplasms of the thyroid in patients treated for hyperthyroidism: a report of cooperative thyrotoxicosis therapy follow-up study. J. Clin. Endocrinol. Metab., 38, 976–998

Franceschi, S., Fassina, A., Talamini, R., Mazzolini, A., Vianello, S., Bidoli, E., Serraino, D. & La Vecchia, C. (1989) Risk factors for thyroid cancer in northern Italy. *Int. J. Epidemiol.*, **18**, 578–584

Franceschi, S., Fassina, A., Talamini, R., Mazzolini, A., Vianello, S., Bidoli, E., Cizza, G. & La Vecchia, C. (1990) The influence of reproductive and hormonal factors on thyroid cancer in women. *Rev. Epidemiol. Santé Publ.*, **38**, 27–34

Franceschi, S., Boyle, P., Maisonneuve, P., La Vecchia, C., Burt, A.D., Kerr, D.J. & MacFarlane, G.J. (1993) The epidemiology of thyroid carcinoma. *Crit. Rev. Oncog.*, **4**, 25–52

Galanti, M.R., Lambe, M., Ekbom, A, Sparen, P. & Pettersson B. (1995a) Parity and risk of thyroid cancer: a nested case-control study of a nationwide Swedish cohort. *Cancer Causes Control*, **6**, 37–44

Galanti, M.R., Sparén, P., Karlsson, A., Grimelius, L. & Ekbom, A. (1995b) Is residence in areas of endemic goiter a risk factor for thyroid cancer? *Int. J. Cancer*, **61**, 615–621

Galanti, M.R., Hansson, L., Bergstrom, R., Wolk, A., Hjartaker, A., Lund, E., Grimelius, L. & Ekbom, A. (1997) Diet and risk of papillary and follicular thyroid carcinoma: a population-based case–control study in Sweden and Norway. *Cancer Causes Control*, **8**, 205–214

Glattre, E. & Kravdal, Ø. (1994) Male and female parity and risk of thyroid cancer. *Int. J. Cancer*, **58**, 616–617

Glattre, E., Haldorsen, T., Berg, J.P., Stensvold, I. & Solvoll, K. (1993) Norwegian case-control study testing the hypothesis that seafood increases the risk of thyroid cancer. *Cancer Causes Control*, **4**, 11–16

Goldman, M.B., Monson, R.R. & Maloof, F. (1990) Cancer mortality in women with thyroid disease. *Cancer Res.*, **50**, 2283-2289

Goodman, M.T., Yoshizawa, C.N. & Kolonel, L.N. (1988) Descriptive epidemiology of thyroid cancer in Hawaii. *Cancer*, **61**, 1272–1281

Goodman, M.T., Kolonel, L.N. & Wilkens, L.R. (1992) The association of body size, reproductive factors and thyroid cancer. *Br. J. Cancer*, **66**, 1180–1184

Hallquist, A., Hardell, L., Degerman, A. & Boquist, L. (1993) Occupational exposures and thyroid cancer: results of a case-control study. *Eur. J. Cancer Prev.*, **2**, 345–349

Hallquist, A., Hardell, L., Degerman, A. & Boquist, L. (1994) Thyroid cancer: reproductive factors, previous diseases, drug intake, family history and diet. A case–control study. *Eur. J. Cancer Prev.*, **3**, 481–488

Kolonel, L.N., Hankin, J.H., Wilkens, L.R., Fukunaga, F.H. & Hinds, M.W. (1990) An epidemiologic study of thyroid cancer in Hawaii. *Cancer Causes Control*, **1**, 223–234

La Vecchia, C., Tavani, A., Franceschi, S. & Parazzini, F. (1996) Oral contraceptives and cancer. A review of the evidence. *Drug Saf.*, **14**, 260–272

Levi, F., Franceschi, S., La Vecchia, C., Negri, E., Gulie, C., Duruz, G. & Scazziga, B. (1991) Previous thyroid disease and risk of thyroid cancer in Switzerland. *Eur. J. Cancer*, **27**, 85–88

Levi, F., Franceschi, S., Gulie, C., Negri, E. & La Vecchia, C. (1993) Female thyroid cancer: the role of reproductive and hormonal factors in Switzerland. *Oncology*, **50**, 309–315

Levi, F., Lucchini, F. & La Vecchia, C. (1994) Worldwide patterns of cancer mortality, 1985–89. *Eur. J. Cancer Prev.*, **3**, 109–143

Li, M., Liu, D.R., Qu, C.Y., Zhang, P.Y., Qian, Q.D., Zhang, C.D., Jia, Q.Z., Wang, H.X., Eastman, C.J., Boyages, S.C., Collins, J.K., Jupp, J.J. & Maberly, G.F. (1987) Endemic goitre in central China caused by excessive iodine intake. *Lancet*, **ii**, 257–259

Lipworth, L. (1995) Epidemiology of breast cancer. *Eur. J. Cancer Prev.*, **4**, 7–30

McTiernan, A.M., Weiss, N.S. & Daling, J.R. (1984a) Incidence of thyroid cancer in women in relation to reproductive and hormonal factors. *Am. J. Epidemiol.*, **120**, 423–435

McTiernan, A.M., Weiss, N.S. & Daling, J.R. (1984b) Incidence of thyroid cancer in women in relation to previous exposure to radiation therapy and history of thyroid disease. *J. Natl Cancer Inst.*, **73**, 575–581

McTiernan, A.M., Weiss, N.S. & Daling, J.R. (1987) Incidence of thyroid cancer in women in relation to known or suspected risk factors for breast cancer. *Cancer Res.*, **47**, 292–295

Miki, H., Oshimo, K., Inoue, H., Morimoto, T. & Monden, Y. (1990) Sex hormone receptors in human thyroid tissues. *Cancer*, **66**, 1759–1762

Munoz, J.M., Gorman, C.A., Elveback, L.R. & Wentz, J.R. (1978) Incidence of malignant neoplasms of all types in patients with Graves' disease. *Arch. Intern. Med.*, **138**, 944–947

Okamura, K., Nakashima, T., Ueda, K., Inoue, K., Omae, T. & Fujishima, M. (1987) Thyroid disorders in the general population of Hisayama, Japan, with special reference to prevalence and sex differences. *Int. J. Epidemiol.*, **16**, 545–549

Olen, E. & Klinck, G.H. (1966) Hyperthyroidism and thyroid cancer. *Arch. Pathol.*, **81**, 531–535

Pacchiarotti, A., Martino, E., Bartalena, L., Buratti, L., Mammoli, C., Strigini, F., Fruzetti,F., Melis, G.B. & Pinchera. A. (1986) Serum thyrotropin by ultrasensitive immunoradiometric assay and serum free thyroid hormones in pregnancy. *J. Endocrinol. Invest.*, 9, 185–189

Parkin, D.M., Muir, C.S., Whelan, S.L., Gao, Y.T., Ferlay, J. & Powell, J., eds (1992) *Cancer Incidence in Five Continents*, Vol. VI (IARC Scientific Publications No. 120), Lyon, IARC

Pettersson, B., Coleman, M.P., Ron, E. & Adam, H.-O. (1996) Iodine supplementation in Sweden and regional trends in thyroid cancer incidence by histopathologic type. *Int. J. Cancer*, 65, 13–19

Phillips, D.I.W. (1997) Iodine, milk, and the elimination of endemic goitre in Britain: the story of an accidental public heatlh triumph. *J. Epidemiol. Community Health*, 51, 391–393

Preston-Martin, S., Bernstein, L., Pike, M.C., Maldonado, A.A. & Henderson, B.E. (1987) Thyroid cancer among young women related to prior thyroid disease and pregnancy history. *Br. J. Cancer*, 55, 191–195

Preston-Martin, S., Jin, E., Duda, M.J. & Mack, W.J. (1993) A case-control study of thyroid cancer in women under age 55 in Shanghai (People's Republic of China). *Cancer Causes Control*, 4, 431–440

Robbins, S.L., Cotram, R.S. & Kumar, V. (1984) Pathologic Basis of Disease, Philadelphia, W.B. Saunders, pp. 1201–1225

Rolon, P.A. (1986) Cancer of the thyroid in an area of endemic goiter. 'Papillarization' with prophylactic iodization. *Ann. Pathol.*, 6, 170–175

Ron, E. (1996) Thyroid cancer. In: Schottenfeld, D. & Fraumeni, J.F., Jr, eds, Cancer Epidemiology and Prevention, 2nd Ed., New York, Oxford University Press, pp. 1000–1021

Ron, E., Kleinerman, R.A., Boice, J.D., Jr, LiVolsi, V.A., Flannery, J.T. & Fraumeni, J.F., Jr (1987) A population-based case-control study of thyroid cancer. *J. Natl Cancer Inst.*, 79, 1–12

Ron, E., Lubin, J.H., Shore, R.E., Mabuchi, K., Modan, B., Pottern, L.M., Schneider, A.B., Tucker, M.A. & Boice, J.D., Jr (1995) Thyroid cancer after exposure to external radiation: a pooled analysis of seven studies. *Radiat. Res.*, 141, 259–277

Surks, M.I., Chopra, I.J., Mariash, C.N., Nicoloff, J.T. & Solomon, D.H. (1990) American Thyroid Association guidelines for use of laboratory tests in thyroid disorders. *J. Am. Med. Assoc.*, 263, 1529–1532

Suzuki, H., Higuchi, T., Sawa, K., Ohtaki, S. & Horiuchi, Y. (1965) "Endemic coast goitre" in Hokkaido, Japan, *Acta Endocrinol. Copenh.*, 50, 161–176

Talamini, R., Franceschi, S., La Vecchia, C., Negri, E., Borsa, L., Montella, M., Falcini, F., Conti, E. & Rossi, C. (1996) The role of reproductive and menstrual factors in cancer of the breast before and after menopause. *Eur. J. Cancer*, 32A, 303–310

Thoresen, S.Ø., Myking, O., Glattre, E., Rootwelt, K., Andersen, A. & Foss, O.P. (1988) Serum thyroglobulin as a preclinical tumour marker in subgroups of thyroid cancer. *Br. J. Cancer*, 57, 105–108

Wartofsky, L. (1994) Diseases of the thyroid. In: Isselbacher, K.J., Braunwald, E., Wilson, J.D., Martin, J.B., Fauci, A.S. & Kasper, D.L., eds, Harrison's Principles of Internal Medicine, 13th Ed., Vol. 2, Part 13, *Endocrinology and Metabolism*, New York, McGraw-Hill, pp. 1930–1953

Wegelin, C. (1928) Malignant disease of the thyroid gland and its relation to goiter in man and animals. *Cancer Rev.*, 3, 297–313

Williams, E.D. (1977) The epidemiology of thyroid cancer. *Ann. Radiol.* (Paris), 20, 722–724

Williams, E.D., Doniach, I., Bjarnason, O. & Michie, W. (1977) Thyroid cancer in an iodine rich area: a histopathological study. *Cancer*, 39, 215–222

Wingren, G., Hatschek, T. & Axelson, O. (1993) Determinants of papillary cancer of the thyroid. *Am. J. Epidemiol.*, 138, 482–491

Wynder, E.L. (1952) Some practical aspects of cancer prevention (concluded). *New Engl. J. Med.*, 246, 573–582

Zhu, X.Y., Lu, T.Z., Song, X.K., Li, X.T., Gao, S.M., Yang, H.M., Ma, T., Li, Y.Z. & Zhang, W.Q. (1984) Endemic goiter due to iodine rich salt and its pickled vegetables. *Chin. Med. J.*, 97, 545–548

Corresponding author

S. Franceschi
Servizio di Epidemiologia, Centro di Riferimento Oncologico, Via Pedemontana Occ. 12, 33081 Aviano (PN), Italy

Species Differences in Thyroid, Kidney and Urinary Bladder Carcinogenesis
C.C. Capen, E. Dybing, J.M. Rice and J.D. Wilbourn, eds
IARC Scientific Publications No. 147
International Agency for Research on Cancer, Lyon, 1999

Thyroid stimulating hormone (TSH)-associated follicular hypertrophy and hyperplasia as a mechanism of thyroid carcinogenesis in mice and rats

G.A. Thomas and E.D. Williams

Introduction

The mammalian thyroid is composed of two types of epithelial cell: the follicular cells, which line the lumen of the colloid-filled follicles and are responsible for the production of thyroid hormones, and the C cells, which are derived from the neuroectoderm, are parafollicular in position in most mammals and are responsible for the production of calcitonin. In both humans and rodents, the cells lie between the follicular cells and the basement membrane, while in dogs they form islands that lie in the interfollicular space. In humans there is no great change in either follicular or C cells with age, but laboratory rats show an age-related increase in the number of C cells. This may correlate with the fact that tumours of the C cells are a relatively common finding in aged rats, although the frequency varies with sex and strain from 0% to 47%, with the highest frequency in the male WAG/Rij rat (DeLellis, 1994). In contrast, C cell number does not increase with age in the mouse, and the incidence of C cell tumours is very low (DeLellis et al., 1996). In humans, C cell numbers are relatively much lower than in the laboratory rodent, and spontaneous C cell tumours (medullary carcinomas) form less than 10% of all thyroid malignancies. They can occur as part of a multiple endocrine neoplasia syndrome, which is associated with a germline mutation in the ret proto-oncogene. C cell tumours and differentiated tumours derived from the follicular cells can usually be easily distinguished by the use of immuno-cytochemical techniques for calcitonin and thyroglobulin.

In contrast to C cell tumours, spontaneous tumours of the follicular cell are rare in both rats and mice. In mice, the frequency in all strains studied is of the order of 1% (Thomas & Williams, 1996); in rats, some variation has been noticed with strain, but the incidence is still lower than 3% (Thomas & Williams, 1994), and such tumours usually occur only in aged animals. The majority of spontaneous tumours are benign. However, the incidence of follicular cell tumours (both benign and malignant) is greatly increased when animals are maintained on a diet which is low in iodide or contains substances known to interfere with thyroid hormone homeostasis (goitrogens). Administration of a mutagen followed by long-term goitrogen treatment can increase the incidence of follicular cell tumours still further.

Pathology of thyroid follicular proliferative lesions

The majority of proliferative lesions found in both man and animals are benign. Two types of benign lesion can be distinguished: the nodule and the adenoma. Adenomas are defined as being solitary, encapsulated and having a relatively uniform internal architecture and cytology, differing from the surrounding thyroid. They commonly compress the adjacent gland. Nodules are typically less well circumscribed, have a more variable architecture and cytology, which may in part be similar to background thyroid, are unencapsulated and do not compress adjacent tissue. In toxicological studies, multiple lesions are often observed in a background of follicular cell hyperplasia, and distinction between nodule and adenoma can be difficult.

Distinction between nodule and adenoma has been made not only on grounds of morphology but also on differences in clonal origin in a study in mice. Nodules, in addition to the similarities in their morphology to background thyroid, are polyclonal in origin, whereas adenomas, which show distinct morphological changes from background normal or hyperplastic thyroid, are monoclonal in origin (Thomas *et al.*, 1989).

Nodules and adenomas also occur in humans, where the same morphological criteria are applied for their distinction, and the same difficulties occur in making this distinction in some lesions. Multiple nodules are particularly common in areas of iodide deficiency.

Carcinomas of the thyroid follicular cells in man may be differentiated or, more rarely, undifferentiated. The differentiated types fall into two main groups, named after the dominant architectural pattern in the classical lesions — papillary or follicular. The separation of these two types is now recognized to correlate with a different pattern of oncogene change, different clinical behaviour and different epidemiological associations. The diagnostic importance of the architectural pattern is now considered less specific, but the names remain. Attempts have been made to separate carcinomas in rodents into the same groups as in humans, but while there are architectural differences between tumours, the evidence that these correlate with biologically different entities, as they do in humans, is lacking. In practice carcinomas in rodents show morphologically similar characteristics to adenomas, but are distinguished from them by the evidence of invasion through the capsule into veins and surrounding tissue.

Thyroid hormone homeostasis

The induction of thyroid follicular cell tumours in rodents is greatly influenced by the level of growth stimulation from thyroid-stimulating hormone (TSH). It is therefore important in considering mechanisms of carcinogenesis in the thyroid to bear in mind some of the steps involved in thyroid hormone synthesis, secretion and metabolism.

Thyroid hormone homeostasis utilizes a variety of mechanisms, many of which have been shown to be affected by diet and xenobiotic agents. Synthesis of the thyroid hormones tri-iodothyronine (T3) and tetra-iodothyronine (thyroxine, T4) is dependent upon the dietary supply of iodine. Briefly, iodide is taken via a

symporter into the thyroid follicular cell, where it is quickly oxidized by the thyroid-specific enzyme thyroid peroxidase and bound at the apical membrane to tyrosyl residues on the thyroid-specific protein, thyroglobulin. The newly iodinated thyroglobulin molecule lies next to the apical membrane, just within the follicular lumen, where the iodide is bound in the form of mono-iodotyrosine (MIT) and di-iodotyrosine (DIT). These two compounds are then coupled (again under the influence of thyroid peroxidase) to give T3 and T4, which remain bound to thyroglobulin in the follicular lumen. Thyroglobulin is taken up from the lumen by a follicular cell by pinocytosis, and MIT, DIT, T3 and T4 are released. T3 and T4 pass into the circulation, where they are bound to plasma proteins, whereas MIT and DIT are enzymatically deiodinated in the follicular cell to release iodine for more hormone production.

Thyroid-binding globulin (TBG) is the main plasma protein which binds thyroid hormones in humans. It has a greater affinity for T4 than T3. Two other human proteins are known to bind thyroid hormones, TBPA (which is responsible for 15% of bound plasma thyroid hormone) and albumin. In the rat, the majority of thyroid hormone in plasma is bound to albumin. Only low levels of a protein showing 70% homology to human TBG are present (Shuji, 1991). However, the level of TBG in the rat is upregulated by thyroidectomy, suggesting that it may play some physiological role (Nanno *et al.*, 1986). More T4 than T3 is released from the thyroid, but T4 is metabolized peripherally to give local production of T3, the more active hormone.

Metabolism of thyroid hormones

Thyroid hormones are taken up into the liver, where most conversion to T3 takes place, by an active process (Krenning *et al.*, 1978) and are then metabolized by deiodination. There are three distinct deiodinases which show different tissue distribution. 5'-Deiodinase I is found in most tissues, including thyroid itself, but is most abundant in liver and kidney. It is capable of both outer-ring deiodination to give T3 and inner-ring deiodination to give rT3, which is not produced by the thyroid, and as yet has no known function. 5'-Deiodinase II, a selenium-containing protein, occurs in the central nervous system, anterior pituitary and in brown adipose tissue. It deiodinates the outer ring only and its preferred substrate is T4. 5'-Deiodinase III is found only in the brain, skin and placenta and deiodinates only the inner ring. It shows a high affinity for both T3 and T4. The latter two deiodinases are thought to give rise only to local T3 and rT3 production; in the pituitary thyrotroph cells, this locally produced T3 is very important in regulating the level of TSH secretion.

Apart from local peripheral tissue production of the more active hormone, T3, deiodination is the major route of catabolism of the thyroid hormones in humans, resulting ultimately, after stepwise deiodination, in the production of thyronine. Thyroid hormones are also sulfated by the action of phenol sulfotransferases, and this process is believed to facilitate deiodination. In addition, they are subject to glucuronidation. This pathway is less important in humans, but in rat it is the major route for catabolism of thyroid hormones.

The circulating T4 level is monitored by the thyrotrophs of the anterior pituitary, which are responsible for the production of the major trophic hormone involved in both thyroid function and growth, TSH. T4 is metabolized to T3 by 5'-deiodinase II in the thyrotroph: T3 then binds to nuclear receptors in the cell. A decrease in T3 receptor occupancy results in increased synthesis of TSH. A higher tier of control exists in the hypothalamus, which secretes thyrotropin-releasing hormone (TRH), which also stimulates release of TSH from the thyrotrophs.

Xenobiotic effects on thyroid hormone homeostasis

The complexity of both the production and the catabolism of thyroid hormones provides many mechanisms with which xenobiotics can interact. Broadly, these agents can be divided into five categories (Table 1). Class 1 comprises directly acting agents, such as those which interfere with thyroid hormone production either by inhibiting iodine uptake or by inhibiting the thyroid peroxidase stimulated organification of iodide. Class 2 compounds stimulate T4 clearance, predominantly through an effect on the liver. 2A compounds induce hepatic microsomal enzymes, leading to increased biliary clearance of T4, while 2B compounds affect the hepatic transport of thyroid

hormones. Class 3 compounds influence the deiodination of thyroid hormones, either by inhibiting 5'-deiodinase II (e.g., iopanoic acid) or by stimulating 5'-deiodinase I (e.g. phenobarbital). Class 4 includes compounds which affect the plasma binding of thyroid hormones and Class 5 certain neurotransmitters including dopamine which have been implicated in the control of TSH output via TRH. Virtually all compounds which induce thyroid follicular tumours in animals in the long term have been shown to interfere with thyroid hormone homeostasis in the short term. The majority are restricted to classes 1 and 2. A more exhaustive list can be found in Atterwill *et al.* (1992).

Interaction of compounds with thyroid hormone homeostasis has been shown by a variety of different methods, both *in vitro* and *in vivo*. Substances belonging to Class 1 lead to thyroid hyperplasia but reduced thyroid uptake of radioiodine, while substances belonging to Classes 2, 3 and 5 induce thyroid hyperplasia and increased uptake of radioiodine. Substances belonging to Class 4 may, like the other groups, lower total serum levels of T3 and T4. This is followed by transient alterations in circulating TSH and thyroid hormone clearance. These transient effects lead to a new equilibrium and complete adjustment in terms of circulating thyroid hormone and TSH usually occurs. Exceptions to this are compounds, such as polychlorinated biphenyls, which have additional effects on thyroid hormone catabolism (Atterwill *et al.*, 1992). Further tests using assessment of radioactive uptake of iodide or organification of iodide can be carried out using cultured thyroid cells, to separate direct effects on thyroid hormone synthesis from those on catabolism. Where a direct effect on thyroid hormone synthesis has been excluded, further tests to study the effect of xenobiotics on the clearance of radiolabelled T4 *in vivo* can be carried out. The exact mechanism by which compounds increase T4 metabolism can be elucidated by measuring the activity of deiodinases, of uridine diphosphate glucuronyl transferase (UDT-GT) or of β-glucuronidase *in vitro*. Finally, effects on the active uptake of thyroid hormones into the hepatocyte can be separated from the effects on glucuronidation using cultured hepatocytes. The Gunn rat carries a germline point mutation in the gene that

Class	Action	Example	Tumour induction in animals	Reference
1	Direct action on thyroid (inhibition of either iodine uptake or thyroid peroxidase)	Propylthiourea	Yes	Taurog (1976)
2	Stimulation of T4 clearance	Phenobarbital	Yes	McClain (1989)
3	Affect deiodinase action	Iopanoate	No	Cavalieri & Pitt-Rivers (1981)
4	Affect binding of thyroid hormone to plasma proteins	Salicylates	No	Cavalieri & Pitt-Rivers (1981)
5	Receptor-mediated	Clomiphene	No	Wenzel (1981)

Table 1. Classes of xenobiotics which interfere with thyroid hormone homeostasis, divided according to their mode of interaction

An exhaustive list can be found in Atterwill et al. (1992)

encodes a transcript which is preferentially spliced to give rise to UDT-GT I and II, the enzymes responsible for glucuronidation of T4 and rT3. T3 is glucuronidated by the action of UDT-GT III, which is deficient in Waj rats (Matsui & Hakozaki, 1979). Using hepatocytes isolated from the Gunn or the Waj rat, it is therefore possible to distinguish between effects on glucuronidation of thyroid hormones and active uptake of T3 and T4 into the hepatocyte. The mechanism of antithyroid action of two H2 antagonists, temelastine and lupitidine, was carefully dissected in a series of papers by Atterwill and colleagues, a study involving many of these in-vitro techniques (Brown et al., 1986, 1987, 1988; Atterwill et al., 1989).

The role of mutagens in thyroid carcinogenesis
A number of different mutagens have been used in regimes specifically designed to induce thyroid tumours in rodents. Aromatic amines such as acetylaminofluorene (Doniach, 1950), azo dyes such as 4,4'-methylene-bis-(N,N-dimethyl)-benzylamine (Murthy, 1980), nitrosamines, e.g. diisopropanolnitrosamine (DHPN) (Mohr et al., 1977), N-bis-(2-hydroxypropyl)-nitrosamine (Hiasa et al., 1982) and the nitrosoureas, e.g.,

methylnitrosourea (MNU) (Schäffer & Müller, 1980; Milmore et al., 1982; Tsuda et al., 1983) have all been shown to induce a low frequency of thyroid tumours in rats. In at least two of these studies, an effect of the mutagen concerned on thyroid homeostasis has been identified (DHPN: Hiasa et al., 1982; MNU: Milmore et al., 1982) evidenced by either a transient rise in TSH or a decrease in circulating T4. Whether this is related to a cytotoxic effect of these compounds on follicular cells, with a resultant decrease in T4 production, or to other actions is not clear. Chemical mutagens are rarely used alone in studies of thyroid tumorigenesis; combination regimes of mutagen plus a goitrogen or mutagen plus a low-iodide diet are much more effective than mutagen alone (Milmore et al., 1982; Tsuda et al., 1983; Doniach, 1950). Agents which demethylate DNA, such as 5-azacytidine, can also potentiate goitrogen-induced thyroid carcinogenesis, although such agents do not show the marked effect of the combination of a mutagen and goitrogen (Thomas & Williams, 1992).

Irradiation, whether external (X-ray) or internal (by administration of isotopes of iodine), has been used extensively in experimental studies of thyroid tumorigenesis. However, it is important to realize that radiation has two effects on thyroid: a mutagenic effect and a growth stimulatory effect. Experiments with rats have shown a bell-shaped rather than a linear dose–response curve for the tumorigenic effect of radiation in the thyroid, with 30 µCi giving the highest frequency of thyroid tumours in adult rats (Doniach, 1953). This dose lies within a range which demonstrably interferes with thyroid function (Maloof et al., 1952). Further evidence of a second component to radiation-induced thyroid carcinogenesis comes from studies in which one thyroid lobe was shielded from X-irradiation. Tumours developed in both lobes, but were more frequent in the unshielded lobe (Nichols et al., 1965). In addition, radiation-induced carcinogenesis can be inhibited by hypophysectomy (Nadler et al., 1970) or by long-term T4 administration (Doniach, 1974), suggesting that release of TSH from the pituitary plays a key role in radiation-induced thyroid carcinogenesis.

The bell-shaped dose–response curve to radiation with respect to thyroid carcinogenesis can easily be explained. Low doses of radiation cause little thyroid cytotoxicity and therefore little if any rise in TSH, and they give a low frequency of mutations in the DNA of follicular cells, and therefore a low rate of thyroid tumorigenesis. As the dose of radiation increases, the cytotoxicity of radiation increases, resulting in a loss of functioning thyroid follicular cells, as well as an increase in mutation frequency in those cells which survive. The increased cytotoxicity results in a decrease in T4 and an increase in TSH, which stimulates the remaining thyroid follicular cells to grow. At the peak combination of mutation frequency and TSH-induced follicular cell growth, follicular tumours occur at a high frequency. Higher doses of radiation reduce the number of cells which retain the ability to divide, both through direct cytotoxic effects and through mutation overload, so that the frequency of tumours drops. At very high doses, all or virtually all follicular cells die, and no tumours occur. The morphological type of carcinoma induced in animals by radiation does not differ from that induced by goitrogens alone, but combination of mutagens and goitrogens leads to an increase in the number of carcinomas compared to adenomas.

The role of radiation exposure in carcinoma of the thyroid has recently become more prominent following the exposure of a large population to isotopes of iodine, in fallout from the Chernobyl nuclear accident which occurred in 1986 (Baverstock et al., 1992; Kazakov et al., 1992; Likhtarev et al., 1995). The age distribution and morphology of the cases of thyroid cancer which have so far occurred in the population of southern Belarus and northern Ukraine, the areas closest to the reactor, provide interesting information regarding the role of factors other than mutagens in thyroid tumorigenesis in humans. Firstly, there is an age-related susceptibility to the development of thyroid carcinoma following radiation exposure, with the youngest children (under four years) at the time of exposure being very much more susceptible than older children or adults (Williams et al., 1996a). This has also been observed in studies of age of exposure to radiation for therapeutic or diagnostic purposes (Schneider et al., 1986; Ron et al., 1987, 1989; Akiba et al., 1991). There are few reports of age-related susceptibility to radiation-induced experimental thyroid carcinogenesis, but these too suggest that exposure to radioiodine early in life increases the risk of thyroid neoplasia (Walinder, 1972; Walinder & Sjöden, 1972). Secondly, in contrast to the results of animal studies, there appears to be a specific link between exposure to radioiodine in fallout and the morphological type of thyroid cancer induced in humans. The majority (> 95%) of thyroid cancers that can be linked to exposure to radioactive fallout have been papillary carcinomas.

TSH and the mechanism of induction of thyroid tumours in humans and animals

There is overwhelming evidence to suggest that TSH-induced growth of the thyroid epithelial cell plays a critical role in thyroid tumorigenesis in animals and in one type of human thyroid carcinoma. The majority of agents which induce experimental thyroid tumours, usually after prolonged administration, interfere with thyroid hormone homeostasis (Hill et al., 1989). The xenobiotic induction of both thyroid hyperplasia and neoplasia can be inhibited by either hypophysectomy or concomitant T4 administration (Nadler et al., 1970; Doniach, 1974). The importance of TSH-induced growth can also be demonstrated by the observation that multiple tumours occur in a background of generalized thyroid hyperplasia in those types of congenital hypothyroidism where one of the key steps of thyroid hormone synthesis is absent (dyshormonogenesis). Congenital hypothyroidism from this cause is rare, and occurs in both humans and animals most commonly as a result of mutations in either the thyroid peroxidase or the thyroglobulin genes (Falconer *et al.*, 1965; van Jaarsfeld *et al.*, 1972; de Vijlder *et al.*, 1978; Salvatore *et al.*, 1980). In patients with dyshormonogenesis, the elevated TSH is present from birth, and is now used to detect these cases by neonatal screening. In the untreated severe cases, the continuous high level of TSH leads to diffuse hyperplasia, and multiple benign thyroid tumours commonly develop after some years (often 10 years or more). Carcinoma has been described in patients with dyshormonogenesis, but is very rare (Vickery, 1981).

Thyroid tumours are also more common in man in areas of iodide deficiency (Medeiros-Neto, 1995), and can be induced by iodide deficiency in animals (Axelrad & Leblond, 1955; Schaller & Stevenson, 1966). The effect of iodide deficiency can be exacerbated by the presence of goitrogens in either the diet or drinking water (Ekpechi *et al.*, 1966; Gaitan, 1988). Both iodide deficiency and goitrogen administration cause levels of TSH to rise, and TSH controls not only thyroid cell function, but also growth. When the decrease in the level of circulating T4 is small or short-lived, the deficiency may be redressed by an increase in thyroid cell function alone. However, if the decrease is more severe or prolonged and cannot be redressed by an increase in function alone, an increase in number of units of thyroid hormone production (i.e., the follicular cells) is required. This leads to thyroid follicular cell hyperplasia with the development of a goitre. However, the thyroid follicular cell in the rat posseses only a limited growth potential. Sustained high-dose goitrogen administration results in a rapid increase in follicular cell mitotic activity over 7 to 14 days, but this then falls to relatively low levels after about three months, while the level of TSH remains high. If the goitrogen administration is maintained, tumours of the follicular cell are observed after about eight months (Wynford-Thomas *et al.*, 1982). A similar observation has been made for the mouse (Peter *et al.*, 1991).

The majority of the tumours induced by prolonged goitrogen administration in rodents, in the absence of mutagen, are benign. The finding by several authors (Jemec, 1977; Todd 1986) that follicular tumours regressed on withdrawal of goitrogen administration has led to some confusion over the distinction between hyperplastic and neoplastic lesions. However, more recent studies have demonstrated that monoclonal lesions induced in mice by a combination of radiation and goitrogen (including carcinomas that clearly showed capsular and vascular invasion), regressed on withdrawal of the goitrogen (Thomas *et al.*, 1991). The clonal nature of these lesions suggests that they are truly neoplastic and derive by clonal evolution from a single cell, but their regression suggests that they retain dependence, at least in part, on TSH for growth. One earlier study using serial transplantation of thyroid tissue from rats maintained for 18 months on a low-iodide diet suggested that the tumour phenotype was lost on transplantation to euthyroid rats, but re-emerged when a serial transplantation was made to a hypothyroid rat (Matovinovic *et al.*, 1970). These results suggest that thyroid follicular epithelial cells can undergo a heritable change resulting in tumour formation in animals with sustained high TSH levels, but the heritable change is insufficient to support the tumour phenotype in the absence of the TSH growth stimulus.

The mechanism by which goitrogen-induced thyroid tumours arise is far from clearly understood. We suggest that three key steps are important in spontaneous thyroid carcinogenesis. First, as the normal follicular cell possesses a growth-limiting mechanism, the continued growth of tumour cells implies that any such mechanism must be deactivated in neoplasia. Second, development of TSH-independent growth is likely to be essential for spontaneous thyroid carcinogenesis. Thirdly, cells must acquire the ability to invade – an essential ingredient for malignancy. Each of these steps may involve alteration in more than one gene; for example, loss of tumour-suppressor gene function may require mutation in both copies of the gene, and gain of independent growth could involve successive mutations in different growth control genes.

The development of these successive defects that lead to neoplasia can be considered as a process of natural selection at a cellular level: manipulation of the environment in which selection takes place may alter the selection process. In experimental thyroid carcinogenesis, the induction of persistently high TSH levels creates an environment in which any cell that suffers a mutation or mutations leading to loss of its growth-limiting mechanism will give rise to a clone of cells which will continue to grow and therefore continue to be at risk of further gene alteration in the progeny of that cell. If the cell is exposed to maximal growth stimulation from a very high TSH level, mutation in growth control genes may not lead to any additional growth, and may not therefore confer any selective advantage. When invasiveness develops in a cell that has not acquired TSH-independent growth, the resulting carcinomas retain TSH-dependence and will regress when TSH stimulation is withdrawn (Thomas et al., 1991).

Further evidence for the requirement of thyroid follicular cell growth in thyroid neoplasia can be found from the increase in thyroid cancer after radiation. The greatest risk appears to be to those who were young children at the time of exposure. There appears to be little or no increased risk after exposure to radiation as an adult. Tumour incidence following radiation in animals can be increased either by exposure of neonatal animals or by combination of radiation exposure with goitrogen administration. Developmental thyroid growth continues in the mouse until about six weeks of age and in the human until adulthood. In addition to the arguments for greater uptake of radioiodine in the immature thyroid, two other factors may contribute to the higher risk of thyroid neoplasia following radiation early in life. Carcinogenesis is a multistep phenomenon and requires the acquisition of multiple mutations in a clone of cells. Mutation is more likely to occur at S phase. The immature thyroid has a higher proportion of dividing cells compared with the adult, and is therefore more likely to be susceptible to the mutational effects of radiation. In addition, the phase of developmental growth which occurs results in cells that have been exposed to radiation

and therefore possibly harbour mutations which are deleterious to growth regulation, undergoing several more rounds of cell division, thus increasing the probability of acquiring additional deleterious mutations. It is therefore not surprising that exposure to a mutagen during thyroid developmental growth carries an increased risk of development of thyroid tumours later in life.

Recent research has thrown light on some of the molecular events involved in thyroid carcinogenesis. However, much of the work has centred on identification of oncogene mutations in human thyroid tumours rather than in those tumours generated by long-term xenobiotic administration. In humans, the two different morphological types of thyroid carcinoma are associated with different molecular biological events. Papillary carcinomas are associated with gene rearrangements involving either ret (a tyrosine kinase-linked receptor for glial-derived neurotrophic factor) or trk (a tyrosine kinase-linked receptor for nerve growth factor) oncogenes (Greco et al., 1992; Santoro et al., 1992). However, the frequency of these rearrangements varies between studies (Ishizaka et al., 1991; Jhiang et al., 1994; Zou et al., 1994); this may partly reflect different sex ratios in the study groups, as we have recently identified a sex difference in papillary carcinomas associated with a ret rearrangement (Williams et al., 1996b), or differences in the methodology used to identify ret activation. Follicular carcinomas are more frequently associated with point mutations in the ras oncogene family, although the absolute frequency of ras mutation may vary with the technique used to identify mutation (Lemoine et al., 1989; Manenti et al., 1994). A proportion of benign nodules, which can be demonstrated to possess higher than normal uptake of radioiodine (so called 'hot' nodules) have been shown to be associated with mutation in the TSH receptor, leading to constitutive activation (Parma et al., 1993). The majority of oncogene studies carried out in animals have been those using thyroid-specific expression of specific oncogenes in transgenic animals. These have provided interesting results, with thyroid-specific expression of one of the ret rearrangements associated with papillary carcinoma (PTC1) leading to the induction of discrete tumours which possess some of the features of human papillary carcinoma; these differ morphologically from other experimental tumours (Jhiang et al., 1996; Santoro et al., 1996). Thyroid-specific expression of mutated ras oncogenes has produced two differing pathologies, depending on the species of thyroglobulin promoter used in the transgene construct. Only a low yield of discrete benign tumours was produced in transgenic mice carrying an activated Ki-ras gene on a rat thyroglobulin promoter (Santelli et al., 1993), whereas mice carrying a mutated Ha-ras on a bovine thyroglobulin promoter showed a series of different thyroid pathologies ranging from papillary carcinomas to hyperplasia (Rochefort et al., 1996). This latter study also gave rise to mice which presented with primary lung tumours with papillary morphology, which is slightly surprising as the transgene construct would be predicted to be expressed only in thyroid, suggesting that the use of the bovine promoter may lead to ectopic expression of the transgene. The use of viral genes which have been shown to block p53 and Rb gene action, either separately (p53: E6, Rb: E7), or both together (SV40 large T) has produced a variety of phenotypes, ranging from severe thyroid hyperplasia and neoplasia (SV40; Ledent et al., 1991), or the development of large colloid goitres and malignant poorly differentiated tumours after about one year (E7; Ledent et al., 1995) to nothing more than a slightly enlarged thyroid gland at six months of age (E6; Ledent et al., 1994). This is perhaps in keeping with the observation that, in humans, mutation of p53 is not involved in differentiated thyroid carcinoma, but only plays a role in the transition from differentiated to undifferentiated thyroid carcinoma. A role for activation of the TSH receptor pathway in potentiation of carcinogenic activity has been shown by crossing yet another transgenic line, which shows constitutive activation of the adenosine A2 receptor (and therefore of the cyclic AMP cascade which is also activated by the TSH receptor) with the E7 line. The offspring show rapid development of thyroid neoplasia with early and frequent metastases (Coppée et al., 1996). However, care must be exercised in generalizing from these transgenic experiments, as the mechanism of tumour production may differ fundamentally from that in normal animals. In transgenic mice, the oncogene is expressed from the time at which the thyroglobulin promoter is active (around day 18 of gestation in rodents), whereas in

xenobiotic-induced neoplasia, oncogenes are activated by somatic rather than germline mutation, and factors which are expressed in different development time frames may also contribute to development of a thyroid tumour. Further information on the molecular biology of xenobiotic-induced thyroid tumours will be required in order to examine mechanistic differences between mouse and man with respect to thyroid tumours.

Evidence for species specificity

There is an increasing body of evidence that there are differences in key steps of thyroid hormone synthesis and catabolism between species. Biochemical assays of the inhibitory effect of sulfamethoxazole on thyroid peroxidase in various species have shown that, compared with the rat enzyme, monkey thyroid peroxidase shows significantly less inhibition at the same concentration (Takayama et al., 1986).

Clinically significant antithyroid effects in humans following the use of this and structurally related compounds are lacking (McLaren & Alexander 1979), suggesting that, not surprisingly, humans may be more like monkey than rat, at least with regard to the effect of sulfamethoxazole. In addition, other studies have shown that the H2 antagonists temelastine and lupitidine increase thyroid hormone uptake in isolated rat hepatocytes, but not in a human hepatoblastoma cell line (Aylward, 1995). This suggests that there may be differences in the transporter proteins involved in liver T3 and T4 uptake between rat and human. More evidence of this type is required. However, one should always be aware of the genetic diversity of humans and the limits on the availability of human tissues. Established cell lines are usually derived from cancer cells and have been maintained in culture for long periods. It is therefore possible that some of the effects observed with respect to species differences may be epiphenomena due to the carcinogenic process which occurred in vivo or artefacts induced by prolonged maintenance in culture. Wherever possible, studies utilizing cell culture should involve some performed on primary cultures, with adequate controls for sex, age and pre-existing disease of the donor. Such studies will provide interesting data to help dissect the mechanisms by which xenobiotics interfere with thyroid hormone homeostasis and whether such a mechanism is likely to be relevant to the human.

In addition to biochemical differences, differences in exposure of humans to such compounds should be taken into account. A good case has already been made for the existence of a threshold effect in thyroid carcinogenesis (Paynter et al., 1988). The majority of compounds induce thyroid tumours only after prolonged, high-dose administration in animals, and for most compounds it is unlikely that human exposure would reach such levels (even if the human system involved is as sensitive as that in the test animal). Human exposure more frequently involves a small dose of several different compounds rather than prolonged exposure to a large dose of one. However, little work has been done to study the interaction of compounds which affect different steps in hormone synthesis or catabolism.

General hypothesis for thyroid carcinogenesis

To conclude, we summarize some of the discussion and in particular put forward a specific hypothesis for the development of thyroid neoplasia. Tumours in any stable tissue require a growth rate that is higher than that of the tissue of origin. The increased growth can result from loss of tumour-suppressor genes, gain-of-function mutations in oncogenes or both. Malignant tumours in addition require a genetic defect or defects conferring the ability to invade and or metastasize. The thyroid, unlike organs such as the skin or intestine, is not a stem-cell tissue; the normal follicular cell has a limited growth capacity, and the normal level of growth stimulation in the adult animal is extremely low. The principal conclusions that we can draw are the following:

(i) Sporadic tumours of the follicular cells in rodents or humans require both tumour-suppressor gene and oncogene mutations. Such tumours are very infrequent and a significant proportion are malignant or may progress to malignancy.

(ii) Tumours of the follicular cells induced by exposure to substances inducing a high level of TSH may arise as a result of tumour-suppressor gene mutations, for example in the gene or genes which control the mechanism that desensitizes growth of the thyroid follicular cell in response to TSH stimulation. Such tumours may develop at a relatively high frequency in long-term exposed animals, but retain at least partial dependence on a high level of TSH for continued growth, and show a low rate of progression to malignancy.

(iii) Tumours of the follicular cells occur less frequently with xenobiotic exposure at levels that lead to less lowering of thyroid hormone levels, and therefore lesser degrees of TSH elevation. The importance of acquiring oncogene as well as tumour-suppressor gene mutations increases, but the chance of acquiring these decreases as the level of growth stimulation decreases. Under these conditions, exposure to a mutagen becomes increasingly important for thyroid carcinogenesis. The increase in incidence of follicular cell tumours, including malignant tumours, which follows administration of mutagens to rodents, requires follicular cell growth, is enhanced by a sustained stimulus to growth and is reduced or abolished by diminished post-mutagen growth.

(iv) Nodules, which are polyclonal and not true tumours, occur relatively frequently as a consequence of exposure to high levels of TSH; they do not show any detectable progression to malignancy, retain dependence on TSH for continued growth, and may result from stromal changes, as evidenced by the increased content of stroma in nodules induced in the mouse.

(v) There is a threshold in the carcinogenic response to xenobiotics which are not mutagens, but lead to thyroid follicular cell tumours through their effect on thyroid hormone synthesis or metabolism. This threshold can be related to either the buffering capacity within the complex system that maintains constant thyroid hormone levels or changes in thyroid hormone levels that are sufficiently small that they can be remedied by a very minor increase in TSH, leading to an increase in follicular cell function, but not growth.

The evidence for the involvement of oncogenes in sporadic adenomas or carcinomas of the follicular cells is derived largely from human studies, where mutations in the three ras genes, in ret and in trk have all been described in either adenomas or carcinomas. They have not been found in nodules. Mutations in genes of the TSH receptor pathway, including the receptor itself have also been described in human thyroid tumours. Evidence of their involvement in TSH-induced tumours is limited; mutations in the *ras* genes have been found in rat thyroid tumours induced by radiation followed by goitrogen, and in a much smaller proportion of those induced by goitrogen alone (Lemoine *et al.*, 1988). Recent studies have suggested that the frequency of *ras* involvement in human adenomas was over-estimated in earlier studies (Manenti *et al.*, 1994); the rat studies need therefore to be repeated.

Evidence for involvement of tumour-suppressor genes in both sporadic and TSH-induced tumours of the follicular cell is circumstantial. Transgenic mice carrying oncogenic mutations in either *ret* or *ras*, with targeted expression in the thyroid, do not show widespread carcinogenic change, only a relatively small number of tumours arising in adult mice. This shows that at least one further event is needed for these genes to lead to thyroid tumour formation.

Evidence that continual follicular cell growth stimulation is required for the carcinogenic process in thyroid follicular cells has been provided. In brief, many studies have shown that the frequency of thyroid tumour formation, including carcinoma formation, after mutagen administration is greatly enhanced by increased growth stimulation by TSH and abolished if TSH stimulation is suppressed by hypophysectomy or suppressive thyroid hormone therapy immediately following administration of the mutagen. The importance of post-mutagen growth is that it allows the possible development of further mutations; these occur much more commonly in dividing than intermitotic cells.

Comparison of mechanisms of carcinogenesis of follicular cells in rodents and humans

The evidence suggests that essentially the same mechanism of carcinogenesis exists in both rodents and humans, but there are major quantitative differences. In addition, there are species differences in metabolism of some of the xenobiotics which influence thyroid hormone breakdown. The frequency with which long-term prolonged high levels of TSH in rodents leads to nodules, adenomas and carcinomas is well known

and even hemithyroidectomy was associated with an increase in thyroid carcinogenesis (Doniach & Williams, 1962). In contrast, in humans, while nodules and adenomas are relatively common, carcinoma is very rare. Patients with dyshormonogenesis commonly develop multiple nodules and adenomas; these may occur as early as 7–10 years of age in severe cases, but more commonly they are first noticed in the teens or later. This shows that several years of exposure to very high levels of TSH in infancy will produce benign thyroid tumours. The progression to malignancy, however, is very rare. In a review in 1981, only 17 cases had been reported (Cooper *et al.*, 1981). The development of malignancy after exposure of follicular cells to high levels of growth stimulation in adult life is extremely rare if it occurs at all. Drugs which block thyroid such as carbimazole are very widely used in the treatment of thyrotoxicosis; even when they are used in combination with a mutagen (^{131}I) in patients with Graves disease, no detectable increase in thyroid cancer has been found (Holm *et al.*, 1980, 1988).

Surveys of populations living in areas of iodine deficiency show that nodular goitres and adenomas are significantly more common than in areas with normal iodide intake. The incidence of thyroid cancer is either slightly increased or unchanged. What does change is the type of thyroid cancer, with follicular carcinoma relatively more common in areas of iodide deficiency, while papillary carcinomas are relatively more common in areas of iodide excess (Williams *et al.*, 1977). Here again, exposure to iodide deficiency in the early years of life is probably important.

In our opinion, the risk of development of thyroid carcinoma as a result of exposure to any cause leading to an increase of TSH is very much lower in humans than in animals, requires exposure for several years, is dose-dependent and very probably age-dependent. The risk of human thyroid carcinogenesis following exposure to xenobiotics leading to a small perturbation in thyroid homeostasis is negligible.

One difference between rodents and humans which has been suggested as a cause of different carcinogenic susceptibility is the way in which thyroid hormones are bound in the plasma. In humans, the main circulating protein that binds both thyroxine and tri-iodothyronine is thyroid-binding globulin (TBG); prealbumin binds a much smaller proportion. In rodents, although TBG is present, prealbumin is the main binding protein; it has a much lower affinity for thyroid hormones than TBG. The level at which the thyroid pituitary axis functions is dependent upon the level of free thyroid hormones; under normal circumstances the system adjusts to maintain a normal free thyroid hormone level. Interspecies variations in binding protein may affect the rate at which adjustment takes place, but we do not think it likely that they will alter the normal steady state, or the long-term response to a consistent change. Humans who have a congenital complete deficiency in TBG appear otherwise normal, with no clinical thyroid abnormalities.

Gaps in our knowledge

The tumour-suppressor genes involved in the restriction of thyroid follicular cell growth are not known. It seems unlikely that the genes which predispose to retinoblastoma and familial adenomatous polyposis coli play any major role, as thyroid tumours are not a frequent component of the clinical syndromes that accompany human inherited syndromes when these genes are affected. There is more evidence for a link between thyroid and breast cancer, so that the role of BRCA1 and BRCA2 and the PTEN gene need to be explored, and a further search made for other possibly thyroid-specific tumour-suppressor genes. The PTEN gene is of particular interest, as germline mutations of this gene have been shown to be associated with Cowden's syndrome, in which patients present with breast cancers, hamartomas and thyroid disorders (goitre, adenomas and carcinomas), and the gene encodes a receptor tyrosine kinase and is located in a region where loss of heterozygosity has been previously described in thyroid tumours (Li et al., 1997; Liaw et al., 1997). Very little work has been reported on the oncogenes involved in experimentally induced thyroid tumours (as opposed to the use of known oncogenes in thyroid-specific expression in transgenic animals), and this gap needs to be filled using modern methods.

The comparison between the frequency of development of thyroid tumours in response to elevated TSH in humans and animals could be further studied, for example by developing transgenic dyshormonogenetic mice or rats.

The tumour incidence in these animals, which like human patients with dyshormonogenesis will have elevated TSH from birth if not before, could then be compared to that observed in humans.

The dose–effect relationship in nongenotoxic thyroid carcinogenesis needs further study, including varying length of time of exposure as well as dose, together with measurements of TSH and careful estimation of the numbers of tumours induced.

In conclusion, we consider that there is effectively no risk of thyroid carcinogenesis in man from limited exposure to low doses of a compound that has been shown to produce thyroid tumours in rodents only when administered for long periods of time at high doses, providing that the substance has been shown not to be mutagenic, and that it has been shown to interfere with thyroid hormone homeostasis by a defined mechanism.

References

Akiba, S., Lubin, J., Ezaki, H. et al. (1991) Thyroid Cancer Incidence Among Atomic Bomb Survivors in Hiroshima and Nagasaki 1958–79 (Technical Report TR 5-91), Hiroshima, Japan, Radiation Effects Foundation

Atterwill, C.K., Poole, A., Jones, C., Jones, R. & Brown, C. (1989) Mechanistic investigation of species-specific thyroid lesions induced by treatment with the histamine H_1 antagonist Temelastine (SK&F 93944) in rats. Food Chem. Toxicol., 27, 681–690

Atterwill, C.K., Jones, C. & Brown, C.G. (1992) Thyroid gland II — mechanisms of species dependent thyroid toxicity, hyperplasia and neoplasia induced by xenobiotics. In: Atterwill, C.K. & Flack, J.D., eds, Endocrine Toxicology, Cambridge, Cambridge University Press, pp. 137–182

Axelrad, A.A. & Leblond, C.P. (1955) Induction of thyroid tumors in rats by a low iodine diet. Proc. Am. Assoc. Cancer Res., 1, 2

Aylward, S.P. (1995) Xenobiotic Modulation of Thyroxine Uptake in Cultured Hepatocytes in Relation to Thyroid Gland Toxicology. Ph.D. Thesis, University of Hertfordshire

Baverstock, K., Egloff, B., Pinchera, A., Ruchti, C. & Williams, D. (1992) Thyroid cancer after Chernobyl. Nature, 359, 21–22

Brown, C.G., Fowler, K. & Atterwill, C.K. (1986) Assessment of thyrotoxicity using in vitro cell culture systems. Food Chem. Toxicol., 24, 557–566

Brown, C.G., Harland, R.F., Major, I.R. & Atterwill, C.K. (1987) Effects of toxic doses of a novel histamine (H_2) antagonist on the rat thyroid gland. *Food Chem. Toxicol.*, 25, 787–794

Brown, C.G., Lee, D.M., Jones, C.A. & Atterwill, C.K. (1988) Comparison of the effects of SK&F 93479 and phenobarbitone (PB) treatment on thyroid toxicity and hepatic thyroid hormone metabolizing enzymes in the rat. *Arch. Toxicol., Suppl. 12,* 23–29

Cavalieri, R.R. & Pitt-Rivers, R. (1981) The effects of drugs on the distribution and metabolism of thyroid hormones. *Pharmacol. Rev.*, 33, 55–80

Cooper, D.S., Axelrod, L., DeGroot, L.J., Vickery, A.L., Jr & Maloof, F. (1981) Congenital goitre and the development of metastatic follicular carcinoma with evidence for a leak of nonhormonal iodide: clinical, pathological, kinetic and biochemical studies and a review of the literature. *J. Clin. Endocrinol. Metab.*, 52, 294–306

Coppée, F., Gérard, A.C., Denef, J.F., Ledent, C., Vassart, G., Dumont, J.E. & Parmentier, M. (1996) Early occurrence of metastatic differentiated thyroid carcinomas in transgenic mice expressing the A2a adenosine receptor and the human papillomavirus type 16 E7 oncogene. *Oncogene*, 13, 1471–1482

DeLellis, R.A. (1994) Changes in structure and function of thyroid C cells. In: Mohr, U., Dungworth, D.L. & Capen, C.C., eds, *Pathobiology of the Aging Rat*, Washington DC, ILSI, pp. 285–300

DeLellis, R.A., Sheldon, W.G. & Bucci, T.J. (1996) Changes in thyroid C cells. In: Mohr, U., Dungworth, D.L., Capen, C.C., Sundberg, J.P. & Ward, J.M., eds, *Pathobiology of the Aging Mouse*, Washington DC, ILSI, pp. 103–108

de Vijlder, J.M., van Voorthuizen, W.F., van Dijk, J.E., Rijnberk, A. & Telegaers, W.H.H. (1978) Hereditary congenital goiter with thyroglobulin deficiency in a breed of goats. *Endocrinology*, 102, 1214–1222

Doniach, I. (1950) The effect of radioactive iodine alone and in combination with methylthiourea and acetyl-aminofluorene upon tumour production in the rats thyroid gland. *Br. J. Cancer*, 4, 223–234

Doniach, I. (1953) The effect of radioactive iodine alone and in combination with methylthiouracil upon tumour production in the rat thyroid gland. *Br. J. Cancer*, 7, 181–202

Doniach, I. (1974) Carcinogenic effect of 100, 200, 250 and 500 rad X-rays on the rat thyroid gland. *Br. J. Cancer*, 30, 487–495

Doniach, I. & Williams, E.D. (1962) The development of thyroid and pituitary tumours in the rat two years after partial thyroidectomy. *Br. J. Cancer*, 16, 222–231

Ekpechi, O.L., Dimitriadou, A. & Fraser, R. (1966) Goitrogenic activity of cassava (a staple Nigerian food). *Nature*, 210, 1137–1138

Falconer, I.R., Roitt, I.M., Seamark, R.F. & Torrigiani, G. (1965) Studies of the congenitally goitrous sheep. Iodoproteins of the goitre. *Biochem. J.*, 117, 417–424

Gaitan, E. (1988) Goitrogens. *Balliere's Clin. Endocrinol. Metab.*, 2, 683–702

Greco, A., Pierotti, M.A., Bongarzone, I., Pagliardini, J., Lanzi, C. & Della Porta, G. (1992) Trk-T1 is a novel oncogene formed by the fusion of TPR and Trk genes in human papillary cancer. *Oncogene*, 7, 237–242

Hiasa, Y., Ohshima, M., Kiathori, Y., Yuasa, T., Fujita, T. & Iwata, C. (1982) Promoting effects of 3-amino-1,2,4-triazole on the development of thyroid tumours in rats treated with N-bis-(2-hydroxypropyl)-nitrosamine. *Carcinogenesis*, 3, 381–384

Hill, R.N., Erdreich, L.S., Paynter, O.E., Roberts, P.A., Rosenthal, S.L. & Wilkinson, C.F. (1989) Thyroid follicular cell carcinogenesis. *Fund. Appl. Toxicol.*, 12, 629–697

Holm, L.E., Dahlquist, I., Israelsson, A. & Lundell, G. (1980) Malignant thyroid tumours after iodine 131 therapy, a retrospective cohort study. *New Eng. J. Med.*, 303, 188–191

Holm, L.E., Wiklund, K., Lundell, G., Bergman, N.A., Bjelkengren, G., Cederquist, E.S., Eicsson, U.B., Larsson, L.G., Lidberg, M.E. & Lindberg, R.S. (1988) Thyroid cancer after diagnostic doses of iodine 131. *J. natl Cancer Inst.*, 80, 1132–1138

Ishizaka, Y., Kobayashi, S., Ushijima, T., Hirohashi, S., Sugimura, T. & Nagao, M. (1991) Detection of ret TPC/PTC transcripts in thyroid adenomas and adenomatous goiter by an RT-PCR method. *Oncogene*, 6, 1667–1672

Jemec, B. (1977) Studies on the goitrogenic and tumorigenic effect of two goitrogens. *Cancer*, 40, 2188–2202

Jhiang, S.M., Caruso, D.R., Gilmore, E., Ishizaka, Y., Tahira, Y. & Nagao, M. (1994) Detection of the PTC/retTPC oncogene in human thyroid cancers. *Oncogene*, 7, 1331–1337

Jhiang, S.M., Sagartz, J.E., Tong, Q., Parker, T.J., Capen, C.C., Cho, J.Y., Xing, S. & Ledent, C. (1996) Targeted expression of the ret/PTC1 oncogene induces papillary thyroid carcinomas. *Endocrinology*, 137, 375–378

Kazakov, V.S., Demidchik, E.P. & Astakhova, L.N. (1992) Thyroid cancers after Chernobyl. *Nature*, 359, 21

Krenning, E.P., Docter, R., Bernard, B., Visser, T.J. & Henneman, G. (1978) Active transport of triiodothyronine into isolated liver cells. *FEBS Letts*, 91, 113–116

Ledent, C., Dumont, J.E., Vassart, G. & Parmentier, M. (1991) Thyroid adenocarcinomas secondary to tissue-specific expression of simian virus-40 large T antigen in transgenic mice. *Endocrinology*, **129**, 1391–1401

Ledent, C., Coppee, F. & Parmentier, M. (1994) Transgenic models of metastatic differentiated thyroid carcinomas. *J. Endocrinol. Invest.*, **17** (suppl), 1–6

Ledent, C., Marcotte, A., Dumont, J.E., Vassart, G. & Parmentier, M. (1995) Differentiated carcinomas develop as a consequence of the thyroid specific expression of a thyroglobulin-human papillomavirus type 16 E7 transgene. *Oncogene*, **10**, 1789–1797

Lemoine, N.R., Mayall, E.S., Williams, E.D., Thurston, V. & Wynford-Thomas, D. (1988) Agent specific ras oncogene activation in rat thyroid. *Oncogene*, **3**, 541–544

Lemoine, N.R., Mayall, E.S., Wyllie, F.S., Williams, E.D., Goyns, M., Stringer, B.M.J. & Wynford-Thomas, D. (1989) High frequency of ras oncogene activation in all stages of human thyroid tumourigenesis. *Oncogene*, **2**, 159–164

Li, J., Yen, C., Liaw, D., Podyspanina, K., Bose, S., Wang, S.I., Puc, J., Milaresis, C., Rodgers, L., McCombie, R., Bigner, S.H., Giovanelli, B.C., Ittmann, M., Tycko, B., Hibshoosh, H., Wigler, M.H. & Parsons, R. (1997) PTEN, a putative tyrosine phosphatase gene mutated in human brain, breast and prostate cancer. *Science*, **275**, 1943–1947

Liaw, D., Marsh, D.J., Li, J., Dahia, P.L., Wang, S.I., Zheng, Z., Bose, S., Call, K.M., Tsou, H.C., Peacocke, M., Eng, C. & Parsons, R. (1997) Germline mutations of the PTEN gene in Cowden disease, and inherited thyroid and breast cancer syndrome. *Nature Genet.*, **16**, 64–67

Likhtarev, I.A., Sobolev, B.G., Kairo, I.A., Tronko, N.D., Bogdanova, T.I., Oleinic, V.A., Ephstein, E.V. & Beral, V. (1995) Thyroid cancer in the Ukraine. *Nature*, **375**, 365

Maloof, F., Dobyns, B. & Vickery, A.L. (1952) The effects of various doses of radioactive iodine on the function and structure of the thyroid of the rat. *Endocrinology*, **50**, 612–638

Manenti, G., Pilotti, S., Re, F.C., Della Porta, G. & Pierotti, M.A. (1994) Selective activation of ras oncogenes in follicular and undifferentiated thyroid carcinomas. *Eur. J. Cancer*, **30A**, 987–993

Matovinovic, J., Nishiyama, R.H. & Poissant, G. (1970) Transplantable thyroid tumours in the rat: development of normal appearing thyroid follicles in the differentiated tumours, and development of differentiated tumours from iodide deficient, thyroxine involuted goiters. *Cancer Res.*, **30**, 504–514

Matsui, M. & Hakozaki, M. (1979) Discontinuous variation in hepatic uridine diphosphate glucuronyltransferase toward androsterone in Wistar rats. *Biochem. Pharmacol.*, **28**, 411–415

McClain, R.M. (1989) The significance of hepatic microsomal enzyme induction and altered thyroid function in rats: implications for thyroid gland neoplasia. *Toxicol. Pathol.*, **17**, 294–306

McLaren, E.H. & Alexander, W.D. (1979) Goitrogens. *Clin. Endocrinol. Metab.*, **8**, 129–144

Medeiros-Neto, G. (1995) Iodide deficiency disorders. In: de Groot, L., ed., *Endocrinology*, Volume 1, Philadelphia, W.B. Saunders, pp. 821–833

Milmore, J.E., Chandraskaran, V. & Weisburger, J.H. (1982) Effects of hypothyroidism on development of nitrosomethylurea-induced tumors of the mammary gland, thyroid gland and other tissues. *Proc. Soc. Exp. Biol. Med.*, **169**, 487–493

Mohr, U., Reznik, G. & Pour, P. (1977) Carcinogenic effect of diisopropanolnitrosamine in Sprague-Dawley rats. *J. Natl Cancer Inst.*, **58**, 361–366

Murthy, A.S.K. (1980) Morphology of the neoplasms of the thyroid gland in Fischer 344 rats treated with 4,4′-methylene-bis-(N,N′-dimethyl)-benzylamine. *Toxicol. Lett.*, **6**, 391–397

Nadler, N.J., Mandavia, M. & Goldberg, M. (1970) The effect of hypophysectomy on the experimental production of rat thyroid neoplasia. *Cancer Res.*, **30**, 1909–1911

Nanno, M., Ohtska, R., Kikuchi, N., Oki, Y., Ohgo, S., Kurahachi, H., Yoshimi, T. & Hamada, S. (1986) In: Medeiros-Neto, G. & Gaitan, E., eds, *Frontiers in Thyroidology*, Vol. 1, pp. 481–484

Nichols, C.W., Lindsay, S., Sheline, G.E. & Chaikoff, I.L. (1965) Induction of neoplasms in rat thyroid glands by X-irradiation of a single lobe. *Arch. Pathol.*, **80**, 177–183

Parma, J., Duprez, L., Van Sande, J., Cochaux, P., Gervy, C, Mockel, J. & Dumont Vassart, G. (1993) Somatic mutations in the thyrotropin receptor gene cause hyperfunctioning thyroid adenomas. *Nature*, **365**, 649–651

Paynter, O.E., Burin, G.J., Jaeger, R.B. & Gregorio, C.A. (1988) Goitrogens and thyroid follicular cell neoplasia: evidence for a threshold process. *Regul. Toxicol. Pharmacol.*, **8**, 102–109

Peter, H.J., Gerber, H., Studer, H., Groscurth, P. & Zakarija, M. (1991) Comparison of FRTL-5 cell growth in vitro with that of xenotransplanted cells in the thyroid of the recipient mouse. *Endocrinology*, **128**, 211–219

Rochefort, P., Caillou, B., Michiels, F.M., Ledent, C., Talbot, M., Schlumberger, M., Lavelle, F., Monier, R. & Feunteun, J. (1996) Thyroid pathologies in transgenic mice expressing a human activated Ras gene driven by a thyroglobulin promoter. *Oncogene*, **12**, 111–118

Ron, E., Kleinerman, R., Boice, J., LiVolsi, V., Flannery, J. & Fraumeni, J. (1987) A population based case–control study of thyroid cancer. *J. Natl Cancer Inst.*, **79**, 1–12

Ron, E., Modan, B., Preston, D., Alfandary, E., Stovall, M. & Boice, J. (1989) Thyroid neoplasia following low dose irradiation in childhood. *Radiat. Res.*, **120**, 516–531

Salvatore, G., Stanbury, J.B. & Rall, J.E. (1980) Inherited defects of thyroid hormone biosynthesis. In: De Visscher, M., ed., *Comprehensive Endocrinology: The Thyroid Gland*. New York, Raven Press, pp. 443–487

Santelli, G., de Franciscis, V., Portella, G., Chiappetta, G., D'Alessio, A., Galifano, D., Rosati, R., Mineo, A., Monoaco, C., Manzo, G., Pozzi, L. & Vecchio, G. (1993) Production of transgenic mice expressing the Ki-ras oncogene under the control of a thyroglobulin promoter. *Cancer Res.*, **53**, 5523–5527

Santoro, M., Carlomango, F. & Hay, I.D. (1992) Ret oncogene activation in human thyroid neoplasms is restricted to the papillary cancer subtype. *J. Clin. Invest.*, **89**, 1517–1522

Santoro, M., Chiappetta, G., Cerrato, A., Salvatore, D., Zhang, L., Manzo, G., Picone, A., Portella, G., Santelli, G., Vecchio, G. & Fusco, A. (1996) Development of thyroid papillary carcinomas secondary to tissue-specific expression of the RET/PTC1 oncogene in transgenic mice. *Oncogene*, **12**, 1821–1826

Schäffer, R. & Müller, H.A. (1980) On the development of metastasizing tumors of the thyroid gland after combined administration of nitrosomethylurea and methylthiouracil. *J. Cancer Res. Clin. Oncol.*, **96**, 281–285

Schaller, R.T., Jr & Stevenson, J.K. (1966) Development of carcinoma of the thyroid in iodine deficient rats. *Cancer*, **19**, 1063–1080

Schneider, A., Shore-Freedman, E. & Weinstein, R. (1986) Radiation induced thyroid and other head and neck tumors: occurrence of multiple tumors and analysis of risk factors. *J. Clin. Endocrinol. Metab.*, **63**, 107–112

Shuji, I. (1991) Molecular cloning of the primary structure of rat thyroxine binding globulin. *Biochem. J.*, **3**, 22–27

Takayama, S., Aihara, K., Onodera, T. & Akimoto, T. (1986) Antithyroid effects of phenylthiourea and sulfamonomethoxine in rats and monkeys. *Toxicol. Appl. Pharmacol.*, **82**, 191–199

Taurog, A. (1976) The mechanism of action of the thiourylene antithyroid drugs. *Endocrinology*, **98**, 1031–1046

Thomas G.A. & Williams, E.D. (1992) Production of thyroid tumours in mice by demethylating agents. *Carcinogenesis*, **13**, 1039–1042

Thomas, G.A. & Williams, E.D. (1994) Changes in structure and function of thyroid follicular cells. In: Mohr, U., Dungworth, D.L. & Capen, C.C., eds, *Pathobiology of the Aging Rat*, Washington DC, ILSI, pp. 269–284

Thomas, G.A. & Williams, E.D. (1996) Changes in structure and function of thyroid follicular cells. In: Mohr, U., Dungworth, D.L., Capen, C.C., Sundberg, J.P. & Ward, J.M., eds, *Pathobiology of the Aging Mouse*, Washington DC, ILSI, pp. 87–102

Thomas, G.A., Williams, D. & Williams, E.D. (1989) The clonal origin of thyroid nodules and adenomas. *Am. J. Pathol.*, **134**, 141–147

Thomas, G.A., Williams, D. & Williams, E.D. (1991) The reversibility of the malignant phenotype in monoclonal thyroid tumours in the mouse. *Br. J. Cancer*, **63**, 213–216

Todd, G.C. (1986) Induction and reversibility of thyroid proliferative changes in rats given an antithyroid compound. *Vet. Pathol.*, **23**, 110–117

Tsuda, H., Fukushima, S., Imaida, K., Kurata, Y. & Ito, N. (1983) Organ specific promoting effect of phenobarbital and saccharin in induction of thyroid, liver and bladder tumours in rats after initiation with N-nitrosomethylurea. *Cancer Res.*, **43**, 3292–3296

van Jaarsfeld, P., van der Walt, B. & Theron, C.N. (1972) Afrikander cattle congenital goiter: purification and partial identification of the complex iodoprotein pattern. *Endocrinology*, **91**, 470–482

Vickery, A.L. (1981) The diagnosis of malignancy in dyshormonogenetic goitre. *Clin. Endocrinol. Metab.*, **10**, 317–335

Walinder, G. (1972) Late effects of irradiation on the thyroid gland in mice. I. Irradiation of adult mice. *Radiol. Ther. Phys. Biol.*, **11**, 433–451

Walinder, G. & Sjöden, A.-M. (1972) Late effects of irradiation on the thyroid gland in mice. II. Irradiation of mouse fetuses. *Acta Radiol. Ther. Phys. Biol.*, **11**, 577–589

Wenzel, K.W. (1981) Pharmacological interference with in vitro tests of thyroid function. *Metabolism*, **30**, 717–732

Williams, E.D., Doniach, I., Bjarnason, O. & Michie, W. (1977) Thyroid cancer in an iodide rich area. A histopathological study. *Cancer*, **39**, 215–222

Williams, E.D., Cherstvoy, E., Egloff, B., Höfler, H., Vecchio, G., Bogdanova, T., Bragarnik, M. & Tronko, N.D. (1996a) Interaction of pathology and molecular characterisation of thyroid cancers. In: Karaoglou, A., Desmet, G., Kelly, G.N. & Menzel, H.G., eds, *The Radiological Consequences of the Chernobyl Accident*, European Commission EUR 16544 EN, pp. 785–789

Williams, G.H., Thomas, G.A., Voscoboinik, L., Bogdanova, T., Tronko, N.D., Nerovnya, A., Chestervoy, E.D. & Williams, E.D. (1996b) Rearrangement of the ret oncogene in papillary carcinoma and gender. J. Endocrinol. Invest., 19, (Suppl. 6),11A

Wynford-Thomas, D., Stringer, B.M.J. & Williams, E.D. (1982) Dissociation of growth and function in the rat thyroid during prolonged goitrogen administration. *Acta Endocrinol.*, **101**, 210–216

Zou, M., Shi, Y. & Farid, N.R. (1994) Low rate of ret proto-oncogene activation (PTC/retTPC) in papillary thyroid carcinomas from Saudi Arabia. *Cancer*, **73**, 176–180

Corresponding authors

G.A. Thomas & E.D. Williams
Thyroid Carcinogenesis Group, Strangeways Research Laboratory, Wort's Causeway, Cambridge CB1 4RN, United Kingdom

Species Differences in Thyroid, Kidney and Urinary Bladder Carcinogenesis
C. C. Capen, E. Dybing, J. M. Rice and J. D. Wilbourn, eds
IARC Scientific Publications No. 147
International Agency for Research on Cancer, Lyon, 1999

A Mechanistic Relationship between Thyroid Follicular Cell Tumours and Hepatocellular Neoplasms in Rodents

R. M. McClain and J. M. Rice

Introduction

Thyroid follicular cell neoplasms have been reported to be the most common endocrine tumour response observed in carcinogenicity bioassays of pharmaceutical agents, and neoplasms of liver parenchyma and thyroid follicular epithelium often occur together in rodent carcinogenicity studies (Huff et al., 1991; McConnell, 1992; Haseman & Lockhart, 1993). In one analysis of the United States National Toxicology Program (NTP) database, it was noted that chemicals that produced thyroid proliferative changes were more likely than other chemicals to produce hepatocellular neoplasms, in the same or other species. The correlation is not perfect, since many chemicals that produce liver tumours do not produce thyroid tumours, and vice versa (McConnell, 1992). For chemicals that do produce tumours at both these organ sites, microsomal enzyme induction has been suggested to be a mechanistic link that connects pathogenesis of thyroid follicular tumours with that of hepatocellular neoplasms (McClain, 1989).

When chemicals are tested at high dosages in subchronic and chronic toxicity tests in rats and mice, increased liver weight and centrilobular hepatocellular hypertrophy are commonly observed. These observations are indicative of microsomal enzyme induction, which can be confirmed by biochemical measurement of tissue levels of enzyme protein, enzyme-specific mRNA, and rates of metabolic conversion of substrates specifically acted upon by these enzymes. Two important classes of enzyme inducers are the phenobarbital-like inducers and the polynuclear aromatic hydrocarbon-like inducers. Phenobarbital and many other substances that comprise the first group induce biosynthesis of a wide variety of enzymes, including P450s CYP2B1 and CYP2B2 (Lubet et al.,

1992) and are located principally or exclusively in the liver. The second group includes compounds like 2,3,7,8-tetrachlorodibenzo-para-dioxin (TCDD), which act through a cytoplasmic receptor (the Ah receptor), induce predominantly CYP1A1 and CYP1A2 together with other non-P450 genes, and are widely distributed in many tissues and organs (Conney, 1967; Poland & Knutson, 1982). Chemicals that belong to each of these two classes of enzyme inducers have been shown to produce both hepatocellular and thyroid follicular cell neoplasms in rodents.

The short-term consequences of hepatic microsomal enzyme induction in laboratory animals are relatively minor from a toxicologic point of view. Histologic and functional changes may be observed in the liver, and since microsomal enzymes metabolize a variety of endogenous hormones, vitamins and cofactors as well as many xenobiotic substances, reversible, adaptive functional changes in various endocrine organs can occur. However, the long-term consequences of microsomal enzyme induction can be of greater significance, since alterations in tumour incidence in certain organs may result.

Carcinogenesis and tumour promotion in liver and thyroid gland by phenobarbital

Phenobarbital (PB), the classic example of an inducer of hepatic CYP2B1 and CYP2B2, has been extensively studied as a hepatic tumour promoter following initiating exposures to various DNA-reactive (genotoxic) carcinogens, in rats and to a lesser extent in mice and other rodents and in non-rodent species (Whysner et al., 1996). PB has been shown to promote hepatocarcinogenesis in rats following initiation with 2-acetylaminofluorene (Peraino et al., 1975, 1980), N-nitrosodiethylamine (NDEA; Goldsworthy et al., 1984; Pereira et al., 1986;

Pitot *et al.*, 1987), and other agents (Kitagawa *et al.*, 1984; Diwan *et al.*, 1985a). PB is also a hepatocellular tumour promoter in mice (Diwan *et al.*, 1990; Fullerton *et al.*, 1990; Rumsby *et al.*, 1991) and in *Erythrocebus patas* monkeys (Rice *et al.*, 1989) initiated with NDEA, but does not promote in Syrian golden hamsters, at least at doses comparable to those that are effective for tumour promotion in other species (Diwan *et al.*, 1986a).

PB has also been shown to be a tumour promoter for thyroid follicular cell tumours in rats. Hiasa *et al.* (1982a) gave rats N-nitrosodihydroxypropylamine (DHPN) for a period of four to six weeks followed by PB at 500 parts per million (ppm) in the diet, and observed a marked increase in thyroid follicular cell neoplasms in male rats given DHPN followed by PB, compared to rats that received DHPN alone. The incidence of thyroid tumours was later shown to increase with duration of treatment with PB (Hiasa *et al.*, 1984) and to be much more pronounced in male than in female rats (Hiasa *et al.*, 1985). This sex difference in susceptibility to thyroid tumour promotion by PB in rats was independently confirmed in another laboratory (McClain *et al.*, 1988). PB has also been shown to promote thyroid tumorigenesis in rats initiated with N-nitrosomethylurea (Tsuda *et al.*, 1983; Diwan *et al.*, 1985a) or NDEA (Diwan *et al.*, 1985b).

Prolonged feeding of PB alone, in the absence of an initiating agent, also results in increased hepatocellular tumour incidence in rats (Rossi *et al.*, 1977; Saito *et al.*,1990) and mice (Peraino *et al.*, 1973; Thorpe & Walker, 1973; Jones & Butler, 1975; Ponomarkov *et al.* 1976; Butler & Jones, 1978; Becker, 1982; Evans *et al.*, 1992) that have not received an initiating dose of a genotoxic agent. PB is thus carcinogenic, by the empirical definition of the term. Although PB alone has not been shown to produce thyroid follicular cell tumours in rats, a number of other PB-like inducers have (Hill *et al.*, 1989; McClain, 1989*).

Mechanism of tumour promotion by phenobarbital in thyroid follicular epithelium

It is widely accepted that there are two basic mechanisms whereby chemicals produce thyroid gland neoplasms in rodents (see Thomas & Williams, this volume). One mechanism involves chemicals that exert a direct, genotoxic, carcinogenic effect on the thyroid gland. The other involves chemicals which, through a variety of mechanisms, disrupt thyroid gland function and produce thyroid gland neoplasms by processes involving persistent hormone imbalance.

The latter was originally formulated to explain pathogenesis of thyroid tumours produced in rodents treated with antithyroid drugs (Furth, 1959, 1969). Antithyroid compounds initially cause hormonal imbalance by interfering with thyroid hormone production. A sustained increase in synthesis and secretion of thyroid stimulating hormone (TSH) to stimulate the thyroid occurs via negative feedback stimulation of the pituitary gland. Increased TSH stimulation produces a variety of morphological and functional changes in thyroid follicular cells including follicular cell hypertrophy and progressing, in the rodent, to enlargement of the gland (goitre) and eventually to neoplasia. That excessive and prolonged secretion of endogenous TSH alone in mice and rats, in the absence of any chemical treatment, will produce a high incidence of thyroid tumours has been clearly established by experiments in which rats were fed diets deficient in iodine (Axelrad & Leblond, 1955; Leblond *et al.*, 1957; Isler *et al.*, 1958; Ohshima & Ward, 1986) or in which TSH-secreting pituitary tumours were transplanted into mice with normal thyroids (Furth, 1954).

The effect of chemicals on various aspects of thyroid hormone metabolism has an important impact on thyroid hormone economy in rodents (Cavalieri & Pitt-Rivers, 1981). The monodeiodinases are quantitatively the most important path in the disposition of thyroxine. These enzymes metabolise T4 to the active form of thyroid hormone, T3, and catalyse subsequent monodeiodinations in the catabolism of thyroid hormone. In addition, thyroxine is glucuronidated by microsomal thyroxine UDP-glucuronyl transferase and the glucuronide is subsequently excreted in the bile (Robbins, 1981). Many chemicals are hepatic microsomal enzyme inducers at high dosages and are known to alter thyroid function in rodents by increasing the rate of hepatic disposition of thyroid hormone (Oppenheimer *et al.*, 1968; Bastomsky & Murthy, 1976; Comer *et al.*, 1985; Sanders *et al.*, 1988; Hill *et al.*, 1989; McClain *et al.*, 1989; Curran & DeGroot, 1991; Bookstaff *et al.*, 1996; Waritz *et al.*, 1996). Decreased serum thyroid hormone due to increased hepatic disposition results in a compensatory increase in pituitary TSH which can exert a tumour promoting effect in initiation-promotion model systems (Hiasa *et al.*, 1982a,b) or an increase in thyroid gland neoplasia in two-year carcinogenicity studies (Hill *et al.*, 1989; McClain, 1989).

In rats, PB has been shown to induce hepatic microsomal thyroxine UDP-glucuronyl transferase, increase the biliary excretion of thyroxine glucuronide, decrease serum levels of T3 and T4, and produce a compensatory increase in the plasma level of TSH (McClain, 1989; McClain *et al.*, 1989). In an initiation-promotion model, the tumour promoting effect of PB for the rat thyroid gland was found to be directly proportional to the increased plasma level of TSH. Supplemental administration of thyroxine, at dosages that normalized but did not suppress TSH, completely blocked the tumour promoting effect of PB in the thyroid, but had no inhibitory effect on liver hypertrophy resulting from PB administration (Table 1; McClain *et al.*, 1988; McClain, 1989). The tumour-promoting effect of PB in the thyroid gland thus appears to be mediated by pituitary TSH as a compensatory response to the increased rate of hepatic disposition of thyroid hormone, as opposed to a direct tumour-promoting or carcinogenic effect in thyroid follicular epithelium.

Hepatocellular tumour promotion by phenobarbital

The conclusion that the mode of action for hepatocarcinogenesis by PB is tumour promotion is widely accepted and is based on a large body of evidence accumulated during the last two decades (Pitot & Sirica, 1980; Peraino *et al.*, 1973, 1980). There is no evidence that PB causes DNA damage in the liver, or that it can initiate carcinogenesis. Tumour promoters exert their effect on initiated cells and on preexisting preneoplastic lesions (Schulte-Hermann *et al.*, 1983) and tumour promotion can be operationally defined as preferential enhancement of growth of altered foci of cells that ultimately evolve to become neoplasms. PB has been shown to enhance selectively the nuclear labeling index of cells within eosinophilic hepatocellular foci in mice given NDEA, resulting in development of eosinophilic hepatocellular adenomas (Pereira, 1993). PB had little or no effect on the nuclear labeling index in hepatocytes in surrounding histologically normal liver or in basophilic hepatocellular foci, which corresponded to lack of enhancement by PB of development of basophilic hepatocellular adenomas (Pereira, 1993).

Although the mode of action of PB on development of liver tumours is clearly by promotion of

Table 1. Effect of dietary thyroxine on promotion by phenobarbital of nitrosamine-induced thyroid follicular tumours in male rats (modified from McClain *et al.*, 1988).

Treatment group	% Adenomas (rats affected/rats examined)		Number of tumour foci
Control	0%	(0/20)	0
DHPN[a]	37%	(6/16)	20
DHPN + PB[b]	83%	(15/18)[d]	107
DHPN + PB + T4[c]	25%	(5/20)	11
T4	0%	(0/20)	0
PB	0%	(0/20)	0
PB + T4	0%	(0/20)	0

[a] DHPN: *N*-Nitrosodihydroxypropylamine, 700 mg/kg bw/week subcutaneously for 5 weeks (experimental weeks 1-5).

[b] PB: phenobarbital, fed as the sodium salt, mixed in diet at 500 ppm, for 15 weeks (experimental weeks 6-20).

[c] T4: L-thyroxine, fed as the sodium salt pentahydrate, mixed in diet to provide a dose of 50 µg/kg bw/day for 15 weeks (experimental weeks 6-20).

[d] Fisher's exact test vs. DHPN group, $p \leq 0.05$.

neoplastic development, its mechanism of action in hepatocytes is not well understood. Evidence is accumulating, however, that the process involves stimulation of expression of certain peptide growth factors that control cell replication in hepatocytes.

Hepatocytes isolated from the livers of rats that had previously received an initiating dose of a genotoxic hepatocarcinogen require PB in the culture medium for selective outgrowth *in vitro* (Kaufmann *et al.*, 1988). Initiated hepatocytes proliferate and form colonies in primary culture in the presence of PB, under conditions where hepatocytes from control animals degenerate and die. It has recently been shown that tumour growth factor-α (TGF-α) can substitute for PB in culture medium. Either PB or TGF-α can support colony formation by initiated cells; when combined at optimal concentrations, the response appeared to be saturated, and when these factors were tested in combination at suboptimal concentrations, the two substances were additive for supporting colony formation (Kaufmann *et al.*, 1997).

In rats, PB produces a burst of DNA synthesis in hepatocytes followed by increased mitotic activity and hyperplasia. After the initial burst of DNA synthesis, there is a decrease in the rate of cell proliferation and inhibition of apoptosis in normal hepatocytes (Bursch & Schulte-Hermann, 1983). This corresponds to an increase in tumour growth factor-β (TGF-β) in periportal hepatocytes. TGF-β is a potent inhibitor of cell proliferation and plays a role in apoptosis (Jirtle & Meyer, 1991). After long-term exposure to PB some hepatocytes lose the ability to take up TGF-β. The loss of inhibition of cell proliferation by TGF-β provides a growth advantage over normal hepatocytes (Jirtle & Meyer, 1991). In addition, the inhibition of apoptosis in preneoplastic foci could cause a rapid expansion of foci without a persistent increase in cell proliferation (Bursch & Schulte-Hermann, 1983).

Recent research suggests that in strains of mice that are sensitive to tumour promotion the balance between liver cell mitosis and programmed cell death (apoptosis) is disrupted (Böhm & Moser, 1976; Bursch & Schulte-Hermann, 1983). Furthermore, altered DNA methylation may play a variety of roles in carcinogenesis (Counts & Goodman, 1995). In mice, there is a marked strain difference in the spontaneous incidence of hepatocellular tumours and susceptibility to hepatic

tumour promotion (Drinkwater & Ginsler, 1986). This correlates with the observation that the relatively resistant strain is better able to maintain the normal methylation status of DNA in the face of a higher level of cell proliferation (Counts *et al.*, 1996).

Carcinogenesis and tumour promotion in liver and thyroid gland by TCDD

TCDD binds with exceptionally high affinity to the Ah receptor (reviewed in IARC, 1997). It causes induction of gene expression of CYP1A1 and many other enzymes and modulates expression of many growth factors, transcription factors, and related peptide factors in many tissues. TCDD has significant effects on the thyroid gland and on blood levels of thyroid hormones. TCDD is not genotoxic.

The effects of TCDD on tumour incidence in treated animals are complex, vary markedly with the genetic background of the subjects, and are not confined to the liver and thyroid in all studies (IARC, 1997). Osborne-Mendel rats of both sexes and female B6C3F$_1$ mice given TCDD by gavage twice weekly for 104 weeks developed both thyroid follicular cell adenomas and hepatocellular adenomas; the mice also developed lymphomas and soft-tissue sarcomas. Male mice developed liver tumours and lung tumours (United States National Toxicology Program, 1982).

The relationship of enzyme inducers of the TCDD type to tumour promotion in liver and thyroid is much less well studied than that of PB-type inducers.

Correlation of microsomal enzyme induction with tumour promotion in liver and thyroid gland

A correlation has been well established between potency for hepatic microsomal enzyme induction and capacity for tumour promotion in rat liver and thyroid gland by enzyme inducers of the PB type. Studies of a structurally related series of barbiturates that included non-inducers, weak inducers, and strong inducers have shown a highly significant correlation between microsomal enzyme induction and hepatic tumour promotion in rats (Lubet *et al.*, 1989). For example, the strong enzyme inducers PB (5-ethyl-5-phenylbarbituric acid) and barbital (5,5-diethylbarbituric acid) are effective hepatic tumour promoters, while non-inducers such as either 5-ethyl- or 5-phenyl-barbituric acid are not. Furthermore, within the barbiturate series, the potency for enzyme induction correlates quite well with potency for hepatocellular tumour promotion (Lubet *et al.*, 1989; Rice *et al.*, 1994). This observation extends to other species: PB neither induces microsomal enzymes nor promotes hepatocellular tumorigenesis in the Syrian golden hamster (Diwan *et al.*, 1986a).

The same relationship holds true for hydantoin compounds. 5-Ethyl-5-phenylhydantoin (EPH) was an efficient inducer of hepatic CYP2B1 and other microsomal enzymes in rats and was also an effective promoter of hepatocellular tumours induced by NDEA. In contrast, 5,5-diethylhydantoin (EEH) was ineffective either as an enzyme inducer or as a hepatocellular tumour promoter (Diwan *et al.*, 1986b).

An even more striking interspecies comparison is provided by 1,4-bis[2-(3,5-dichloropyridyl-oxy)]benzene (TCPOBOP), which is quantitatively much more potent (by orders of magnitude) as a microsomal enzyme inducer in mice than in rats. TCPOBOP was shown to be both a potent inducer and a hepatocellular tumour inducer in mice initiated with NDEA, but at 10-fold higher dosage it had neither effect in rats (Diwan *et al.*, 1992). When the dose-response relationship for enzyme induction was fully explored in Fischer 344 rats, however, which required thousand-fold higher dosages, a level of exposure that was effective for hepatic microsomal enzyme induction was established, and at that much higher dosage level, TCPOBOP was also an effective liver tumour promoter (Diwan *et al.*, 1996).

Similar relationships between potency for hepatic microsomal enzyme induction and for tumour promotion in thyroid follicular epithelium have also been established. In addition to PB and several other barbiturates, other PB-like enzyme inducers have been shown to promote carcinogenesis in the thyroid. These include EPH which, like PB, promoted both hepatocellular and thyroid follicular cell tumorigenesis in NDEA-initiated rats at doses that were effective for hepatocellular microsomal enzyme induction, but not its non-enzyme inducing homologue, EEH (Diwan *et al.*, 1988). TCPOBOP also promoted thyroid follicular cell carcinogenesis in NDEA-initiated Fischer 344 rats at doses that caused maximal induction of CYP2B1 (Diwan *et al.*, 1996).

Conclusions

The physiological consequences of microsomal enzyme induction are important in the pathogenesis of hepatic and thyroid follicular neoplasia in rodent bioassays for carcinogenicity. This is most likely the consequence of the known effects of microsomal enzyme inducers (hepatocellular and thyroid follicular cell hypertrophy and hyperplasia) which under certain experimental conditions exert a tumour promoting effect in hepatic parenchyma and thyroid follicular epithelium in susceptible species and strains of animals. The modes of action that are involved for individual chemicals need to be thoroughly understood and incorporated into the processes of hazard identification and risk assessment for chemical carcinogens.

References

Axelrad, A.A. & Leblond, C.P. (1955) Induction of thyroid tumors in rats by a low iodine diet. *Cancer*, **8**, 339–367

Bastomsky, C.M. & Murthy, P.V.N. (1976) Enhanced in vitro glucuronidation of thyroxine in rats following cutaneous application or ingestion of polychlorinated biphenyls. *Can. J. Physiol. Pharmacol.*, **54**, 23–26

Becker, F.F. (1982) Morphological classification of mouse liver tumors based on biological characteristics. *Cancer Res.*, **42**, 3918–3923

Böhm, N. & Moser, B. (1976) Reversible hyperplasia and hypertrophy of the mouse liver induced by a functional charge with phenobarbital. *Beitr. Pathol.*, **157**, 283–300 (in German)

Bookstaff, R.C., Murphy, V.A., Skare, J.A., Minnema, D., Sanzgiri, U. & Parkinson, A. (1996) Effects of doxylamine succinate on thyroid hormone balance and enzyme induction in mice. *Toxicol. Appl. Pharmacol.*, **141**, 584–594

Bursch, W. & Schulte-Hermann, R. (1983) Synchronization of hepatic DNA synthesis by scheduled feeding and lighting in mice treated with the chemical inducer of liver growth α-hexachlorocyclohexane. *Cell Tissue Kinet.*, **16**, 125–134

Butler, W.H. & Jones, G. (1978) Pathological and toxicological data on chlorinated pesticides and phenobarbital. *Ecotoxicol. Environ. Safety*, **1**, 503–509

Cavalieri, R.R. & Pitt-Rivers, R. (1981) The effects of drugs on the distribution and metabolism of thyroid hormones. *Pharmacol. Rev.*, **33**, 55–80

Comer, C.P., Chengelis, C.P., Levin, S. & Kotsonis, F.N. (1985) Changes in thyroidal function and liver UDP-glucuronosyltransferase activity in rats following administration of a novel imidazole. *Toxicol. Appl. Pharmacol.*, **80**, 427–436

Conney, A.H. (1967) Pharmacological implications of microsomal enzyme induction. *Pharmacol. Rev.*, **19**, 317–366

Counts, J.L. & Goodman, J.I. (1995) Alterations in DNA methylation may play a variety of roles in carcinogenesis. *Cell*, **83**, 13–15

Counts, J.L., Sarmiento, J.I., Harbison, M.L., Downing, J.C., McClain, R.M. & Goodman, J.I. (1996) Cell proliferation and global methylation status changes in mouse liver after phenobarbital and/or choline-devoid, methionine-deficient diet administration. *Carcinogenesis*, **17**, 1251–1257

Curran, P.G. & DeGroot, L.J. (1991) The effect of hepatic enzyme-inducing drugs on thyroid hormones and the thyroid gland. *Endocrinol. Rev.*, **12**, 135–150

Diwan, B.A., Rice, J.M., Ohshima, M., Ward, J.M. & Dove, L.F. (1985a) N-Nitroso-N-methylurea initiation in multiple tissues for organ-specific tumor promotion in rats by phenobarbital. *J. Natl Cancer Inst.*, **75**, 1099–1105

Diwan, B.A., Rice, J.M., Ohshima, M., Ward, J.M. & Dove, L.F. (1985b) Comparative tumor-promoting activities of phenobarbital, amobarbital, barbital sodium, and barbituric acid on livers and other organs of male F344/NCr rats following initiation with N-nitrosodiethylamine. *J. Natl Cancer Inst.*, **74**, 509–516

Diwan, B.A., Ward, J.M., Anderson, L.M., Hagiwara, A. & Rice, J.M. (1986a) Lack of effect of phenobarbital on hepatocellular carcinogenesis initiated by N-nitrosodiethylamine or methylazoxymethanol acetate in male Syrian golden hamsters. *Toxicol. Appl. Pharmacol.*, **86**, 298–307

Diwan, B.A., Rice, J.M. & Ward, J.M. (1986b) Tumor-promoting activity of benzodiazepine tranquilizers, diazepam and oxazepam in mouse liver. *Carcinogenesis*, **7**, 789–794

Diwan, B.A., Rice, J.M., Nims, R.W., Lubet, R.A., Hu, H. & Ward, J.M. (1988) P-450 enzyme induction by 5-ethyl-5-phenylhydantoin and 5,5-diethylhydantoin, analogues of barbiturate tumor promoters phenobarbital and barbital, and promotion of liver and thyroid carcinogenesis initiated by N-nitrosodiethylamine in rats. *Cancer Res.*, **48**, 2492–2497

Diwan, B.A., Rice, J.M. & Ward, J.M. (1990) Strain dependent effects of phenobarbital on liver tumor promotion in inbred mice. In: *Mouse Liver Carcinogenesis: Mechanisms and Species Comparisons*. Stevenson, D.E., McClain, R.M., Popp, J.A., Slaga, T.J., Ward, J.M. & Pitot, H.C., eds, Wiley-Liss, New York, pp. 69–83

Diwan, B.A., Lubet, R.A., Ward, J.M., Hrabie, J.A. & Rice, J.M. (1992) Tumor-promoting and hepatocarcinogenic effects of 1,4-bis[2-(3,5-dichloropyridyloxy)]benzene (TCPOBOP) in DBA/2NCr and C57BL/6NCr mice and an apparent promoting effect on nasal cavity tumors but not on hepatocellular tumors in F344/NCr rats initiated with N-nitrosodiethylamine. *Carcinogenesis*, **13**, 1893–1901

Diwan, B.A., Henneman, J.R., Rice, J.M. & Nims, R.W. (1996) Enhancement of thyroid and hepatocarcinogenesis by 1,4-bis[2-(3,5-dichloropyridyloxy)]benzene in rats at doses that cause maximal induction of CYP2B. *Carcinogenesis*, **17**, 37–43

Drinkwater, N.R. & Ginsler, J.J. (1986) Genetic control of hepatocarcinogenesis in C57Bl/6J and C3H/HeJ inbred mice. *Carcinogenesis*, **7**, 1701–1707

Evans, J.G., Collins, M.A., Lake, B.G. & Butler, W.H. (1992) The histology and development of hepatic nodules and carcinoma in C3H/He and C57BL/6 mice following chronic phenobarbitone administration. *Toxicol. Pathol.*, **20**, 585–594

Fullerton, F.R., Hoover, K., Mikol, Y.B., Creasia, D.A. & Poirier, L.A. (1990) The inhibition by methionine and choline of liver carcinoma formation in male C3H mice dosed with diethylnitrosamine and fed phenobarbital. *Carcinogenesis*, **11**, 1301–1305

Furth, J. (1954) Morphologic changes associated with thyrotrophin secreting pituitary tumors. *Am. J. Pathol.*, **30**, 421–463

Furth, J. (1959) A meeting of ways in cancer research: Thoughts on the evolution and nature of neoplasms. *Cancer Res.*, **19**, 241–258

Furth, J. (1969) Pituitary cybernetics and neoplasia. *Harvey Lect.*, **63**, 47–71

Goldsworthy, T., Campbell, H.A. & Pitot, H.C. (1984) The natural history and dose-response characteristics of enzyme-altered foci in rat liver following phenobarbital and diethylnitrosamine administration. *Carcinogenesis*, **5**, 67–71

Haseman, J.K. & Lockhart, A.M. (1993) Correlations between chemically related site-specific carcinogenic effects in long-term studies in rats and mice. *Environ. Health Perspect.*, **101**, 50–54

Hiasa, Y., Kitahori, Y., Ohshima, M., Fujita, T., Yuasa, T., Konishi, N. & Miyashiro, A. (1982a) Promoting effects of phenobarbital and barbital on development of thyroid tumors in rats treated with N-bis(2-hydroxypropyl)-nitrosamine. *Carcinogenesis*, **3**, 1187–1190

Hiasa, Y., Ohshima, M., Kitahori, Y., Yuasa, T., Fujita, T. & Iwata, C. (1982b) Promoting effects of 3-amino-1,2,4-triazole on the development of thyroid tumors in rats treated with N-bis(2-hydroxypropyl)nitrosamine. *Carcinogenesis*, **3**, 381–384

Hiasa, Y., Kitahori, Y., Konishi, N., Enoki, N. & Fujita, T. (1984) Promoting effrect of phenobarbital on N-bis(2-hydroxypropyl)nitrosamine thyroid tumorigenesis in rats. Effect of varying duration of exposure to phenobarbital. In: *Models, Mechanisms and Etiology of Tumour Promotion*. Börzönyi, M., Lapis, K., Day, N.E. & Yamasaki, H., eds, IARC, Lyon, pp. 77–82

Hiasa, Y., Kitahori, Y., Konishi, N., Shimoyama, T. & Lin, J.C. (1985) Sex differential and dose dependence of phenobarbital promoting activity in N-bis(2-hydroxypropyl)nitrosamine-initiated thyroid tumorigenesis in rats. *Cancer Res.*, **45**, 4087–4090

Hill, R.N., Erdreich, L.S., Paynter, O.E., Roberts, P.A., Rosenthal, S.L. & Wilkinson, C.F. (1989) Thyroid follicular cell carcinogenesis. *Fund. Appl. Toxicol.*, **12**, 629–697

Huff, J., Cirvello, J., Haseman, J. & Bucher, J. (1991) Chemicals associated with site-specific neoplasia in 1394 long-term carcinogenesis experiments in laboratory rodents. *Environ. Health Perspect.*, **93**, 247–270

IARC (1997) *IARC Monographs on the Evaluation of Carcino-genic Risks to Humans, Vol. 69: Polychlorinated Dibenzo-para-dioxins and Dibenzofurans*. IARC, Lyon, pp. 33–343

Isler, H., Leblond, C.P & Axelrad, A.A. (1958) Influence of age and of iodine intake on the production of thyroid tumors in the rat. *J. Natl Cancer Inst.*, **21**, 1065–1081

Jirtle, R.L. & Meyer, S.A. (1991) Liver tumor promotion: effect of phenobarbital on EGF and protein kinase C signal transduction and transforming growth factor-beta 1 expression. *Dig. Dis. Sci.*, **36**, 659–668

Jones, G. & Butler, W.H. (1975) Morphology of spontaneous and induced neoplasia. In: *Mouse Hepatic Neoplasia*. Butler, W.H. & Newberne, P.M., eds, Elsevier, Amsterdam, pp. 21–59

Kaufmann, W.K., Ririe, D.G. & Kaufman, D.G. (1988) Phenobarbital-dependent proliferation of putative initiated rat hepatocytes. *Carcinogenesis*, **9**, 779–782

Kaufmann, W.K., Byrd, L.L., Palmieri, D., Nims, R.W. & Rice, J.M. (1997) TGF-α sustains clonal expansion by promoter-dependent, chemically initiated rat hepatocytes. *Carcinogenesis*, **18**, 1381–1387

Kitagawa, T., Hino, O., Nomura, K. & Sugano, H. (1984) Dose-response studies on promoting and anticarcinogenic effects of phenobarbital and DDT in the rat hepatocarcinogenesis. *Carcinogenesis*, **5**, 1653–1656

Leblond, C.P., Isler, H. & Axelrad, A.A. (1957) Induction of thyroid tumors by a low iodine diet. *Can. Cancer Conf.*, **2**, 248–266

Lubet, R.A., Nims, R.W., Ward, J.M., Rice, J.M. & Diwan, B.A. (1989) Induction of cytochrome P450$_b$ and its relationship to liver tumor promotion. *J. Am. Coll. Toxicol.*, **8**, 259–268

Lubet, R.A., Dragnev, K.H., Chauhan, D.P., Nims, R.W., Diwan, B.A., Ward, J.M., Jones, C.R., Rice, J.M. & Miller, M.S. (1992) A pleiotropic response to phenobarbital-type enzyme inducers in the F344/NCr rat. Effects of chemicals of varied structure. *Biochem. Pharmacol.*, **43**, 1067–1078

McClain, R.M. (1989) The significance of hepatic microsomal enzyme induction and altered thyroid function in rats: implications for thyroid gland neoplasia. *Toxicol. Pathol.*, **17**, 294–306

McClain, R.M., Posch, R.C., Bosakowski, T. & Armstrong, J.M. (1988) Studies on the mode of action for thyroid gland tumor promotion in rats by phenobarbital. *Toxicol. Appl. Pharmacol.*, **94**, 254–265

McClain, R.M., Levin, A.A., Posch, R. & Downing, J.C. (1989) The effect of phenobarbital on the metabolism and excretion of thyroxine in rats. *Toxicol. Appl. Pharmacol.*, **99**, 216–228

McConnell, E.E. (1992) Thyroid follicular cell carcinogenesis: Results from 343 2-year carcinogenicity studies conducted by the NCI/NTP. *Regul. Toxicol. Pharmacol.*, **16**, 177–188

Ohshima, M. & Ward, J.M. (1986) Dietary iodine deficiency as a tumor promoter and carcinogen in male F344/NCr rats. *Cancer Res.*, **46**, 877–883

Oppenheimer, J.H., Bernstein, G. & Surks, M.I. (1968) Increased thyroxine turnover and thyroidal function after stimulation of hepatocellular binding of thyroxine by phenobarbital. *J. Clin. Invest.*, **47**, 1399–1406

Peraino, C., Fry, R.J. & Staffeldt, E. (1973) Enhancement of spontaneous hepatic tumorigenesis in C3H mice by dietary phenobarbital. *J. Natl Cancer Inst.*, **51**, 134–1350

Peraino, C., Fry, R.J.M. & Staffeldt, E. (1973) Brief communication: enhancement of spontaneous hepatic tumorigenesis in C3H mice by dietary phenobarbital. *J. Natl Cancer Inst.*, **51**, 1349–1350

Peraino, C., Fry, R.J., Staffeldt, J.M. & Christophen, J.P. (1975) Comparative enhancing effects of phenobarbital, amobarbital, diphenylhydantoin and dichlorodiphenyltrichloroethane on 2-acetylaminofluorene-induced hepatic tumorigenesis in the rat. *Cancer Res.*, **35**, 2884–2890

Peraino, C., Staffeldt, E.F., Haugen, D.A., Lombard, L.S., Stevens, F.J. & Fry, R.J. (1980) Effects of varying the dietary concentration of phenobarbital on its enhancement of 2-acetylaminofluorene-induced hepatic tumorigenesis. *Cancer Res.*, **40**, 3268–3273

Pereira, M.A. (1993) Comparison in C3H and C3B6F1 mice of the sensitivity to DEN-initiation and phenobarbital-promotion to the extent of cell proliferation. *Carcinogenesis*, **14**, 299–302

Pereira, M.A., Herren-Freund, S.L. & Long, R.E. (1986) Dose response relationship of phenobarbital promotion of diethylnitrosamine initiated tumors in rat liver. *Cancer Lett.*, **32**, 305–311

Pitot, H.C. & Sirica, A.E. (1980) The stages of initiation and promotion in hepatocarcinogenesis. *Biochim. Biophys. Acta*, **605**, 191–215

Pitot, H.C., Goldsworthy, T.L., Moran, S., Kennan, W., Glauert, H.P., Maronpot, R.R. & Campbell, H.A. (1987) A method to quantitate the relative initiating and promoting potencies of hepatocarcinogenic agents in their dose-response relationships to altered hepatic foci. *Carcinogenesis*, **8**, 1491–1499

Poland, A. & Knutson, J.C. (1982) 2,3,7,8-Tetrachlorodibenzo-p-dioxin related halogenated aromatic hydrocarbons: Examination of the mechanism of toxicity. *Annu. Rev. Pharmacol. Toxicol.*, **22**, 517–554

Ponomarkov, V., Tomatis, L. & Turusov, V. (1976) The effect of long term administration of phenobarbitone in CF-1 mice. *Cancer Lett.*, **1**, 165–172

Rice, J.M., Rehm, S., Donovan, P.J. & Perantoni, A.O. (1989) Comparative transplacental carcinogenesis by directly acting and metabolism-dependent alkylating agents in rodents and nonhuman primates. In: *Perinatal and Multigeneration Carcinogenesis*. Napalkov, N.P., Rice, J.M., Tomatis, L. & Yamasaki, H., eds, IARC, Lyon, pp. 17–34

Rice, J.M., Diwan, B.A., Hu, H., Ward, J.M., Nims, R.W. & Lubet, R.A. (1994) Enhancement of hepatocarcinogenesis and induction of specific cytochrome P450-dependent monooxygenase activities by the barbiturates allobarbital, aprobarbital, pentobarbital, secobarbital, and 5-phenyl- and 5-ethylbarbituric acids. *Carcinogenesis*, **15**, 395–402

Robbins, J. (1981) Factors altering thyroid hormone metabolism. *Environ. Health Perspect.*, **38**, 65–70

Rossi, L., Ravra, M., Repetti, G. & Santi, L. (1977) Long-term administration of DDT or phenobarbital-Na in Wistar rats. *Int. J. Cancer*, **19**, 179–185

Rumsby, P.C., Barrass, N.C., Phillimore, H.E. & Evans, J.G. (1991) Analysis of the Ha-ras oncogene in C3H/He mouse liver tumors derived spontaneously or induced with diethylnitrosamine or phenobarbitone. *Carcinogenesis*, 12, 2331–233

Saito, R., Chandar, N., Janosky, J.E.& Lombardi, B. (1990) No enhancement by phenobarbital of the hepatocarcinogenicity of a choline-devoid diet in the rat. *Res. Commun. Chem. Pathol. Pharmacol.*, **69**, 197–207

Sanders, J.E., Eigenberg, D.A., Bracht, L.J., Wang, W.R. & van Zwieten, M.J. (1988) Thyroid and liver trophic changes in rats secondary to liver microsomal enzyme induction by an experimental leukotriene antagonist (L-649,923). *Toxicol. Appl. Pharmacol.*, **95**, 378–387

Schulte-Hermann, R., Timmermann-Troisener, I. & Schuppler, J. (1983) Promotion of spontaneous preneoplastic cells in rat liver as a possible explanation of tumor production by nonmutagenic compounds. *Cancer Res.*, **43**, 839–844

Thorpe, E. & Walker, A.I.T. (1973) The toxicology of dieldrin (HEOD*). II. Comparative long-term oral toxicity studies in mice with dieldrin, DDT, phenobarbitone, β-BHC, and γ-BHC. *Food Cosmet. Toxicol.*, **11**, 433–442

Tsuda, H., Fukushima, S., Imaida, K., Kurata, Y. & Ito, N. (1983) Organ-specific promoting effect of phenobarbital and saccharin in induction of thyroid, liver, and urinary bladder tumors in rats after initiation with N-nitrosomethylurea. *Cancer Res.*, **43**, 3292–3296

United States National Toxicology Program (1982) *Carcinogenesis Bioassay of 2,3,7,8-Tetrachlorodibenzo-p-dioxin (CAS No. 1746-01-6) in Osborne-Mendel Rats and B6C3F1 Mice (Gavage Study)*. Technical Report Series No. 209; DHEW Publication No. (NIH) 82-1765, Research Triangle Park, NC

Waritz, R.S., Steinberg, M., Kinoshita, F.K., Kelly, C.M. & Richter, W.R. (1996) Thyroid function and thyroid tumors in toxaphene-treated rats. *Regul. Toxicol. Pharmacol.*, **24**, 184–192

Wilson, A.G., Thake, D.C., Heydens, W.E., Brewster, D.W. & Hotz, K.J. (1996) Mode of action of thyroid tumor formation in the male Long-Evans rat administered high doses of alachlor. *Fund. Appl. Toxicol.*, **33**, 16–23

Whysner, J., Ross, P.M. & Williams, G.M. (1996) Phenobarbital mechanistic data and risk assessment: Enzyme induction, enhanced cell proliferation, and tumor promotion. *Pharmacol. Ther.*, **71**, 153–191

Corresponding authors

R. McClain
Hoffmann-La Roche, Inc.
340 Kingsland St.
Nutley,
NJ 07110, USA

J. Rice
International Agency for Research on Cancer
150 cours Albert Thomas
Lyon 69372 Cedex 08
France

Species Differences in Thyroid, Kidney and Urinary Bladder Carcinogenesis
C.C. Capen, E. Dybing, J.M. Rice and J.D. Wilbourn, eds
IARC Scientific Publications No. 147
International Agency for Research on Cancer, Lyon, 1999

Human renal-cell carcinoma — epidemiological and mechanistic aspects

A. Mellemgaard

Introduction

Renal-cell carcinoma (RCC), also known as adeno-carcinoma of the kidney, hypernephroma or Grawitz tumour, is the most frequent type of kidney cancer. Other frequent types of kidney cancer include tumours derived from the urothelium in the pelvis and ureter and Wilm's tumour in children.

RCC was first described by König (1826). The erroneous assumption that the tumour originated from the fatty adrenal tissue led to the term hypernephroma, but it later became clear that RCC originates in the mature renal tubular epithelium. Early studies of RCC focused on histology, staging and prognostic factors as well as descriptive epidemiology. In the 1960s and 1970s, studies of risk factors with systematic data collection were published. In the 1980s and 1990s, several specific hypotheses were tested in case–control and follow-up studies, including studies of the roles of tobacco, occupation and medication.

This paper summarizes current knowledge on the etiology of RCC and the possible mechanisms of action of the risk factors so far identified. Reference is made to a selection of the studies of RCC that were particularly well executed or provided new insight.

Descriptive epidemiology of renal-cell carcinoma

The incidence rates of RCC vary greatly from high-incidence areas in northern Europe and North America, where the incidence is up to 10 per 100 000 (standardized to the world standard population) to low-incidence areas in Asia, Africa and South America where the incidence rates are from 1 to 3 per 100 000. RCC accounts for approximately 2% of all non-skin cancer in the western world (Parkin et al., 1997).

The incidence rate of RCC has been increasing in most countries that have population-based cancer registries. In Denmark, where nationwide cancer incidence figures have been available since 1943, the incidence doubled among men between the 1950s and 1970s and has remained stable since then, at about 8 per 100 000. Among Danish women, the incidence increased slightly from 3 to 4 per 100 000 in the same period (Mellemgaard et al., 1993). The data from the Connecticut Cancer Registry for the period 1935–89 indicate that rates in the USA increased among men from 1.6 to 9.6 per 100 000 and among women from 0.7 to 4.2 per 100 000. Just in the period 1974–90, the incidence has increased by 38% in the USA (Katz et al., 1994). Throughout this period, the male : female incidence ratio has remained close to 2, a ratio which is similar in all high-incidence areas, and the incidence is uniformly increasing with age. Incidence rates of RCC are consistently higher among urban than rural dwellers.

Two risk factors, cigarette smoking and obesity, have consistently been linked with RCC in epidemiological studies. For a number of other risk factors such as drugs, occupation, diet, medical and reproductive history and socioeconomic status, there is some evidence of an association.

Cigarette smoking

In a hospital-based case–control study, Wynder et al. (1974) found that the relative risk (RR) for RCC among cigarette smokers was 2 compared with nonsmokers. A dose–response relationship was observed for the number of cigarettes smoked per day. Use of other types of tobacco smoking (pipe and cigar) was weakly associated with risk for RCC. In contrast, another hospital-based case–control study found no association between tobacco smoking and RCC, although chewing tobacco increased the risk four-fold (Goodman *et al.*, 1986). A case–control study, in which cases were restricted to subjects 55 years of age or under and controls were sampled from the neighbourhoods of cases, found an RR of 2 for RCC among men but not among women (Yu *et al.*, 1986). A hospital-based case–control study, in which controls were sampled from patients without cancer or urological disease, found an association and a dose–effect relationship for cigarette smoking (La Vecchia *et al.*, 1990). Statistically insignificant associations were observed in a case–control study in which controls were individuals with non-tobacco-, non-alcohol- and non-hormone-related diseases (Talamini *et al.*, 1990). A number of population-based studies have confirmed the association. In the study by McLaughlin *et al.* (1984), an association among both men and women was found for cigarette smoking, including a dose–response relationship. In a case–control study that included hospital and population-based controls, a weak nonsignificant association was found (Asal *et al.*, 1988a). A two-fold risk was found for smokers in a Canadian study which also investigated passive smoking, for which a nonsignificant association was observed (Kreiger *et al.*, 1993). A study based in Shanghai found an RR of 2.3 for subjects who had ever versus never smoked cigarettes. The risk among heavy smokers of non-filtered cigarettes was particularly high (McLaughlin *et al.*, 1992a). Although use of smokeless tobacco has generally been found not to increase the risk for RCC, a recent study found an RR of more than 3 among men using chewing tobacco (Muscat *et al.*, 1995). An international multicentre study found a significant, but modest, increase in risk among cigarette smokers (RR, 1.4). Furthermore, an increasing risk was found with increased consumption and duration of smoking. Use of other types of tobacco was not associated with RCC (McLaughlin *et al.*, 1995a). Findings in a cohort study confirmed the association, including a dose–response relationship (McLaughlin *et al.*, 1990).

The few studies which have not found this association have either been small or have used hospital controls, which might lead to underestimation of the true relative risk. In most studies, heavy cigarette smoking was associated with a two- to three-fold increase in risk; the attributable fraction may be as high as one-third.

Obesity

Wynder *et al.* (1974) observed an excess of overweight female cases and prompted subsequent studies to examine the role of weight. Although some case–control studies confirmed the association in women only (Lew & Garfinkel, 1979; McLaughlin *et al.*, 1984; Chow et al., 1996), other studies found the effect to be present in men also (Goodman *et al.*, 1986; Yu *et al.*, 1986; Asal *et al.*, 1988a,b; Maclure & Willett, 1990; McLaughlin *et al.*, 1992b; Benhamou *et al.*, 1993; Kreiger *et al.*, 1993). One study found a nonsignificant reduction in risk for individuals with a high body mass index (BMI) (Talamini *et al.*, 1990). The international multicentre study found a significant effect in both sexes, but the effect was stronger in women. Among the top 5% women, the odds ratio was 3.6 compared with the lowest quartile. The rate of weight change appeared to be an independent risk factor in women but not in men and there was no association with height or physical activity. The association remained after adjustment for socioeconomic status, smoking and diet (protein and fat) (Mellemgaard *et al.*, 1994a). A cohort study of individuals discharged from Danish hospitals with a diagnosis of obesity found an increased risk for RCC in both sexes (Mellemgaard *et al.*, 1991).

Although there is no direct evidence of the mechanism, the differences found between men and women and other indications of a possible role of hormones in RCC (reproductive factors, receptors on tumour cells) are compatible with a mechanistic pathway involving the formation of oestrogens in fatty tissue which then stimulate the malignant cell. The evidence is sufficient to categorize obesity as a likely risk factor for RCC, with increased peripheral oestrogen formation as a possible mechanism.

Socioeconomic status

Early reports on the epidemiology of RCC were suggestive of an increased mortality in higher socioeconomic strata (Case, 1964). In the majority of case–control studies, no association has been found, but a French study found that the risk for RCC was higher among individuals with longer education (Benhamou *et al.*, 1993). However, recent studies have found an inverse association in some countries, such as the USA (Asal *et al.*, 1988a,b; Muscat *et al.*, 1995) and Denmark

(Mellemgaard et al., 1994b). The increased risk in lower socioeconomic strata is not caused by the suspected occupational risk factors, obesity or cigarette smoking and may indicate the existence of yet unidentified occupational or other lifestyle factors. The current evidence is not strong enough to label socioeconomic factors as a risk factor for RCC and the underlying reason for the effects observed is unknown.

Medical history

It has been known for many years that the risk for RCC is increased in individuals with polycystic kidney disease and kidney failure (Ishikawa et al., 1990). In case–control studies of medical history, an association has been observed for previous diagnosis of thyroid and kidney disease, particularly infections (McLaughlin et al., 1984; Schlehofer et al., 1996), as well as circulatory disease in men and digestive disease in women (Asal et al., 1988a). A cohort study of diabetics found an increased risk for RCC in women, but findings from case–control studies offer only limited support for this hypothesis (Adami et al., 1991; Schlehofer et al., 1996). The role of hypertension has attracted special attention because diuretics have been suspected of increasing the risk for RCC (see below). A cohort study of individuals discharged with hypertension, heart failure or oedema showed a two-fold increase in relative risk irrespective of diagnosis. Based on a random sample, 70% of the discharged individuals were treated with diuretics (Mellemgaard et al., 1992a). A similar register-linkage study from Sweden confirmed an increased risk in men and women discharged with a diagnosis of heart failure or oedema (Lindblad et al., 1993). The cohort studies, however, were unable to adjust for the effect of other risk factors such as smoking and obesity. In a large follow-up study of Seventh Day Adventists, an increased risk was found for individuals who reported hypertension (RR, 4.5) or taking antihypertensive medications (RR, 2.9) (Fraser et al., 1990). A prospective study of blood pressure and cancer incidence found an increased RR of 1.2–1.5 for kidney cancer among hypertensive Japanese men in Hawaii. No other cancer site showed an elevated RR (Grove et al., 1991). A follow-up study of thyroid disorders revealed significantly increased risks of kidney cancer in women

discharged from a Danish hospital with a diagnosis of myxoedema (RR, 1.8) or thyrotoxicosis (RR, 1.3). The risk among men was unchanged (Mellemgaard, unpublished). Several case–control studies have found an association between RCC and hypertension (Kreiger et al., 1993; Muscat et al., 1995). In the international multicentre study, the odds ratio for hypertension was 1.4 after adjustment for medication (McLaughlin et al., 1995b).

There is thus some evidence that hypertension and polycystic kidney disease are risk factors for RCC, while the evidence for thyroid disorders is limited.

Drugs

Two kinds of drug have attracted much attention: diuretics and weak analgesics (Mellemgaard et al., 1992a, 1992b). A case–control study found a five-fold increase in risk for RCC among users of diuretics (Yu et al., 1986). The association was noted in both hypertensive and non-hypertensive individuals. Subsequent studies have shown divergent findings. Apart from the findings in cohort studies of users or suspected users of diuretics described above, one case–control study found the association only in non-hypertensive women (McLaughlin et al., 1988) and another in women irrespective of the presence of hypertension (Kreiger et al., 1993). A screening study, in which prescription information was linked with cancer incidence data, did not find a significant association between furosemide, spironolactone or thiazides and RCC (Selby et al., 1989). In contrast, a case–control study nested in a health plan cohort found a three-fold increase in risk for RCC among individuals who had filled prescriptions for diuretics. The association remained after adjustment for hypertension (Finkle et al., 1993). A similarly designed study found an odds ratio of 4 in female users of thiazide, but no dose–response effect was detected. No other diuretics were studied (Hiatt et al., 1994). Finally, a third study nested in a health plan found an association with several types of diuretic such as thiazides (odds ratio, 1.9), loop diuretics (odds ratio, 3.1) and potassium sparing (odds ratio, 2.1). Other antihypertensive agents and hypertension itself were so closely associated with diuretic use that it was difficult to separate the effect of one from the other (Weinmann et al., 1994). The fact that all types of diuretic collectively have been linked with risk for RCC weakens the plausibility of the association because diuretics have different modes of action.

The other extensively studied drugs are analgesics. It is known that phenacetin causes kidney failure and is involved in urothelial cancers, but the association with RCC is less well established. Several case–control studies have found moderately increased risks among users of phenacetin (McLaughlin et al., 1984; Maclure & MacMahon, 1985; McCredie et al., 1988; Kreiger et al., 1993), as well as non-phenacetin-containing analgesics (Asal et al., 1988a). Two cohort studies of hospital discharge records from patients with painful chronic diseases such as rheumatoid arthritis both found a weak association in women (Mellemgaard et al., 1992b; Lindblad et al., 1993). In these studies, there was no information on the type of drug or other risk factors. A cohort study found a six-fold increase in risk, but the observation was based on only nine cases, all male (Paganini-Hill et al., 1989). The international multicentre study found no effect of any of the commonly used analgesics on the risk of RCC (McCredie et al., 1995). A recent study of acetaminophen (paracetamol), a phenacetin metabolite, found a more than two-fold increase in risk for renal cancer among subjects who filled 40 or more prescriptions compared to no prescriptions (Derby & Jick, 1996).

In conclusion, there is some evidence that phenacetin increases the risk for RCC, while the evidence is insufficient with regard to other analgesics and diuretics.

Diet

An early correlation study of international consumption figures and cancer mortality data showed significant correlations between RCC and animal fat and protein (Wynder et al., 1974). Later case–control studies have provided some support for the suspected association with animal protein. A particularly strong association was seen in a study from Shanghai, where men with high meat consumption were at a four-fold increased risk for RCC. The effect among women was insignificant and weak (McLaughlin et al., 1992a). A case–control study of diet and RCC found some indication of an effect of a high intake of animal protein and fat, but the findings were not consistent over case groups (incident/prevalent) and generally this

study was hampered by a very low participation rate (Maclure & Willett, 1990). Other US studies have found no association with meat intake (McLaughlin et al., 1984; Yu et al., 1986; Kreiger et al., 1993). An Italian case–control study found a positive association with fat intake, especially oils and margarine (Talamini et al., 1990). The international multicentre study, which included a wide range of dietary questions, found an odds ratio of 1.7 for the highest quartile for total energy consumption. However, it was not possible to identify one energy source as more important than others (Wolk et al., 1996).

A protective effect has been suggested for vegetables (Maclure & Willett, 1990; Talamini et al., 1990; McLaughlin et al., 1992a; Wolk et al., 1996) and fruits (McLaughlin et al., 1992a; Wolk et al., 1996). For micronutrients, the international multicentre study found an increased risk of RCC associated with low intake of vitamin E and magnesium (Wolk et al., 1996). In one of the participating centres in this study (Denmark), a striking association was seen for dairy products, with increased risks particularly among women associated with a high intake of milk with a high fat content and thick butter spread (Mellemgaard et al., 1996). An association with milk had previously been observed (McCredie et al., 1988) but the majority of studies did not confirm this association (Kreiger et al., 1993; Wolk et al., 1996).

An association between intake or exposure to d-limonene and risk of RCC in man has not been studied. The primary dietary source of d-limonene, citrus fruits and juice, is not associated with an increase in risk (Chow et al., 1994; Wolk et al., 1996).

In spite of the wide international variation in incidence, there is thus little evidence that dietary factors play a role in RCC.

Reproductive factors

The clinical observation that oestrogens may interfere with the course of RCC and the existence of steroid receptors in RCC cells prompted a search for epidemiological evidence of an association. A role for reproductive factors in RCC has been suggested in several case–control studies. An increased risk was found in women taking oestrogens at menopause (Asal et al., 1988a) and another study found an increased risk among women who had experienced a fetal loss and also had three or more live births. In women who reported no fetal loss, there was no effect of number of live births (Kreiger *et al.*, 1993). The international multicentre study, which collected information on a number of reproductive variables, found an increased risk (odds ratio, 1.8) among women who reported six or more births compared with those reporting one birth. Furthermore, the data suggested a decrease in risk with increasing age at menarche and age at first birth. There was no association with age at menopause, but women who took oral contraceptives were at half the risk of those who did not (Lindblad *et al.*, 1995).

For reproductive factors, it thus appears that although there is a plausible mechanism, the evidence of an association with RCC is limited.

Coffee, tea and alcohol

The international consumption figures for coffee and renal cancer mortality have a correlation coefficient of 0.79 (Shennan, 1973), and the association has been evaluated in several case–control studies, without positive findings (Asal *et al.*, 1988a; McCredie *et al.*, 1988; Maclure & Willett, 1990; Talamini *et al.*, 1990; Kreiger *et al.*, 1993) with two exceptions. One case–control study found an association with decaffeinated coffee (Goodman *et al.*, 1986) and another found an increased risk among female coffee drinkers (Yu *et al.*, 1986). In neither study was a dose–response relationship observed. In the international multicentre study, no clear trend was seen, but women with the highest consumption (more than 41 cups per week) had a significantly increased risk of 2.1 (Wolk *et al.*, 1996).

There are very few data on tea use and risk of RCC. McLaughlin *et al.* (1984) found a three-fold increased risk among women who drank more than three cups a day. No effect was seen in men. In contrast, an inverse association was found in another case–control study (Yu *et al.*, 1986). The international multicentre study found no effect of tea drinking (Wolk *et al.*, 1996).

Most studies on alcohol–drinking have found no association with the risk for RCC (Wynder *et al.*, 1974; McLaughlin *et al.*, 1984; Yu *et al.*, 1986; Asal *et al.*, 1988a; Maclure & Willett, 1990; Kreiger *et al.*, 1993; Muscat *et al.*, 1995). However, the international multicentre study found a protective

effect of alcohol among women. The risk for women with a high intake of alcohol, especially wine, was reduced to half the risk of teetotallers (Wolk *et al.*, 1996).

In conclusion, these beverages are probably not risk factors for RCC, and the evidence that alcohol protects against RCC is inconclusive.

Occupation

Occupational risk factors for RCC have been studied more than any other type of risk factor. Several occupations or exposures are under suspicion.

Human exposure to gasoline is particularly interesting in the light of these agents' ability to induce α_{2u}-globulin nephropathy and renal tumours in male rats. A number of cohort studies of refinery workers, truck drivers and gas station attendants have found either no increase, or a very moderate increase in risk (Schottenfeld *et al.*, 1981; Hanis *et al.*, 1982; Thomas *et al.*, 1982; Wen *et al.*, 1983; McLaughlin *et al.*, 1987; Poole *et al.*, 1993; Lynge *et al.*, 1997). Cohort studies are usually not able to separate the effect of gasoline from that of other hydrocarbons and other substances which may affect risk of renal cell carcinoma such as asbestos or cigarette smoking. Case–control studies, which can adjust for the effects of other factors, have either given negative results or found moderate and statistically non-significant increases in risk, and a trend with duration of exposure is often absent (McLaughlin *et al.*, 1985; Asal *et al.*, 1988a; Siemiatycki *et al.*, 1988; Sharpe *et al.*, 1989; Partanen *et al.*, 1991; Mandel *et al.*, 1995) (Table 1).

An excess risk has been reported among workers exposed to asbestos, and asbestos fibres have been found in kidneys (Smith *et al.*, 1989). Cohort studies of workers in asbestos production, insulation and shipyards have shown increased risks (Selikoff *et al.*, 1979; Maclure, 1987). The international multicentre study found an increased risk among workers who reported being exposed to asbestos (Mandel *et al.*, 1995), but other studies that have examined the role of asbestos have found no association (McLaughlin *et al.*, 1984; Asal *et al.*, 1988a; Partanen *et al.*, 1991).

Employment in coke-ovens and exposure to aviation fuels and possibly other hydrocarbons were associated with RCC in some studies (Redmond *et al.*, 1972; McLaughlin *et al.*, 1984;

Table 1. Studies on the association between exposure to gasoline (vapour or engine exhausts) and renal cell carcinoma		
Case-control studies		
McLaughlin *et al.* (1985)	USA	OR=1.0
Asal *et al.* (1988a)	USA	OR=4.3 for men, 1.6 for women
Siemiatycki *et al.* (1988)	Canada	OR=1.2
Sharpe *et al.* (1989)	Canada	OR=1.1
Partanen *et al.* (1991)	Finland	OR=1.7
Mandel *et al.* (1995)	International	OR=1.6
Cohort studies		
Schottenfeld (1981)	USA	95701 petroleum industry employees: SIR =1.0 among refinery workers: SIR=0.9
Hanis *et al.* (1982)	USA	8666 refinery workers: SMR=1.6
Thomas *et al.* (1982)	USA	2509 refinery workers: SMR=1.4
Wen *et al.* (1983)	USA	16880 refinery workers: SMR =1.1
McLaughlin *et al.* (1987)	USA	7405 gas station attendants/refinery workers: SIR <1.0
Poole *et al.* (1993) (nested case-control)	USA	100 000 refinery workers: OR =1.0
Lynge *et al.* (1997)	Scandinavia	19000 gas station attendants: SIR=1.3

OR= Odds ratio, SIR= Standardized incidence rate, SMR= Standardized mortality rate

Siemiatycki *et al.*, 1987; Asal *et al.*, 1988a; Partanen *et al.*, 1991; Mandel *et al.*, 1995) while other studies found no association (McLaughlin *et al.*, 1987; McCredie & Stewart, 1993; Poole *et al.*, 1993).

Laundry and dry-cleaning workers have been found, in both cohort and case–control studies, to be at increased risk for RCC (Blair *et al.*, 1979; Asal *et al.*, 1988a; McCredie & Stewart, 1993). However, two recent large cohort studies have found no effect of employment in laundry and dry cleaning (Blair *et al.*, 1990; Lynge *et al.*, 1995).

Two heavy metals, cadmium and lead, have come under suspicion as risk factors for RCC. Such an association was first suggested in a small case–control study of RCC (Kolonel, 1976), but later studies have not offered much support for an association between exposure to cadmium and RCC (McLaughlin *et al.*, 1984; Asal *et al.*, 1988a; McCredie & Stewart, 1993). As cigarette smoking was one of the sources of cadmium examined in the original study, it is possible that the association was caused by confounding. Limited support is, however, offered by the international multicentre study, in which an association with self-reported exposure to cadmium was observed (Mandel *et al.*, 1995).

There are several studies of renal tumours in rodents induced by lead in the diet (van Esch & Kroes, 1969). Human data are sparse, and a large register-linkage study of a Danish supplementary pension scheme found no excess risk for RCC in metallic industries (Olsen & Jensen, 1987), while a cohort study of lead smelter workers found an excess mortality from kidney cancer (Steenland et al., 1992). Lead and cadmium content in renal tissue in RCC patients has been examined, but concentrations of both metals were low (Ala-Opas & Tahvonen, 1995).

With the large number of comparisons in screening studies for occupational risk factors in the work environment, it is not surprising that a number of associations have been suggested but not confirmed in subsequent studies. This is the case with newspaper pressmen, lumberjacks, physicians, architects, paperboard printing workers, firefighters, painters and textile workers (Paganini-Hill et al., 1980; McLaughlin et al., 1987; Sinks et al., 1992; Auperin et al., 1994; Delahunt et al., 1995; Henschler et al., 1995).

Miscellaneous

Patients with chronic lymphocytic leukaemia, who are known to have decreased immune function, have been found in one study to have a risk for RCC which is twice that of the background population (Mellemgaard et al., 1994c).

Based on the observation of endemic nephropathy in the Balkans, which may be caused by ochratoxin A or other fungal products, and which has been linked to urothelial cancer, there has been concern that ochratoxins may also be involved in the etiology of RCC. RCC has been induced in mice fed a diet containing ochratoxin A (Kanisawa & Suzuki, 1978). However, there are no human epidemiological data supporting this hypothesis, as occupational groups which may be exposed to fungi, such as bakers and handlers of flour and grain, are not at increased risk for RCC (Mellemgaard et al., 1994d).

Marginally increased risks for RCC have been described in individuals who have received radiation therapy for ankylosing spondylitis (Boice et al., 1988), and an increased incidence has been noted in individuals who were exposed to Thorotrast (an α, β and γ emitter) used for retrograde pyelography (Kauzlaric et al., 1987). However, recent case–control studies have found no association between radiation and risk for RCC (Mellemgaard et al., 1994d).

In summary, the evidence regarding asbestos and polycyclic aromatic hydrocarbons demonstrates a possible association with RCC, while the evidence regarding exposure to gasoline, lead, cad-

mium, radiation and dry-cleaning products is insufficient.

Genetic factors

Examination of RCC tumour tissue has often revealed a characteristic chromosomal defect consisting of deletions of distal chromosome 3p (Zbar et al., 1987). The region involved is in the same area as the defects seen in von Hippel–Lindau disease, in which a tumour–suppressor gene has been identified, and as many as one-third of all those affected may develop RCC (Glenn et al., 1991; Latif et al., 1993; Bailly et al., 1995). Studies of families with many cases of RCC have revealed a balanced translocation between chromosomes 3 and 8 (Wang & Perkins, 1984). However, the proportion of cases with a genetic background is probably small (Mellemgaard et al., 1994b).

Conclusion

Table 2 summarizes the epidemiological evidence concerning the etiology of RCC. It has been established beyond doubt that cigarette smoking causes RCC, and, furthermore, that obesity, in particular in women, is involved in the carcinogenic process, by a process that possibly involves peripheral formation of oestrogens which stimulate tumour cells. The suspected occupational risk factors are responsible for a minor proportion of the RCC cases in the developed countries, but the facts that low socioeconomic status is a risk factor and that the sum of etiological fractions is far from 1.0, particularly among men, suggest that other occupations or exposures which may confer an increased risk are yet to be identified. The effect of diet may be significant but, as for other cancer sites, it is very difficult to identify the responsible food items. A diet rich in protein and fat may lead to RCC, and dairy products may have a special role.

Generally speaking, there is a problem in making inferences from epidemiological data, which by definition are based on observations made in populations rather than individuals (Kaldor, 1992). The difficulties can be illustrated by the very complex nature of the association between reproductive factors and RCC, where the effect of the reproductive factors are intertwined with those of hypertension, obesity and use of oral contraceptives (Chow et al., 1995).

Table 2. Assessment of evidence concerning risk factors for renal cell carcinoma

Risk factor	Evidence of association[a]	Mechanism
Cigarette smoking	3	
Obesity	3	Peripheral oestrogen formation?
Alcohol	0	
Phenacetin	2	
Other analgesics	1	
Protein/fat	2	
Other dietary factors	0	
Diuretics	1	Shared risk factors?
Reproductive factors	2	Oestrogens act as promoters?
Socioeconomic status	1	Indicator of occupational factors? Diet?
Asbestos	2	Direct action on tubular epithelium?
Polycyclic aromatic hydrocarbons	2	
Dry cleaners	1	
Lead/cadmium	1	
Medical history (hypertension, thyroid disorders)	1	

[a] Evidence of association:

0, No evidence

1, Little evidence, i.e. positive and negative studies, too little evidence to draw conclusions

2, Positive association in several studies

3, Positive association in most studies, very likely to increase risk for RCC

Although previous studies have provided valuable information, the etiology of RCC remains incompletely understood and many suspected risk factors, including occupational, warrant further investigation. Information on the molecular epidemiology and on the mechanisms of the risk factors is sparse and much work is needed to provide a better understanding of the pathogenesis of RCC.

References

Adami, H.O., McLaughlin, J., Ekbom, A., Berne, C., Silverman, D., Hacker, D. & Persson, I. (1991) Cancer risk in patients with diabetes mellitus. *Cancer Causes Control*, 2, 307–314

Ala-Opas, M. & Tahvonen, R. (1995) Concentrations of cadmium and lead in renal cell cancer. *J. Trace Elements Med. Biol.*, 9, 176–180

Asal, N.R., Geyer, J.R., Risser, D.R., Lee, E.T., Kadamani, S. & Cherng, N. (1988a) Risk factors in renal cell carcinoma. II. Medical history, occupation, multivariate analysis, and conclusions. *Cancer Detect. Prev.*, 13, 263–279

Asal, N.R., Risser, D.R., Kadamani, S., Geyer, J.R., Lee, E.T. & Cherng, N. (1988b) Risk factors in renal cell carcinoma: I. Methodology, demographics, tobacco, beverage use, and obesity. *Cancer Detect. Prev.*, 11, 359–377

Auperin, A., Benhamou, S., Ory-Paoletti, C. & Flamant, R. (1994) Occupational risk factors for renal cell carcinoma: a case-control study. *Occup. Environ. Med.*, 51, 426–428

Bailly, M., Bain, C., Favrot, M.C. & Ozturk, M. (1995) Somatic mutations of von Hippel-Lindau (VHL) tumor-suppressor gene in European kidney cancers. *Int. J. Cancer*, 63, 660–664

Benhamou, S., Lenfant, M.H., Ory-Paoletti, C. & Flamant, R. (1993) Risk factors for renal-cell carcinoma in a French case-control study. *Int. J. Cancer*, 55, 32–36

Blair, A., Decoufle, P. & Grauman, D. (1979) Causes of death among laundry and dry cleaning workers. *Am. J. Publ. Health*, 69, 508–511

Blair, A., Stewart, P.A., Tolbert, P.E., Grauman, D., Moran, F.X., Vaught, J. & Rayner, J. (1990) Cancer and other causes of death among a cohort of dry cleaners. *Br. J. Ind. Med.*, 47, 162–168

Boice, J.D., Jr, Engholm, G., Kleinerman, R.A., Blettner, M., Stovall, M., Lisco, H., Moloney, W.C., Austin, D.F., Bosch, A., Cookfair, D.L., Krementz, E.T., Larourette, H.B., Merrill, J.A., Peters, L.J., Schulz, M.D., Storm, H.H., Björkholm, E., Petterson, F., Bell, C.M.J., Coleman, M.P., Fraser, P., Neal, F.E., Prior, P., Choi, N.W., Hislop, T.G., Koch, M., Kreiger, N., Robb, D., Robson, D., Thomson, D.H., Lochmüller, H., von Fournier, D., Frischkorn, R., Kjørstad, K.E., Rimpela, A., Pejovic, M.-H., Kirn, V.P., Stankusova, H.., Berrino, F., Sigurdsson, K., Hutchison, G.B. & MacMahon, B. (1988) Radiation dose and second cancer risk in patients treated for cancer of the cervix. *Radiat. Res.*, 116, 3–55

Case, R.A. (1964) Mortality from cancer of the kidney in England and Wales. In: Riches, E., ed., *Tumours of the Kidney and Ureter*, Edinburgh, Livingstone, pp. 9–27

Chow, W.H., Gridley, G., McLaughlin, J.K., Mandel, J.S., Wacholder, S., Blot, W.J., Niwa, S. & Fraumeni, J.F., Jr (1994) Protein intake and risk of renal cell cancer. *J. Natl Cancer Inst.*, **86**, 1131–1139

Chow, W.H., McLaughlin, J.K., Mandel, J.S., Blot, W.J., Niwa, S. & Fraumeni, J.F., Jr (1995) Reproductive factors and the risk of renal cell cancer among women. *Int. J. Cancer*, **60**, 321–324

Chow, W.H., McLaughlin, J.K., Mandel, J.S., Wacholder, S., Niwa, S. & Fraumeni, J.F., Jr (1996) Obesity and risk of renal cell cancer. *Cancer Epidemiol. Biomarkers Prev.*, **5**, 17–21

Delahunt, B., Bethwaite, P.B. & Nacey, J.N. (1995) Occupational risk for renal cell carcinoma. A case-control study based on the New Zealand Cancer Registry. *Br. J. Urol.*, **75**, 578–582

Derby, L.E. & Jick, H. (1996) Acetaminophen and renal and bladder cancer. *Epidemiology*, **7**, 358–362

van Esch, G.J. & Kroes, R. (1969) The induction of renal tumours by feeding basic lead acetate to mice and hamsters. *Br. J. Cancer*, **23**, 765–771

Finkle, W.D., McLaughlin, J.K., Rasgon, S.A., Yeoh, H.H. & Low, J.E. (1993) Increased risk of renal cell cancer among women using diuretics in the United States. *Cancer Causes Control*, **4**, 555–558

Fraser, G.E., Phillips, R.L. & Beeson, W.L. (1990) Hypertension, antihypertensive medication and risk of renal carcinoma in California Seventh-Day Adventists. *Int. J. Epidemiol.*, **19**, 832–838

Glenn, G.M., Daniel, L.N., Choyke, P., Linehan, W.M., Oldfield, E., Gorin, M.B., Hosoe, S., Latif, F., Weiss, G., Walther, M., Lerman, M.I. & Zbar, B. (1991) Von Hippel-Lindau (VHL) disease: distinct phenotypes suggest more than one mutant allele at the VHL locus. *Hum. Genet.*, **87**, 207–210

Goodman, M.T., Morgenstern, H. & Wynder, E.L. (1986) A case-control study of factors affecting the development of renal cell cancer. *Am. J. Epidemiol.*, **124**, 926–941

Grove, J.S., Nomura, A., Severson, R.K. & Stemmermann, G.N. (1991) The association of blood pressure with cancer incidence in a prospective study. *Am. J. Epidemiol.*, **134**, 942–947

Hanis, N.M., Holmes, T.M., Shallenberger, G. & Jones, K.E. (1982) Epidemiologic study of refinery and chemical plant workers. *J. Occup. Med.*, **24**, 203–212

Henschler, D., Vamvakas, S.. Lammert, M., Dekant, W., Kraus, B., Thomas, B. & Ulm, K. (1995) Increased incidence of renal cell tumors in a cohort of cardboard workers exposed to trichloroethene. *Arch. Toxicol.*, **69**, 291–299

Hiatt, R.A., Tolan, K. & Quesenberry, C.P., Jr (1994) Renal cell carcinoma and thiazide use: a historical, case-control study (California, USA). *Cancer Causes Control*, **5**, 319–325

Ishikawa, I., Saito, Y., Shikura, N., Kitada, H., Shinoda, A. & Suzuki, S. (1990) Ten-year prospective study on the development of renal cell carcinoma in dialysis patients. *Am. J. Kidney Dis.*, **16**, 452–458

Kaldor, J. (1992) The role of epidemiological observation in elucidating the mechanisms of carcinogenesis. In: Vainio, H., Magee, P.N., McGregor, D.B. & McMichael, A.J., eds, *Mechanisms of Carcinogenesis in Risk Identification* (IARC Scientific Publications No. 116), Lyon, IARC, pp. 601–608

Kanisawa, M. & Suzuki, S. (1978) Induction of renal and hepatic tumors in mice by ochratoxin A, a mycotoxin. *Gann*, **69**, 599–600

Katz, D.L., Zheng, T., Holford, T.R. & Flannery, J. (1994) Time trends in the incidence of renal carcinoma: analysis of Connecticut Tumor Registry data, 1935-1989. *Int. J. Cancer*, **58**, 57–63

Kauzlaric, D., Barmeir, E., Luscieti, P., Binek, J., Ramelli, F. & Petrovic, M. (1987) Renal carcinoma after retrograde pyelography with Thorotrast. *Am. J. Roentgenol.*, **148**, 897–898

Kolonel, C.L. (1976) Association of cadmium with renal cancer. *Cancer*, **37**, 1782–1787

König, G. (1826) Praktische Abhandlung über die Krankheiten der Nieren, durch Krankheitsfälle erläutert (Practical description of kidney diseases, using some examples of diseases), Leipzig, Knobloch, pp. 246–248

Kreiger, N., Marrett, L.D., Dodds, L., Hilditch, S. & Darlington, G.A. (1993) Risk factors for renal cell carcinoma: results of a population-based case-control study. *Cancer Causes Control*, **4**, 101–110

Latif, F., Tory, K., Gnarra, J., Yao, M., Duh, F.M., Orcutt, M.L., Stackhouse, T., Kuzmin, I., Modi, W., Geil, L., Schmidt, L., Zhou, F., Li, H., Wei, M.H., Chen, F., Glenn, G., Choyke, P., Walther, M.M., Weng, Y., Duan, D.-S.R., Dean, M., Glavac, D., Richards, F.M., Crossey, P.A., Ferguson-Smith, M.A., Le Paslier, D., Chumakov, I., Cohen, D., Chinault, A.C., Maher, E.R., Linehan, W.M., Zbar, B. & Lerman, M.I. (1993) Identification of the von Hippel-Lindau disease tumor suppressor gene. *Science*, **260**, 1317–1320

La Vecchia, C., Negri, E., D'Avanzo, B. & Franceschi, S. (1990) Smoking and renal cell carcinoma. *Cancer Res.*, **50**, 5231–5233

Lew, E.A. & Garfinkel, L. (1979) Variations in mortality by weight among 750,000 men and women. *J. Chron. Dis.*, **32**, 563–576Lindblad, P., McLaughlin, J.K., Mellemgaard, A. & Adami, H.O. (1993) Risk of kidney cancer among patients using analgesics and diuretics: a population-based cohort study. *Int. J. Cancer*, **55**, 5–9

Lindblad, P., Mellemgaard, A., Schlehofer, B., Adami, H.O., McCredie, M., McLaughlin, J.K. & Mandel, J.S. (1995) International renal-cell cancer study. V. Reproductive factors, gynecologic operations and exogenous hormones. *Int. J. Cancer*, **61**, 192–198

Lynge, E., Carstensen, B. & Andersen, O. (1995) Primary liver cancer and renal cell carcinoma in laundry and dry-cleaning workers in Denmark. *Scand. J. Work Environ. Health*, **21**, 293–295

Lynge, E., Andersen, A., Nilson, R., Barlow, L., Pukkala, E., Nordlinder, R., Boffetta, P., Grandjean, P., Heikkilä, P., Hörte, L.-G., Jakobsson, R., Lundberg, I., Moen, B., Partanen, T. & Riise, T. (1997) Risk of cancer and exposure to gasoline vapors. *Am. J. Epidemiol.*, **145**, 449–58

Maclure, M. (1987) Asbestos and renal adenocarcinoma: a case–control study. *Environ. Res.*, **42**, 353–361

Maclure, M. & MacMahon, B. (1985) Phenacetin and cancers of the urinary tract. *N. Engl. J. Med.*, **313**, 1479

Maclure, M. & Willett, W. (1990) A case–control study of diet and risk of renal adenocarcinoma. *Epidemiology*, **1**, 430–440

Mandel, J.S., McLaughlin, J.K., Schlehofer, B., Mellemgaard, A., Helmert, U., Lindblad, P., McCredie, M. & Adami, H.O. (1995) International renal-cell cancer study. IV. Occupation. *Int. J. Cancer*, **61**, 601–605

McCredie, M. & Stewart, J.H. (1993) Risk factors for kidney cancer in New South Wales. IV. Occupation. *Br. J. Ind. Med.*, **50**, 349-354

McCredie, M., Ford, J.M. & Stewart, J.H. (1988) Risk factors for cancer of the renal parenchyma. *Int. J. Cancer*, **42**, 13–16

McCredie, M., Pommer, W., McLaughlin, J.K., Stewart, J.H., Lindblad, P., Mandel, J.S., Mellemgaard, A., Schlehofer, B. & Niwa, S. (1995) International renal cell cancer study. II. Analgesics. *Int. J. Cancer*, **60**, 345–349

McLaughlin, J.K., Mandel, J.S., Blot, W.J., Schuman, L.M., Mehl, E.S. & Fraumeni, J.F., Jr (1984) Population based case–control study of renal cell carcinoma. *J. Natl Cancer Inst.*, **72**, 275–284

McLaughlin, J.K., Blot, W.J., Mehl, E.S., Stewart, P.A., Venable, F.S. & Fraumeni, J.F., Jr (1985) Petroleum-related employment and renal cell cancer. *J. Occup. Med.*, **27**, 672–674

McLaughlin, J.K., Malker, H.S., Stone, B.J., Weiner, J.A.,

Malker, B.K., Ericsson, J.L., Blot, W.J. & Fraumeni, J.F., Jr (1987) Occupational risks for renal cancer in Sweden. *Br. J. Ind. Med.*, **44**, 119–123

McLaughlin, J.K., Blot, W.J. & Fraumeni, J.F. Jr (1988) Diuretics and renal cell cancer. *J. Natl Cancer Inst.*, **80**, 378 [letter]

McLaughlin, J.K., Hrubec, Z., Heinemann, E.F., Blot, W.J. & Fraumeni, J.F., Jr (1990) Renal cancer and cigarette smoking in a 26-year followup of U.S. veterans. *Public Health Rep.*, **105**, 535–537

McLaughlin, J.K., Gao, Y.T., Gao, R.N., Zheng, W., Ji, B.T., Blot, W.J. & Frameni, J.F., Jr (1992a) Risk factors for renal cell cancer in Shanghai, China. *Int. J. Cancer*, **52**, 562–565

McLaughlin, J.K., Malker, H.S., Blot, W.J., Weiner, J.A., Stone, B.J., Ericsson, J.L. & Fraumeni, J.F., Jr (1992b) Renal cell cancer among architects and allied professionals in Sweden. *Am. J. Ind. Med.*, **21**, 873-876

McLaughlin, J.K., Lindblad, P., Mellemgaard, A., McCredie, M., Mandel, J.S., Schlehofer, B., Pommer, W. & Adami, H.O. (1995a) International renal cell cancer study. I. Tobacco use. *Int. J. Cancer*, **60**, 194–198

McLaughlin, J.K., Chow, W.H., Mandel, J.S., Mellemgaard, A., McCredie, M., Lindblad, P., Schlehofer, B., Pommer, W., Niwa, S. & Adami, H.O. (1995b) International renal cell cancer study. VIII. Role of diuretics, other anti-hypertensive medications and hypertension. *Int. J. Cancer*, **63**, 216–221

Mellemgaard, A., Møller, H., Olsen, J.H. & Jensen, O.M. (1991) Increased risk of renal cell carcinoma among obese women. *J. Natl Cancer Inst.*, **83**, 1581-1582

Mellemgaard, A., Møller, H. & Olsen, J.H. (1992a) Diuretics may increase risk of renal cell carcinoma. *Cancer Causes Control*, **3**, 309–312

Mellemgaard, A., Møller, H., Jensen, O.M., Halberg, P. & Olsen, J.H. (1992b) Risk of kidney cancer in analgesics users. *J. Clin. Epidemiol.*, **45**, 1021–1024

Mellemgaard, A., Carstensen, B., Norgaard, N., Knudsen, J.B. & Olsen, J.H. (1993) Trends in the incidence of cancer of the kidney, pelvis, ureter and bladder in Denmark 1943-88. *Scand. J. Urol. Nephrol.*, **27**, 327–232

Mellemgaard, A., Engholm, G., McLaughlin, J.K. & Olsen, J.H. (1994a) Risk factors for renal-cell carcinoma in Denmark. III. Role of weight, physical activity and reproductive factors. *Int. J. Cancer*, **56**, 66–71

Mellemgaard, A., Engholm, G., McLaughlin, J.K. & Olsen, J.H. (1994b) Risk factors for renal cell carcinoma in Denmark. I. Role of socioeconomic status, tobacco use, beverages, and family history. *Cancer Causes Control*, **5**, 105–113

Mellemgaard, A., Geisler, C.H. & Storm, H.H. (1994c)

Risk of kidney cancer and other second solid malignancies in patients with chronic lymphocytic leukemia. *Eur. J. Haematol.*, **53**, 218–222

Mellemgaard, A., Engholm, G., McLaughlin, J.K. & Olsen, J.H. (1994d) Occupational risk factors for renal-cell carcinoma in Denmark. *Scand. J. Work Environ Health*, **20**, 160–165

Mellemgaard, A., McLaughlin, J.K., Overvad, K. & Olsen, J.H. (1996) Dietary risk factors for renal cell carcinoma in Denmark. *Eur. J. Cancer*, **32**, 673–682

Muscat, J.E., Hoffmann, D. & Wynder, E.L. (1995) The epidemiology of renal cell carcinoma. A second look. *Cancer*, **75**, 2552-2557

Olsen, J.H. & Jensen, O.M. (1987) Occupation and risk of cancer in Denmark. An analysis of 93,810 cancer cases, 1970–79. *Scand. J. Work Environ. Health*, **13** (Suppl. 1), 1–91

Paganini-Hill, A., Glazer, E., Henderson, B.E. & Ross, R.K. (1980) Cause-specific mortality among newspaper web pressmen. *J. Occup. Med.*, **22**, 542–544

Paganini-Hill, A., Chao, A., Ross, R.K. & Henderson, B.E. (1989) Aspirin use and chronic diseases: a cohort study of the elderly. *Br. Med. J.*, **299**, 1247–1250

Parkin, D.M., Whelan, S.L., Ferlay, J., Raymond, L. & Young, J., eds (1997) *Cancer Incidence in Five Continents*, Vol. VII (IARC Scientific Publications No. 143), Lyon, IARC

Partanen, T., Heikkila, P., Hernberg, S., Kauppinen, T., Moneta, G. & Ojajarvi, A. (1991) Renal cell cancer and occupational exposure to chemical agents. *Scand. J. Work Environ. Health*, **17**, 231–239

Poole, C., Dreyer, N.A., Satterfield, M.H., Levin, L. & Rothman, K.J. (1993) Kidney cancer and hydrocarbon exposures among petroleum refinery workers. *Environ. Health Perspect.*, **101** (Suppl. 6), 53–62

Redmond, C.K., Ciocco, A., Lloyd, J.W. & Rush, H.W. (1972) Long term mortality study of steelworkers. VI. Mortality from malignant neoplasms among coke oven workers. *J. Occup. Med.*, **14**, 621–629

Schlehofer, B., Pommer, W., Mellemgaard, A., Stewart, J.H., McCredie, M., Niwa, S., Lindblad, P., Mandel, J.S., McLaughlin, J.K. & Wahrendorf, J. (1996) International renal-cell cancer study. VI. The role of medical and family history. *Int. J. Cancer*, **66**, 723-726

Schottenfeld, D., Warshaure, M.E., Zauber, A.G., Meikle, J.G. & Hart, B.R. (1981) A prospective study of morbidity and mortality in petroleum industry employees in the United States – a preliminary report. In: Peto, R. & Schneiderman, M., eds, *Quantification of Occupational Cancer* (Banbury Report 9) Cold Spring Harbor, NY, Cold Spring Harbor Laboratory, pp. 247–260

Selby, J.V., Friedman, G.D. & Fireman, B.H. (1989) Screening prescription drugs for possible carcinogenicity: eleven to fifteen years of follow-up. *Cancer Res.*, **49**, 5736–5747

Selikoff, I.J., Hammond, E.C. & Seidman, H. (1979) Mortality experience of insulation workers in the United States and Canada, 1943–76. *Ann. N.Y. Acad. Sci.*, **330**, 91–116

Sharpe, C.R., Rochon, J.E., Adam, J.M. & Suissa, S. (1989) Case-control study of hydrocarbon exposures in patients with renal cell carcinoma. *Can. Med. Assoc. J.*, **140**, 1309–1318

Shennan, D.H. (1973) Renal carcinoma and coffee consumption in 16 countries. *Br. J. Cancer*, **28**, 473–474

Siemiatycki, J., Dewar, R., Nadon, L., Gerin, M., Richardson, L. & Wacholder, S. (1987) Associations between several sites of cancer and twelve petroleum-derived liquids. Results from a case-referent study in Montreal. *Scand. J. Work Environ. Health*, **13**, 493–504

Siemiatycki, J., Gerin, M., Stewart, P., Nadon, L., Dewar, R. & Richardson, L. (1988) Associations between several sites of cancer and ten types of exhaust and combustion products. Results from a case-referent study in Montreal. *Scand. J. Work Environ. Health*, **14**, 79–90

Sinks, T., Lushniak, B., Haussler, B.J., Sniezek, J., Deng, J.F., Roper, P., Dill, P. & Coates, R. (1992) Renal cell cancer among paperboard printing workers. *Epidemiology*, **3**, 483–489

Smith, A.H., Shearn, V.I. & Wood, R. (1989) Asbestos and kidney cancer: the evidence supports a causal association. *Am. J. Ind. Med.*, **16**, 159–166

Steenland, K., Selevan, S. & Landrigan, P. (1992) The mortality of lead smelter workers: an update. *Am. J. Public Health*, **82**, 1641–1644

Talamini, R., Baron, A.E., Barra, S., Bidoli, E., La Vecchia, C., Negri E., Serraino, D. & Franceschi, S. (1990) A case-control study of risk factor for renal cell cancer in northern Italy. *Cancer Causes Control*, **1**, 125–131

Thomas, T.L., Waxweiler, R.J., Moure-Eraso, R., Itaya, S. & Fraumeni, J.F., Jr (1982) Mortality patterns among workers in three Texas oil refineries. *J. Occup. Med.*, **24**, 135–41

Wang, N. & Perkins, K.L. (1984) Involvement of band 3p14 in t(3;8) hereditary renal carcinoma. *Cancer Genet. Cytogenet.*, **11**, 479–481

Weinmann, S., Glass, A.G., Weiss, N.S., Psaty, B.M., Siscovick, D.S. & White, E. (1994) Use of diuretics and other antihypertensive medications in relation to the risk of renal cell cancer. *Am. J. Epidemiol.*, **140**, 792–804

Wen, C.P., Tsai, S.P., McClellan, W.A. & Gibson, R.L. (1983) Long-term mortality study of oil refinery workers. I. Mortality of hourly and salaried workers. *Am. J. Epidemiol.*, **118**, 526–542

Wolk, A., Gridley, G., Niwa, S., Lindblad, P., McCredie, M., Mellemgaard, A., Mandel, J.S., Wahrendorf, J., McLaughlin, J.K. & Adami, H.O. (1996) International renal cell cancer study. VII. Role of diet. *Int. J. Cancer*, **65**, 67–73

Wynder, E.L., Mabuchi, K. & Whitmore, W.F., Jr (1974) Epidemiology of adenocarcinoma of the kidney. *J. Natl Cancer Inst.*, **53**, 1619–1634

Yu, M.C., Mack, T.M., Hanisch, R., Cicioni, C. & Henderson, B.E. (1986) Cigarette smoking, obesity, diuretic use, and coffee consumption as risk factors for renal cell carcinoma. *J. Natl Cancer Inst.*, **77**, 351–356

Zbar, B., Brauch, H., Talmadge, C. & Linehan, M. (1987) Loss of alleles of loci on the short arm of chromosome 3 in renal cell carcinoma. *Nature*, **327**, 721–724

Corresponding author

A. Mellemgaard
Danish Cancer Society
Division of Cancer Epidemiology
Copenhagen
Denmark

Species Differences in Thyroid, Kidney and Urinary Bladder Carcinogenesis
C.C. Capen, E. Dybing, J.M. Rice and J.D. Wilbourn, eds
IARC Scientific Publications No. 147
International Agency for Research on Cancer, Lyon, 1999

Human renal carcinoma – pathogenesis and biology

J.B. Beckwith

Introduction

In order to relate any animal model to a given human cancer, the model should resemble its putative human counterpart. Renal carcinoma (RC) in the human is characterized by substantial cytohistological diversity, which has led to classification schemes based primarily on microscopic appearance. It is of fundamental importance to establish whether classification schemes that are in use identify biologically distinct entities. Since distinct entities are likely to result from different pathogenetic mechanisms, a classification scheme that reflects true biological diversity provides an indispensable foundation for interspecies comparisons.

The classification of human RC is at present in an uncomfortable but exciting state of transition. Earlier classification schemes were based solely upon cytological (usually cytoplasmic) characteristics, architectural pattern or putative level of origin within the renal tubule. Recent molecular and cytogenetic findings have provoked a re-examination of these criteria. Some morphological features which pathologists had emphasized for decades have been shown to have little or no fundamental significance. Criteria used to distinguish some RC categories may have been spurious. Lines of definition between entities have been drawn inappropriately, and the names applied to entities are often misleading. Distinct entities are being identified within categories hitherto viewed as homogeneous. Those who wish to relate patho-biology of animal models of RC to their human counterparts must be aware of the present transitional state of classification schemes for these tumours, and the central role now being played by cytogenetic and molecular criteria for classification.

Histological categories of RC

For decades, RC was perceived as a single entity with somewhat heterogeneous cytological appearances and growth patterns. Certain cytoplasmic appearances (e.g., clear, granular or basophilic) and architectural patterns (e.g., tubular, papillary, solid) were incorporated into popular classification schemes. However, these descriptive designations seemed to lack clinical or biological significance, and were merely assigned adjectival status in WHO and some other classification systems. With the exception of those rare specimens with predominantly spindle cell ('sarcomatoid') features, which were associated with poor prognosis, these cytohistological features seemed not to identify important clinical or biological characteristics. Nuclear features were more closely related to prognosis, and nuclear grading schemes based on nuclear enlargement and atypia were applied to all morphological variants of RC (Fuhrman *et al.*, 1982). Nuclear grade, though important prognostically, was not used to define biologically distinct neoplastic entities.

The existence of clinically and histologically distinct entities within the RC spectrum became generally accepted in the late 1970s, when renal *oncocytoma* was established as a low-grade or benign entity formerly subsumed under RC (Klein & Valensi, 1976). Oncocytomas were initially thought to be derived from proximal tubules, but subsequent studies suggested an origin from one of the intercalated cell types in collecting ducts of the cortex and outer medulla (Störkel *et al.*, 1988). During the same period, *papillary RC* was recognized as a distinct clinical and biological entity (Mancilla-Jimenez *et al.*, 1976). Though this concept was supported by most workers, the quantitative criteria for assigning the term varied, some authors using 50% papillary structures, while others required up to 100% in order to use this designation (Amin *et al.*,1997a). Recently, positive staining for cytokeratin 7 has been suggested as a phenotypic feature helpful in the diagnosis of papillary RC (Gatalica *et al.*, 1995). Some authors have suggested that all papillary RC are positive for cytokeratin 7 (Gatalica *et al.*, 1995; Amin *et al.*, 1997a), while others have noted that high-grade tumours within this spectrum are often negative for this marker (Delahunt & Eble, 1997). My own experience supports the latter conclusion.

A series of important morphological studies by Thoenes, Störkel, and colleagues (Thoenes *et al.*, 1986; Störkel & van den Berg, 1995) introduced new concepts and excellent analytical approaches to the subject that have proven to be directly related to distinctive cytogenetic anomalies. They added *chromophobe carcinoma* to the list of apparently distinct entities (Thoenes *et al.*, 1985), also derived from an intercalated cell in the outer collecting duct (Störkel *et al.*, 1989). Their studies reinforced the concept that tumours formerly designated as papillary RC might comprise a distinct clinical and biological category, but suggested that cytological features might be more definitive than architectural pattern. They introduced the term *chromophil RC* for tumours formerly termed papillary RC. This departure from emphasis on papillary architecture was justified. Other RC subtypes can have a papillary growth pattern, and some tumours that otherwise fit the papillary carcinoma profile have a predominantly tubular architecture. However, the term 'chromophil' also lacks precision. Oncocytomas and other renal epithelial neoplasms are characterized by strong affinity for histological stains, and some 'papillary' tumours have abundant clear cells. The designation *papillary RC* retains general popularity despite its imperfections.

Another addition to the list of morphological entities is *Bellini duct* (or *collecting duct*) *carcinoma* (Fleming & Lewi, 1986; Rumpelt *et al.*, 1991). The spectrum of Bellini duct carcinoma was more recently expanded by the recognition of a distinctive, highly malignant carcinoma of children and young adults, arising near the papillary end of the collecting duct in patients with the sickle cell trait, and designated as *medullary RC* (Davis *et al.*, 1995a; Eble, 1996). It was proposed that this is triggered by epithelial injury from vascular occlusion in the renal papillary region by sickled erythrocytes. This does not, however, account for the curious fact that medullary RC has to date been reported only in patients with sickle trait. It does not appear that this tumour has ever been reported in a patient known to have had homozygous sickle cell anaemia.

Cytogenetic and molecular correlations

Cytogenetic studies of RC have revolutionized the identification of neoplastic entities, and have confirmed that RC is indeed a collection of pathogenetically distinct neopasms. This has provided a new and potentially more valid basis for distinguishing different diseases that have common morphologic features, which is rapidly becoming incorporated into the definitional criteria for these neoplasms. Cytogenetic and molecular phenotyping is becoming an indispensable diagnostic tool, capable of resolving cytohistological dilemmas and controversies (Kovacs & Hoene, 1987; Störkel & van den Berg, 1995; Bugert & Kovacs, 1996; Motzer *et al.*, 1996; Steiner & Sidransky, 1996; van den Berg *et al.*, 1997a). These techniques show tremendous promise for defining RC subtypes and distinguishing degrees of malignancy within subtypes. However, molecular and cytogenetic studies are now facing the same problem that has bedevilled morphologists, which is the distinction of fundamental changes from those of secondary importance.

Table 1 presents a current cytohistological classification scheme for human RC, and indicates the major cytogenetic characteristics now associated with each entity. This table is necessarily tentative, and subject to revision as new data become available in this rapidly evolving field.

Conventional (or clear cell) renal carcinoma

This is by far the most common pattern of RC in humans, constituting approximately 75–85% of cases. The term 'clear cell' is potentially misleading, since only about 75% of tumours are composed exclusively or predominantly of cells with clear cytoplasm (Figure 1). Most of the remaining tumours are composed mainly, or exclusively, of cells with granular cytoplasm.

As many as 97% of sporadic conventional RC studied to date have shown deletions, mutations or hypermethylation inactivation involving at

Table 1. Renal carcinoma classification[a]

Category (alternative name)	Proposed origin	Cytogenetic features	
		Major	Minor
Conventional RC (clear cell)	Proximal tubule	3p–	5q+,+7,-Y,8p-,9p-,14q-
Papillary RC (chromophil)	Proximal tubule	+7,+17,-Y	3q+,+12,+16,+20
Xp 11.2 RC	? Proximal tubule		t(Xp11.2)
Oncocytoma	Collecting duct (intercalated cell)	Mitochondrial DNA t(11q13)	
Chromophobe RC	Collecting duct (intercalated cell)	–X,–Y,–1	–2,–6,–10,–13,–17,–21
Bellini duct carcinoma (collecting duct)	Collecting duct (principal cell)	?1q32.1–.2	8p–, 13q–
Medullary RC	Collecting duct (distal end)	Unknown	
Miscellaneous, unclassified			

[a] Modified from scheme presented by Motzer et al. (1996).
Cytogenetic data derived primarily from Dijkhuizen et al., 1995; Dijkhuizen, 1997; van der Berg et al., 1997a and Buger & Kovacs (1996). Sarcomatoid RC is not included as an entity, as it apparently represents progression phenomena occurring in most of the other RC subtypes on this table. The designation Xp11.2 RC is suggested here, to emphasize the unique features of this carcinoma, which other authors have included under the heading of papillary RC or conventional RC.

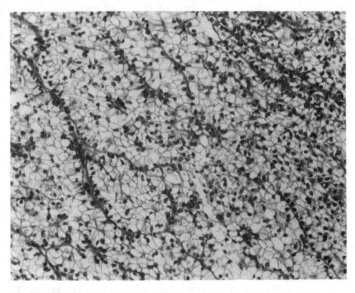

Figure 1. Clear cell renal carcinoma

least one allele of the von Hippel–Lindau (*VHL*) gene at chromosome 3p25 (Linehan *et al.*, 1995; Los *et al.*, 1996; Steiner & Sidransky, 1996). The *VHL* gene is thought to be a classic tumour-suppressor gene that controls gene transcription. The protein it encodes binds to elongins B and C, interfering with the function of RNA polymerase II (Duan *et al.*, 1995; Kibel *et al.*, 1995; Los *et al.*, 1996). Patients with von Hippel–Lindau disease show evidence of loss of the wild-type allele along with retention of the mutated allele not only in established conventional RC, but also in a variety of putative precursor lesions, including microscopic atypical cysts with early epithelial proliferative changes (Lubensky *et al.*, 1996). A recent study of sporadic conventional RC reported a single 3p deletion in renal cell adenomas, suggesting that a second deletion is involved in progression of adenoma to carcinoma (van den Berg *et al.*, 1997b). The potential relevance of this finding to at least one animal model is suggested by the recent report of *VHL* mutations in three conventional RC produced in rats by *N*-nitrosodimethylamine and protein-deprived diet (Shiao *et al.*, 1998).

Because only one allele of *VHL* is altered in some tumours, it is suggested that other genes can be involved in development of sporadic conventional RC, some of which act in coordination with the altered *VHL* allele. Other sites on 3p are involved in many of these tumours. One recently identified site is a breakpoint region centering on 3p14 (van den Berg *et al.*, 1997a). Partial trisomy of 5p is another relatively common finding, and may be involved in progression of adenoma to carcinoma. A variety of other nonrandom chromosomal increases and deletions have been reported in smaller numbers of cases, and probably reflect secondary events in conventional RC (van den Berg *et al.*, 1997a).

The *Rb* gene, often involved in a variety of human neoplasms, is rarely altered or absent in conventional RC (Lai *et al.*, 1997), and *p53* was found to be mutated in only 3/53 RC of unspecified subtypes (Imai *et al.*, 1994). The three cases with mutations were of high grade and stage, suggesting that when present, these mutations were associated with tumour progression. *MDM2* was not amplified in any case in that study. Escape from the growth-suppressing activity of TGFβ$_1$ was observed in 16/30 human RC cell lines, suggesting

that this mechanism may be an especially important progression factor (Ramp *et al.*, 1997). Many other growth factors have been implicated in the progression of conventional RC (Motzer *et al.*, 1996).

Papillary (chromophil) renal carcinoma
Papillary RC comprises approximately 10–15% of human RC, and is typically characterized microscopically by prominent papillary architecture with basophilic or acidophilic epithelial cells surfacing the papillations (Amin *et al.*, 1997a; Delahunt & Eble, 1997) (Figure 2). Clinically, this tumour has a propensity for multifocal and bilateral involvement, and is usually less aggressive than conventional RC. Debate as to whether papillary RC comprised a distinct neoplastic entity was silenced by the discovery that the chromosome 3p abnormalities characteristic for most conventional RC, as well as the commonly observed 5q duplications, were not present in papillary RC. Instead, the latter show consistent polysomies for certain chromosomes (Kovacs, 1989; Dijkhuizen *et al.*, 1996). Chromosomes 17 and 7 are the most important, being increased in number in 80–90% of reported tumours. Loss of the Y chromosome from tumour cells is observed in about 85% of papillary RC in males (Dijkhuizen *et al.*, 1996). Numerical gains of certain other chromosomes, especially 12, 16 and 20, and partial loss of 17p were associated with evidence of progression in papillary RC (Dijkhuizen *et al.*, 1996).

A recent report of trisomy 3 in five of eight papillary RC suggests that this trisomy may be associated with prominent haemosiderin deposits in the neoplastic epithelium, and with low-grade, early-stage tumours (Renshaw & Fletcher, 1997).

Xp11.2 renal carcinoma
This distinctive carcinoma is often characterized by papillary arrangements with prominent clear cell cytological features (Figure 3), showing a consistent chromosomal translocation involving Xp11.2, the most commonly reported one being t(X;1)p11.2;p34 (de Jong *et al.*, 1986; Tomlinson *et al.*, 1991; Meloni *et al.*, 1993; Dijkhuizen *et al.*, 1995; Tonk *et al.*, 1995). Most of the cases showing these features were males whose diagnosis was in early childhood. This tumour probably deserves a separate place in RC classification schemes because of its unique histological and cytogenetic features.

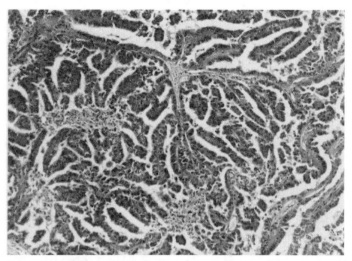

Figure 2. Papillary renal carcinoma

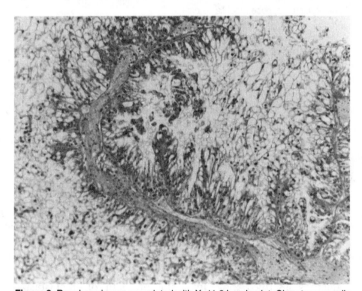

Figure 3. Renal carcinoma associated with Xp11.2 breakpoint. Clear tumour cells identical to those of clear cell renal carcinoma are arranged in prominent papillary formations.

Histologically it shares features of conventional RC and papillary RC, but cytogenetic and clinical distinctions justify its designation as a separate entity.

Chromophobe renal carcinoma
This recently delineated entity (Thoenes *et al.*, 1985) comprises about 4% of cases (Akhtar *et al.*, 1995; Crotty *et al.*, 1995). It is thought to arise from intercalated cells, which are found in collecting ducts within the cortex and outer medulla, and in the junctional region connecting distal convoluted tubules with collecting ducts (Störkel *et al.*, 1989; Kim *et al.*, 1994). Cytologically, chromophobe RC has abundant pale cytoplasm with a pale, finely reticulated cytoplasm, instead of the prominent vacuolated or granular cytoplasmic appearance of conventional RC (Figure 4). Colloidal

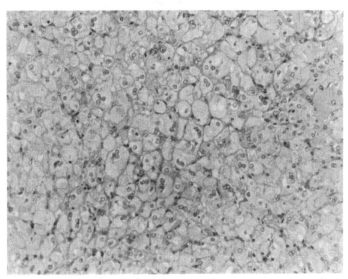

Figure 4. Chromophobe renal carcinoma

iron stains are strongly positive in this entity, in contrast to other recognized variants of RC.

This tumour is distinguished by hypodiploidy, with loss of multiple chromosomes. The most commonly observed deletions are of chromosomes 1, 2, 6, 10, 13, 17, 21 and Y (Bugert *et al.*, 1997). Alterations of mitochondrial DNA have also been described (Horton *et al.*, 1996).

Oncocytoma

Oncocytoma is a distinctive neoplasm with abundant eosinophilic, densely granular cytoplasm and an alveolar growth pattern. Histochemical and ultrastructural studies reveal abundant mitochondria (Amin *et al.*, 1997b). This tumour is thought to arise from an intercalated cell of the distal nephron and outer collecting duct, as described above for chromophobe RC (Störkel *et al.*, 1988). Two categories of intercalated cells are recognized; type A cells have fewer mitochondria than type B (Clapp *et al.*, 1987). Morphological similarities suggest that type A cells may be more closely related to chromophobe RC and type B cells to oncocytoma. Morphological overlap exists between chromophobe RC and oncocytoma, reflecting the closely related nature of the putative cells of origin. Oncocytomas are generally perceived as benign tumours, and it has been suggested that 'metastasizing oncocytomas'

represent other entities (Amin *et al.*, 1997b; Dijkhuizen, 1997). High-grade papillary RC, medullary and collecting duct RC, some chromophobe RC, and possibly other malignant renal epithelial tumours often possess abundant eosinophilic cytoplasm. Nuclear atypia in true oncocytomas do not denote a worse prognosis (Amin *et al.*, 1997b).

Cytogenetic studies indicate considerable heterogeneity among oncocytomas, but suggest the existence of two distinct categories (Neuhaus *et al.*, 1997). One variant is characterized by loss of chromosomes 1 and X/Y, a feature shared with chromophobe RC. It has been suggested that this subset of oncocytomas may in fact belong to the chromophobe category, which could contribute to the problem of 'metastasizing oncocytomas', (Neuhaus *et al.*, 1997). The other subset is characterized by translocations involving 11q13 (Neuhaus *et al.*, 1997). The 11q13 region includes a number of genes potentially involved in oncogenesis. Chromosomes 1 and 11 also contain genes encoding mitochondrial proteins, and oncocytomas contain numerous mitochondria with altered mitochondrial DNA (Welter *et al.*, 1989).

Bellini duct (collecting duct) carcinoma

Bellini duct carcinoma is an uncommon neoplasm, presumably arising from the principal cells of the inner medullary collecting duct (Fleming & Lewi, 1986; Rumpelt *et al.*, 1991). It is characterized by basophilic or acidophilic cells with variably atypical nuclei, and variably distinct tubular or tubulopapillary growth patterns. Papillary formations may be so prominent as to lead to diagnostic confusion with papillary RC at the light microscopic level. These tumours are often associated with nuclear atypia in adjacent non-neoplastic collecting ducts. Few data concerning cytogenetic features of Bellini duct carcinoma are available. One report suggests that loss of 1q32.1-32.2 may be a consistent finding in these tumours (Steiner *et al.*, 1996). Loss of 8p and 13q is also reported to be frequent in these tumours (Dijkhuizen, 1997).

Medullary renal carcinoma (Davis *et al.*, 1995a; Eble, 1996) is of extraordinarily malignant potential, and death within a few months of diagnosis is the rule. It is characterized by pleomorphic acidophilic cells growing as sheets, tubules, or cribiform nodules. It is highly invasive, and intensely desmoplastic. The strong association of this entity with sickle cell trait, and the known tendency for patients with sickle trait or sickle cell anaemia to suffer focal ischaemic damage to this region of the kidney suggests a possible pathogenetic relationship to distal collecting duct injury. To date, no cytogenetic results have been reported for this entity.

Precursor lesions as clues to pathogenesis

The studies outlined above suggest that most RC subtypes have a narrow range of cytogenetic anomalies common to most examples, with an increasingly large number of additional changes associated with tumour progression. It is assumed that high-grade RC of most, if not all, subtypes represents the end of a multistep process, as has been so clearly defined for adenocarcinoma of the colon in humans and certain other neoplastic models in animals.

If multiple discrete steps are involved in progression of most RC, then a search for morphological correlates of various stages in initiation, promotion and progression is reasonable. Small epithelial neoplasms are commonly encountered incidentally during autopsy examination of adult patients. In a careful study of 400 autopsies, in which both kidneys were completely sectioned at 1–2 mm intervals and all grossly visible lesions examined microscopically, a total of 251 tumours were found in 83 patients (Eble & Warfel, 1991; Eble, 1993). There was a linear increase with age in the proportion of patients with these small tumours, from 10% between ages 21–40 to 40% of patients aged 70–90 years. A striking male preponderance (70:13) was observed, but it was not possible to determine whether these lesions were related to potentially carcinogenic exposures. Papillary lesions predominated, and clear cell foci constituted fewer than 10% of these small, presumably early, tumours.

Debate concerning the malignant status of these small lesions has raged for many years, and has been well summarized by Eble (1993). The earlier view that renal tumours below a certain arbitrary size were adenomas, and those above this limit carcinomas has been supplanted by widespread acceptance of the concept that some epithelial nodules are benign adenomas, whereas other lesions of equally small size have already achieved malignant status. Arbitrary definitions based on tumour size are no longer considered valid.

Much of the debate on differentiating adenoma from carcinoma antedates the recognition of cytogenetically defined RC subtypes. In view of their presumably distinct biological nature, it is essential to consider these subtypes individually.

Conventional (or Clear cell) renal carcinoma

Experimental models of carcinogenesis are valuable for studying early cytological anomalies that precede overt proliferative activity in the pathogenesis of conventional RC. The demonstration of comparable sequences in humans, especially those that might be related to particular carcinogenic exposures, would represent a major advance. However, many difficulties lie in the way of achieving this goal, and little information is available concerning early stages in the development of conventional RC.

Mourad *et al.* (1994) evaluated renal tubular cytological changes in 110 kidneys resected for RC, including 66 cases of conventional RC. They observed intratubular epithelial dysplasia, characterized by cytological abnormalities, including nuclear enlargement, enlargement and eosinophilia of nucleoli, and cellular crowding in 21 cases of conventional RC (32%). Such dysplasia was felt to resemble changes reported in kidneys of male Syrian hamsters bearing RC induced by high doses of oestrogen. In one case, the abnormal cells had proliferated to obliterate the lumen of proximal tubules, and was felt to represent intratubular carcinoma *in situ*. Intratubular epithelial dysplasia was found mainly in sections near the tumour, and seemed to occur independently of other abnormalities in the kidney such as inflammation or nephrosclerosis.

Patients with von Hippel–Lindau disease, an autosomal dominant disorder due to mutations in the *VHL* gene, which are also found in a majority of conventional RC, provide a unique opportunity to study early stages in the development of conventional RC. Cystic changes are commonly observed in these patients, and cysts are often lined by clear cells resembling those of low-grade conventional RC (Bernstein *et al.*, 1987). These sometimes form intraluminal nodules of proliferating epithelial cells, suggestive of early neoplasia. A recent study of 26 cysts and microscopic clear cell proliferations in kidneys of two von Hippel–Lindau patients revealed loss of the wild-type and retention of the mutated allele in all but one of the lesions studied. These results suggested that *all* clear cell lesions in the kidneys of von Hippel–Lindau patients represent neoplasms, including cysts lined by a single layer of clear epithelial cells (Lubensky *et al.*, 1996).

Other polycystic renal disorders, including adult polycystic kidney disease and tuberous sclerosis, are associated with increased incidence of RC, including conventional RC, and frequently show epithelial hyperplasia of cyst linings (Bernstein *et al.*, 1987). These authors argued effectively that cystic change itself is an early manifestation of epithelial hyperplasia and may represent an early stage in development of conventional RC.

Papillary (chromophil) renal carcinoma

Putative precursor lesions more commonly encountered in kidneys with papillary RC than with any other category of RC (Kovacs & Kovacs, 1993). A resemblance to nephrogenic rests, the usual precursor of nephroblastoma (Beckwith *et al.*, 1990), was suggested by Kovacs. A potential relationship between papillary RC and nephroblastoma is also supported by our observation (unpublished) that papillary proliferative foci in some nephroblastomas stain positively for cyto-

keratin 7. Monomorphous papillary epithelial neoplasms in infant kidneys may appear identical to tumours deemed to be papillary RC in adults. However, the fact that the incidence of the small papillary lesions encountered incidentally at autopsy increases decade by decade through adult life (Eble & Warfel, 1991; Eble, 1993) suggests that most early papillary 'adenomas' are acquired rather than congenital lesions.

In the last few years, pathologists have become increasingly aware of an adenomatous lesion of the human kidney characterized by basophilic epithelium and variably prominent papillary formations. These lesions are designated 'metanephric adenoma'. It has been suggested that these may be related to nephrogenic rests or nephroblastoma, but some may also be related to papillary RC (Davis *et al.*, 1995b; Jones *et al.*, 1995).

Cytogenetic studies have revealed a relatively consistent pattern (–Y,+7,+17) in papillary adenomas, with additional karyotypic changes being associated with progression to malignancy (Kovacs *et al.*, 1991). Papillary RC would appear to be the subtype most amenable to investigation of early pathogenetic stages in RC.

End-stage kidneys maintained on long-term dialysis are particularly prone to development of papillary RC (Ishikawa & Kovacs, 1993; Hughson *et al.*, 1996). Basophilic epithelial proliferations termed 'embryonal hyperplasia' are frequent in such kidneys (Hughson *et al.*, 1978). The chemical determinants triggering and maintaining the hyperplastic and neoplastic changes in these kidneys have not yet been clearly defined, but may ultimately provide useful clues to chemical induction of papillary RC.

Bellini duct carcinoma and medullary renal carcinoma

Bellini duct carcinoma is often associated with dysplastic changes in cells of adjacent non-neoplastic collecting ducts (Kennedy *et al.*, 1990). This suggests that cytologically detectable precursor changes may be commonly present in this form of malignancy. The variant occurring in patients with sickle cell trait, designated medullary RC, has been suggested to be related pathogenetically to sequelae of microvascular injury caused by the underlying haematological disorder (Davis *et al.*, 1995a).

Oncocytomas and chromophobe renal carcinoma

Patients with tuberous sclerosis may develop onco-cytomas (Srinivas *et al.*, 1985). The cells of these tumours are identical to those lining cysts that sometimes occur in young infants with tuberous sclerosis (Bernstein *et al.*, 1986). It is possible that these cysts represent early stages in oncocytoma formation. We are aware of no description of comparable findings in chromophobe RC. A distinctive form of RC has been reported in patients with tuberous sclerosis, which were considered by the authors to have a clear or granular cell appearance comparable to conventional RC. Their distinguishing feature is consistent positivity for the melanocyte marker HMB-45, and frequently negative findings for cytokeratin (Bjornsson *et al.*, 1996). Though the cases were described as having clear cell RC, the published photomicrographs suggest a similarity to chromophobe RC. It remains to be determined whether these lesions are related, or represent a renal neoplasm unique to patients with tuberous sclerosis.

Transitional cell (urothelial) carcinomas

Urothelial carcinoma of the renal pelvis, like those of the ureter and urinary bladder, has long been associated with known or suspected carcinogenic exposures. Features supporting this association include a male preponderance, increasing incidence with age, and a tendency for multifocal origin with adjacent cellular dysplasia (Corrado *et al.*, 1991). Specific risk factors identified or suspected to date include tobacco and industrial exposures (McLaughlin *et al.*, 1983), phenacetin (Palvio *et al.*, 1987) and Thorotrast, a thorium-containing radiological contrast material (Christensen *et al.*, 1983).

Pathogenetic mechanisms

Pathogenetic mechanisms can be considered at two levels of resolution, cellular and molecular.

Cellular injury and tumour pathogenesis

Cellular injury, and hyperplastic reparative response, are early stages before overt tumorigenesis in animal models of RC pathogenesis. Mellemgaard (this volume) has summarized the epidemiological observations suggesting that environmental factors play a role in pathogenesis of human RC. If it could be shown that a putative human carcinogen was associated with tubular epithelial alterations progressing to neoplasia, powerful support for causal relevance would be established. However, early stages of nephron injury attributable to these putative environmental factors seem not to have been clearly defined to date. A significant difficulty in this type of analysis is that tubular damage in kidneys of ageing adults is extremely common.

The high metabolic rate of most nephron cells predisposes them to injury from many causes. Renal tubular damage and cellular necrosis are common sequelae of anoxia, hypovolaemic shock and a wide variety of metabolic or toxic derangements in patients of all ages. Features specific to individual cell types in the nephron (e.g., protective surface layers, receptors for a given toxic agent, high concentration of organelles that concentrate, detoxify or chemically alter a specific agent) can also determine specific patterns of injury within nephrons.

Renal physiology creates an intriguing scenario for agent-specific patterns of toxic injury to different levels of the nephron, varying with the pattern of excretion, secretion, and reabsorption of the agent in question. The key role of the kidney in excretion of toxins from the circulation exposes renal cells to high concentrations of a wide variety of toxic substances. Some substances are delivered via glomerular filtration, while others are secreted into the lumen, or reabsorbed, at specific levels of the nephron. The concentration of a given toxin will usually change dramatically as it progresses down the nephron. A substance present in the glomerular filtrate that is not reabsorbed by the nephron will be concentrated approximately 100-fold by the time it reaches the distal end of the collecting duct, due to the normal process of urinary concentration. A toxic substance that is filtered by the glomerulus but completely resorbed in the proximal tubule, on the other hand, would be capable of producing direct cellular injury only in the most proximal portion of the nephron. These and other potential scenarios illustrate how different substances might injure specific levels of the nephron. A complete list of therapeutic, environmental and nutritional factors that are known to injure renal tubule cells at some concentration would probably be longer than the list of substances known *not* to injure them. However, the list of agents or factors known or suspected to be involved in RC pathogenesis is relatively short (see Mellemgaard, this volume).

The critical issue would be to identify the cytological and molecular features of tubular cell injury preceding formation of the various types of RC, and to determine if these features are associated with specific exposures to suspected carcinogenic factors. To date, there seems to be virtually no information of this type for humans. One of the most widely available models for study is the end-stage kidney with long-term dialysis support, discussed above. A variety of early hyperplastic changes are seen in these kidneys before the development of overt neoplasia. Most of the tumours appear to be related to papillary RC.

There is a disappointing paucity, if not complete lack, of information concerning renal changes attributable to hydrocarbon exposure, tobacco usage, or other situations suspected or known to be associated with increased RC incidence in humans. A major obstacle in the way of such analyses is the frequency of renal tubular injury from a variety of causes, making it difficult to establish a relationship of tubular damage to any one factor.

Molecular mechanisms

Various molecular mechanisms of RC pathogenesis have been proposed. The best characterized single gene defect associated with RC to date is the *VHL* mutations associated with most cases of clear cell RC, as discussed above. The protein encoded by this gene inhibits the elongation of transcription, by binding to elongins B and C. Lack of this protein facilitates uncontrolled proliferation. Thus, the *VHL* gene is a classic tumour-suppressor gene (Linehan *et al.*, 1995; Los *et al.*, 1996; Lubensky *et al.*, 1996).

A long list of cell cycle regulators and growth factors has been implicated in RC pathogenesis or progression (Motzer *et al.*, 1996). In addition, IL6 and other cytokines have been suggested to play a role, though their importance remains uncertain (Kozlowski, 1997). It is probable that identification of specific genes in addition to *VHL* that are involved in the pathogenesis of various types of RC will rapidly lead to a precise understanding of molecular mechanisms underlying development of these tumours.

Conclusion

Traditional cytohistological criteria for classification of RC are rapidly being supplemented, and in many instances replaced, by definitions based on cytogenetic and molecular features. The distinctive cytogenetic patterns revealed to date show clearly that RC is not a homogeneous entity, and that different mechanisms probably apply to each distinct tumour category. Epidemiological studies of human renal neoplasms and experimental animal models must be related to specific RC phenotypes.

As histological and cytogenetically based tumour definitions become supplanted by specific molecular definitions, it will be possible to address more precisely the fundamental question as to whether the various subtypes of human RC are biologically related to seemingly similar tumours of other species. At the present time this can be addressed only for conventional RC, by inquiring whether similar tumours in experimental models are related to alterations in a gene or gene product comparable to those in the *VHL*-associated tumours in humans.

Acknowledgements

This review is drawn almost entirely from the work of others. The author acknowledges in particular the inspiration he has drawn from the work of Professor Stefan Störkel, Professor Gyula Kovacs, and their colleagues. Dr Eva van den Berg kindly provided a copy of the thesis of Dr T. Dijkhuizen, which contains reprints and preprints of many of the fundamental contributions of the Department of Medical Genetics at the University of Groningen.

References

Akhtar, M., Kardar, H., Linjawi, T., McClintock, J. & Ali, M.A. (1995) Chromophobe cell carcinoma of the kidney: A clinicopathological study of 21 cases. *Am. J. Surg. Pathol.*, 19, 1245–1256

Amin, M.B., Corless, C.L., Renshaw, A.A., Tickoo, C.L., Kubus, J. & Schultz, D.S. (1997a) Papillary (chromophil) renal cell carcinoma: histomorphologic characteristics and evaluation of conventional pathologic prognostic parameters in 62 cases. *Am. J. Surg. Pathol.*, 21, 621–635

Amin, M.B., Crotty, T.B., Tickoo, S.K. & Farrow, G.M. (1997b) Renal oncocytoma: a reappraisal of morphologic features with clinicopathologic findings in 80 cases. *Am. J. Surg. Pathol.*, **21**, 1–12

Beckwith, J.B., Kiviat, N.B. & Bonadio, J.F. (1990) Nephrogenic rests, nephroblastomatosis, and the pathogenesis of Wilms' tumor. *Pediatr. Pathol.*, **10**, 1-36

van den Berg, E., Dijkhuizen, T., Oosterhuis, J.W., Geurts van Kessel, A., de Jong, B. & Störkel, S. (1997a) Cytogenetic classification of renal cell cancer. *Cancer Genet. Cytogenet.*, **95**, 103–107

van den Berg, A., Dijkhuizen, T., Draaijers, T.G., Hulsbeek, M.M.F., Maher, E.R., van den Berg, E., Störkel, S. & Buys, C.H.C. (1997b) Analysis of multiple renal cell adenomas and carcinomas suggests allelic loss at 3p21 to be a prerequisite for malignant development. *Genes Chrom. Cancer*, **19**, 228-232

Bernstein, J., Robbins, T.O. & Kissane, J.M. (1986) The renal lesions of tuberous sclerosis. *Semin. Diagn. Pathol.*, **3**, 97–105

Bernstein, J., Evan, A.P. & Gardner, K.D., Jr (1987) Epithelial hyperplasia in human polycystic kidney diseases. Its role in pathogenesis and risk of neoplasia. *Am. J. Pathol.*, **129**, 92–101

Bjornsson, J., Short, M.P., Kwiatkowski, D.J. & Henske, E.P. (1996) Tuberous sclerosis-associated renal cell carcinoma. Clinical, pathological, and genetic features. *Am. J. Pathol.*, **149**, 1201–1208

Bugert, P. & Kovacs, G. (1996) Molecular differential diagnosis of renal cell carcinomas by microsatellite analysis. *Am. J. Pathol.*, **149**, 2081–2088

Bugert, P., Gaul, C., Weber, K., Herbers, J., Akhtar, M., Ljungberg, B. & Kovacs, G. (1997) Specific genetic changes of diagnostic importance in chromophobe renal cell carcinomas. *Lab. Invest.*, **76**, 203–208

Christensen, P., Madsen, M.R. & Jensen, O.M. (1983) Latency of thorotrast-induced renal tumours. *Scand. J. Urol. Nephrol.*, **17**, 127–130

Clapp, W.L., Madsen, K.M., Verlander, J.W. & Tisher, C.C. (1987) Intercalated cells of the rat inner medullary collecting duct. *Kidney Int.*, **31**, 1080–1087

Corrado, F., Ferri, C., Mannini, D., Corrado, G., Bertoni, F., Bacchini, P., Lelli, G., Lieber, M.M. & Song, J.M. (1991) Transitional cell carcinoma of the upper urinary tract: evaluation of prognostic factors by histopathology and flow cytometric analysis. *J. Urol.*, **145**, 1159–1163

Crotty, T.B., Farrow, G.M. & Lieber, M.M. (1995) Chromophobe renal cell carcinoma: clinicopathological features of 50 cases. *J. Urol.*, **154**, 964–967

Davis, C.J., Jr, Mostofi, F.K. & Sesterhenn, I.A. (1995a) Renal medullary carcinoma. The seventh sickle cell nephropathy. *Am. J. Surg. Pathol.*, **19**, 1–11

Davis, C.J., Jr, Barton, J.H., Sesterhenn, I.A. & Mostofi, F.K. (1995b) Metanephric adenoma. Clinicopathological study of fifty patients. *Am. J. Surg. Pathol.*, **19**, 1101–1104

Delahunt, B. & Eble, J.N. (1997) Papillary renal cell carcinoma: a clinicopathologic and immunohistochemical study of 105 tumors. *Mod. Pathol.*, **10**, 537–544

Dijkhuizen, T. (1997) *Genetic Contributions to the Classification of Renal Cell Cancer*. Ph.D. Thesis, Rijksuniversiteit Groningen

Dijkhuizen, T., van den Berg, E., Wilbrink, M., Weterman, M., Geurts van Kessel, A., Störkel, S., Folkers, R.P., Braam, A. & de Jong, B. (1995) Distinct Xp11.2 breakpoints in two renal cell carcinomas exhibiting X;autosome translocations. *Genes Chrom. Cancer*, **14**, 43–50

Dijkhuizen, T., van den Berg, E., van den Berg, A., Störkel, S., De Jong, B., Seitz, G. & Henn, W. (1996) Chromosomal findings and p53-mutation analysis in chromophilic renal-cell carcinomas. *Int. J. Cancer*, **68**, 47–50

Duan, D.R., Pause, A., Burgess, W.H., Aso, T., Chen, D.Y., Garrett, K.P., Conaway, R.C., Conaway, J.W., Linehan, W.M. & Klausner, R.D. (1995) Inhibition of transcription elongation by the VHL tumor suppressor protein. *Science*, **269**, 1402–1406

Eble, J.N. (1993) Kidney. In: Henson, D.E. & Albores-Saavedra, J., eds, *Pathology of Incipient Neoplasia*, 2nd edition, Philadelphia, W.B. Saunders, pp. 401–419

Eble, J.N. (1996) Renal medullary carcinoma: a distinct entity emerges from the confusion of 'collecting duct carcinoma'. *Adv. Anat. Pathol.*, **3**, 233–238

Eble, J.N. & Warfel, K. (1991) Early human renal cortical epithelial neoplasia. *Mod. Pathol.*, **4**, 45A (Abstract No. 262)

Fleming, S. & Lewi, H.J. (1986) Collecting duct carcinoma of the kidney. *Histopathology*, **10**, 1131–1141

Fuhrman, S.A., Lasky, L.C. & Limas, C. (1982) Prognostic significance of morphologic parameters in renal cell carcinoma. *Am. J. Surg. Pathol.*, **6**, 655–663

Gatalica, Z., Kovatich, A. & Miettinen, M. (1995) Consistent expression of cytokeratin 7 in papillary renal cell carcinomas: an immunohistochemical study in formalin-fixed paraffin-embedded tissues. *J. Urol. Pathol.*, **3**, 205–211

Horton, T.M., Petros, J.A., Heddi, A., Shoffner, J., Kaufman, A.E., Graham, S.D., Jr, Gramlich, T. & Wallace, D.C. (1996) Novel mitochondrial DNA deletion found in a renal cell carcinoma. *Genes Chrom. Cancer*, **15**, 95–101

Hughson, M.D., McManus, J.F. & Hennigar, G.R. (1978) Studies on 'end stage' kidneys. II. Embryonal hyperplasia of Bowman's capsular epithelium. *Am. J. Pathol.*, **91**, 71–84

Hughson, M.D., Meloni, A.M., Silva, F.G. & Sandberg, A.A. (1996) Renal cell carcinoma in an end-stage kidney of a patient with a functional transplant: cytogenetic and molecular genetic findings. *Cancer Genet. Cytogenet.*, **89**, 65–68

Imai, Y., Strohmeyer, T.G., Fleischhacker, M., Slamon, D.J. & Koeffler, H.P. (1994) p53 mutations and MDM-2 amplification in renal cell cancers. *Mod. Pathol.*, **7**, 766–770

Ishikawa, I. & Kovacs, G. (1993) High incidence of papillary renal cell tumours in patients on chronic haemodialysis. *Histopathology*, **22**, 135–139

Jones, E.C., Pins, M., Dickersin, G.R. & Young R.H. (1995) Metanephric adenoma of the kidney. A clinicopathological, immunohistochemical, flow cytometric, cytogenetic, and electron microscopic study of seven cases. *Am. J. Surg. Pathol.*, **19**, 615–626

de Jong, B., Molenaar, I.M., Leeuw, J.A., Idenburg, V.J.S. & Oosterhuis, J.W. (1986) Cytogenetics of a renal adenocarcinoma in a 2-year-old child. *Cancer Genet. Cytogenet.*, **21**, 165–169

Kennedy, S.M., Merino, M.J., Linehan, W.M., Roberts, J.R., Robertson, C.N. & Neumann, R.D. (1990) Collecting duct carcinoma of the kidney. *Hum. Pathol.*, **21**, 449–456

Kibel, A., Iliopoulos, O., DeCaprio, J.A. & Kaelin, W.G., Jr (1995) Binding of the von Hippel-Lindau tumor suppressor protein to Elongin B and C. *Science*, **269**, 1444–1446

Kim, J., Tisher, C.C. & Madsen, K.M. (1994) Differentiation of intercalated cells in developing rat kidney: an immunohistochemical study. *Am. J. Physiol.*, **266**, F977–F990

Klein, M.J. & Valensi, Q.J. (1976) Proximal tubular adenomas of kidney with so-called oncocytic features. A clinicopathologic study of 13 cases of a rarely reported neoplasm. *Cancer*, **38**, 906–914

Kovacs, G. (1989) Papillary renal cell carcinoma. A morphologic and cytogenetic study of 11 cases. *Am. J. Pathol.*, **134**, 27–34

Kovacs, G. & Hoene, E. (1987) Multifocal renal cell carcinoma: a cytogenetic study. *Virchows Arch. A. Pathol. Anat. Histopathol.*, **412**, 79–82

Kovacs, G. & Kovacs, A. (1993) Parenchymal abnormalities associated with papillary renal cell tumors: a morphologic study. *J. Urol. Pathol.*, **1**, 301–312

Kovacs, G., Füzesi, L., Emanual, A. & Kung, H.F. (1991) Cytogenetics of papillary renal cell tumors. *Genes Chrom. Cancer*, **3**, 249–255

Kozlowski, J.M. (1997) Renal cell carcinoma. Tumor markers. In: Raghavan, D., Scher, H.I., Leibel, S.A. & Lange, P., eds, *Principles and Practice of Genitourinary Oncology*, Philadelphia, Lippincott-Raven, pp. 813–822

Lai, S., Benedict, W.F., Silver, S.A. & El-Naggar, A.K. (1997) Loss of retinoblastoma gene function and heterozygosity at the RB locus in renal cortical neoplasms. *Hum. Pathol.*, **28**, 693–697

Linehan, W.M., Lerman, M.I. & Zbar, B. (1995) Identification of the von Hippel-Lindau (VHL) gene. Its role in renal cancer. *J. Am. Med. Assoc.*, **273**, 564–570

Los, M., Jansen, G.H., Kaelin, W.G., Lips, C.J., Blijham, G.H. & Voest, E.E. (1996) Expression pattern of the von Hippel-Lindau protein in human tissues. *Lab. Invest.*, **75**, 231–238

Lubensky, I.A., Gnarra, J.R., Bertheau, P., Walther, M.M., Linehan, W.M. & Zhuang, Z. (1996) Allelic deletions of the VHL gene detected in multiple microscopic clear cell renal lesions in von Hippel-Lindau disease patients. *Am. J. Pathol.*, **149**, 2089–2094

Mancilla-Jimenez, R., Stanley, R.J. & Blath, R.A. (1976) Papillary renal cell carcinoma. A clinical, radiologic, and pathologic study of 34 cases. *Cancer*, **38**, 2469–2480

McLaughlin, J.K., Blot, W.J., Mandel, J.S., Schuman, L.M., Mehl, E.S. & Fraumeni, J.F., Jr (1983) Etiology of cancer of the renal pelvis. *J. Natl Cancer Inst.*, **71**, 287–291

Meloni, A.M., Dobbs, R.M., Pontes, J.E. & Sandberg, A.A. (1993) Translocation (X;1) in papillary renal cell carcinoma. A new cytogenetic subtype. *Cancer Genet. Cytogenet.*, **65**, 1–6

Motzer, R.J., Bander, N.H. & Nanus, D.M. (1996) Renal-cell carcinoma. *New Engl. J. Med.*, **335**, 865–875

Mourad, W.A., Nestok, B.R., Saleh, G.Y., Solez, K., Power, R.F. & Jewell, L.D. (1994) Dysplastic tubular epithelium in 'normal' kidney associated with renal cell carcinoma. *Am. J. Surg. Pathol.*, **18**, 1117–1124

Neuhaus, C., Dijkhuizen, T., van den Berg, E., Störkel, S., Stöckle, M., Mensch, B., Huber, C. & Decker, H.J. (1997) Involvement of the chromosomal region 11q13 in renal oncocytoma: a case report and literature review. *Cancer Genet. Cytogenet.*, **94**, 95–98

Palvio, D.H., Andersen, J.C. & Falk, E. (1987) Transitional cell tumors of the renal pelvis and ureter associated with capillarosclerosis indicating analgesic abuse. *Cancer*, **59**, 972–976

Ramp, U., Jaquet, K., Reinecke, P., Nitsch, T., Gabbert, H.E. & Gerharz, C.-D. (1997) Acquisition of TGFβ$_1$ resistance: an important progression factor in human renal cell carcinoma. *Lab. Invest.*, **76**, 739–749

Renshaw, A.A. & Fletcher, J.A. (1997) Trisomy 3 in renal cell carcinoma. *Mod. Pathol.*, **10**, 481–484

Rumpelt, H.J., Störkel, S., Moll, R., Schärfe, T. & Thoenes, W. (1991) Bellini duct carcinoma: further evidence for this rare variant of renal cell carcinoma. *Histopathology*, **18**, 115–122

Shiao, Y.-H., Rice, J.M., Anderson, L.M., Ward, J.M., Diwan, B.A. & Hard, G.C. (1998) von-Hippel-Lindau gene mutations in *N*-nitrosodimethylamine-induced rat renal epithelial tumors. *J. Natl Cancer Inst.*, **90**, 1720–1723

Srinivas, V., Herr, H.W. & Hajdu, E.O. (1985) Partial nephrectomy for a renal oncocytoma associated with tuberous sclerosis. *J. Urol.*, **133**, 263–265

Steiner, G. & Sidransky, D. (1996) Molecular differential diagnosis of renal carcinoma: from microscopes to microsatellites. *Am. J. Pathol.*, **149**, 1791–1795

Steiner, G., Cairns, P., Polascik, T.J., Marshall, F.F., Epstein, J.I., Sidransky, D. & Schoenberg, M. (1996) High-density mapping of chromosomal arm 1q in renal collecting duct carcinoma: region of minimal deletion at 1q32.1-32.2. *Cancer Res.*, **56**, 5044–5046

Störkel, S. & van den Berg, E. (1995) Morphological classification of renal cancer. *World J. Urol.*, **13**, 153–158

Störkel, S., Pannen, B., Thoenes, W., Steart, P.V., Wagner, S. & Drenckhahn, D. (1988) Intercalated cells as a probable source for the development of renal oncocytoma. *Virchows Arch. B. Cell Pathol.*, **56**, 185–189

Störkel, S., Steart, P.V., Drenckhahn, D. & Thoenes, W. (1989) The human chromophobe cell renal carcinoma: its probable relation to intercalated cells of the collecting duct. *Virchows Arch. B. Cell Pathol.*, **56**, 237–245

Thoenes, W., Störkel, S. & Rumpelt, H.J. (1985) Human chromophobe cell renal carcinoma. *Virchows Archiv. B. Cell Pathol.*, **48**, 207–217

Thoenes, W., Störkel, S. & Rumpelt, H.J. (1986) Histopathology and classification of renal cell tumors (adenomas, oncocytomas, and carcinomas). The basic cytological and histopathological elements and their use for diagnostics. *Pathol. Res. Pract.*, **181**, 125–143

Tomlinson, G.E., Nisen, P.D., Timmons, C.F. & Schneider, N.R. (1991) Cytogenetics of a renal cell carcinoma in a 17-month-old child. Evidence for Xp11.2 as a recurring breakpoint. *Cancer Genet. Cytogenet.*, **57**, 11–17

Tonk, V., Wilson, K.S., Timmons, C.F., Schneider, N.R. & Tomlinson, G.E. (1995) Renal cell carcinoma with translocation (X;1). Further evidence for a cytogenetically defined subtype. *Cancer Genet. Cytogenet.*, **81**, 72–75

Welter, C., Kovacs, G., Seitz, G. & Blin, N. (1989): Alteration of mitochondrial DNA in human oncocytomas. *Genes Chrom. Cancer*, **1**, 79–82

Corresponding author

J.B. Beckwith
Department of Pathology and Human Anatomy,
Loma Linda University,
Loma Linda, California, USA

Species Differences in Thyroid, Kidney and Urinary Bladder Carcinogenesis
C.C. Capen, E. Dybing, J.M. Rice and J.D. Wilbourn, eds
IARC Scientific Publications No. 147
International Agency for Research on Cancer, Lyon, 1999

α_2-Urinary globulin-associated nephropathy as a mechanism of renal tubule cell carcinogenesis in male rats

J.A. Swenberg and L.D. Lehman-McKeeman

Introduction

α_2-Urinary globulin (α_{2u}-globulin) nephropathy is a renal syndrome that occurs exclusively in male rats. To date, a diverse group of chemicals has been shown to cause acute renal changes manifested by accumulation of protein in phagolysosomes of renal proximal tubule cells. The acute toxicity appears to be caused by the accumulation of a single protein, α_{2u}-globulin, that is specific to the male rat. The protein overload causes renal cell injury, compensatory cell proliferation and ultimately a low but significant incidence of renal tubule tumours.

The contribution of α_{2u}-globulin to the species-specificity of the nephropathy has been proven in several ways. It has been determined that rats that do not synthesize α_{2u}-globulin do not develop renal toxicity or tumours. Furthermore, although mice are resistant to this toxicity, transgenic mice engineered to synthesize α_{2u}-globulin do develop the nephropathy. Mechanistic studies have demonstrated that the rate-limiting step in development of the syndrome is the reversible, but specific, binding of a chemical (or its metabolites) to α_{2u}-globulin. A comprehensive survey of structurally-related proteins along with experimental analyses has provided evidence that, although other species including humans synthesize proteins that are similar to α_{2u}-globulin, differences in ligand-binding properties, physiological function and renal handling of these homologues preclude their involvement in this protein droplet nephropathy.

Chemical inducers of α_{2u}-globulin nephropathy

The chemicals currently known to produce α_{2u}-globulin nephropathy, as well as the major molecular events believed to be mechanistically

linked to the syndrome, are summarized in Table 1. Overall, chemical inducers of α_{2u}-globulin nephropathy represent a diverse and ever-growing class. The nephropathy was originally characterized following exposure of rats to a variety of small, branched-chain petroleum hydrocarbons (Carpenter et al., 1975), but it is now recognized that both aliphatic and aromatic compounds representing a variety of solvents, fuels, pesticides, drugs and naturally occurring compounds can produce this toxicity. As noted in Table 1, many chemicals are known to cause the acute syndrome of renal protein overload, but only a small subset has been tested in chronic carcinogenicity bioassays. However, all such chemicals that induced renal tubule tumours exclusively in male rats (Table 1) have also produced the acute nephropathy, suggesting that there is a link between the nephropathy and the carcinogenic outcome. The only exception to this generalization is gabapentin (Dominick et al., 1991), which produced the nephropathy but did not produce renal tumours.

Collectively, the research that underpins the mechanistic understanding of α_{2u}-globulin nephropathy is extensive and highly coherent. Several chemicals and mixtures have been studied in great detail. These include d-limonene, 2,4,4-trimethylpentane (TMP), unleaded gasoline, isophorone, 1,4-dichlorobenzene, 3,5,5-trimethylhexanoic acid and decalin. Many other chemicals that show male-rat-specific nephropathy have been evaluated for morphological and biochemical parameters of the syndrome, albeit to varying, usually lesser, extents. This can create confusion, and critics of the α_{2u}-globulin nephropathy hypothesis have frequently cited data on additional chemicals that clearly do not fit the

Table 1. Biochemical and pathophysiological data for chemicals causing α_{2u}-globulin nephropathy[a]

Substance/chemical	Protein droplets	Increased α_{2u}-globulin	Binding to α_{2u}-globulin	Cell proliferation	Initiation/ promotion	Male rat renal tumours
d-Limonene	+	+	+	+	+	+
Unleaded gasoline	+	+	+	+	+	+
2,2,4-Trimethylpentane	+	+	+	+	+	NR
Sodium barbital	+	+	+	+	+	NR
Diethylacetyl urea	+	+	+	+	+	NR
1,4-Dichlorobenzene	+	+	+	+	+	+
Isophorone	+	+	+	+	NR	+
3,5,5-Trimethyl hexanoic acid derivatives	+	+	+	NR	NR	NR
Decalin	+	+	NR	+b	NR	NR
Tricyclodecane	+	NR	NR	NR	NR	NR
1-Decalone	+	+	+	NR	NR	NR
2-Decalone	+	+	+	NR	NR	NR
Tetrachloroethylene	+	+	NR	+	NR	+
Pentachloroethane	+	+	NR	+	NR	+
C_{10}-C_{12} isoparaffinic solvent (saturated aliphatic hydrocarbons)	+	+	NR	NR	NR	NR
JP-4, JP-5 jet fuel (mixed distillate hydrocarbons)	+	NR	NR	NR	NR	+
Diesel fuel, marine	+	NR	NR	NR	NR	NR
JP-10 synthetic jet fuel (exohexahydro-4,7-methanoindan)	+	NR	NR	NR	NR	+
RJ-5 synthetic jet fuel (hydrogenated dimers of norbornadiene)	+	NR	NR	NR	NR	+
JP-7 distillate jet fuel	+	NR	NR	NR	NR	NR
JP-TS distillate jet fuel	+	NR	NR	NR	NR	NR
Stoddard solvent	+	NR	NR	NR	NR	NR
Naphthas	+	NR	NR	NR	NR	NR
60 Solvent	+	NR	NR	NR	NR	NR
Levamisole	+	+	NR	NR	NR	NR
Gabapentin	+	+	NR	NR	NR	NR

Table 1. (contd)

Substance/chemical	Protein droplets	Increased α_{2u}-globulin	Binding to α_{2u}-globulin	Cell proliferation	Initiation/ promotion	Male rat renal tumours
Tridecyl acetate	+	+	NR	NR	NR	NR
Isopropylcyclohexane	+	+	NR	NR	NR	NR
t-Butyl cyclohexane	+	NR	NR	NR	NR	NR
Tetralin	+	NR	NR	NR	NR	NR
Hexachloroethane	+	NR	NR	NR	NR	+
Dimethyl methylphosphonate	+	NR	NR	NR	NR	+
Methyl isobutyl ketone	+	NR	NR	NR	NR	NR
Methyl isoamyl ketone	+	NR	NR	NR	NR	NR
Diisobutyl ketone	+	NR	NR	NR	NR	NR
1,3,6-Tricyanohexane	+	NR	NR	NR	NR	NR
4-Chloro-α,α,α-trifluorotoluene	+	NR	NR	NR	NR	NR

[a] Compilation of US Environmental Protection Agency, 1991; Swenberg, 1993; Lehman-McKeeman, 1997
[b] Based on cell counts from urine
NR, not reported

mechanistic requirements, in order to cloud the issue. It is also necessary to understand the criteria that exclude a chemical from being considered to work through the α_{2u}-globulin nephropathy mechanism. For instance, a chemical that is considered to be genotoxic or that induces a similar response in male and female rats or in other species may also induce α_{2u}-globulin nephropathy, but the primary mechanism of carcinogenic action would not require α_{2u}-globulin.

Along with the broad spectrum of chemicals listed in Table 1, it is also apparent that chemicals that cause α_{2u}-globulin nephropathy differ in their potency. d-Limonene is one of the most potent members of this class, inducing significant renal disease with all of the pathognomonic lesions and a 25% incidence of renal tumours only in male rats at the end of two year carcinogenicity bioassays (US National Toxicology Program, 1990). In contrast, other less potent chemicals induce increases in hyaline droplets, but no progression to more advanced lesions (Dominick et al., 1991). Chemicals that are genotoxic or produce renal tumours in female rats or in mice are not included in Table 1. Furthermore, if an alternate mechanism has been established, as in the case of potassium bromate-induced oxidative stress, it is not included. While these chemicals may also cause α_{2u}-globulin nephropathy, it cannot be considered the sole mechanism for carcinogenesis. The α_{2u}-globulin nephropathy is likely to change quantitative relationships for dose response. This chapter summarizes the biochemical and pathophysiological mechanisms underlying the renal protein overload and development of renal tubule tumours seen with α_{2u}-globulin nephropathy.

Histopathological features of α_{2u}-globulin nephropathy

The acute, pathognomonic feature of α_{2u}-globulin nephropathy is the rapid accumulation of protein (or hyaline) droplets in the proximal tubule cells following chemical treatment (Alden et al., 1984; Swenberg et al., 1989). Male rats are unique among all species in that they present with a background of spontaneous protein droplets in the proximal tubule, particularly the cells of the P_2 segment. These spontaneous droplets have been attributed to the large amount of filtered protein that is reabsorbed and degraded in the lysosomal com-

partment of these cells (Maunsbach, 1966; Kretchmer & Bernstein, 1974). By light microscopy, these droplets are somewhat difficult to detect with routine haematoxylin and eosin staining, but they can be readily visualized with special stains including the Mallory–Heidenhain stain (Alden et al., 1984; Lehman-McKeeman, 1997), Lee's methylene basic blue fuschin stain (Short et al., 1986) or immunohistochemistry (Burnett et al., 1989; Dietrich & Swenberg, 1991a). Figure 1 (top panel) shows the typical appearance of an untreated male rat kidney prepared with Mallory–Heidenhain staining, in which a few small protein droplets are noted. In contrast, after d-limonene treatment (Figure 1, bottom panel), there is an obvious and significant increase in the number, size and staining intensity of the protein droplets. These droplets contain significant amounts of α_{2u}-globulin, as determined by immunohistochemical detection (Figure 2). At the ultrastructural level (Figure 3), these large droplets are seen to represent phagolysosomes that can be so engorged with protein that they become irregular and polyangular in shape and contain crystalloid inclusions (Stone et al., 1987; Garg et al., 1989).

Whereas the accumulation of protein droplets occurs rapidly, continued chemical treatment results in additional histological changes in the kidney. Thus, 3–13 weeks of dosing leads to progressive renal injury, characterized by single cell degeneration and necrosis in the renal proximal tubule. Dead cells are sloughed into the lumen of the nephron, and while moving through the nephron contribute to the development of granular casts at the cortico-medullary junction. These granular casts stain positively for α_{2u}-globulin, representing a highly specific lesion (Figure 4). As a result of renal cell death and degeneration, there is compensatory cell proliferation in the cortex. This increase in cell proliferation is dose- and time-related and only occurs in male rats (Alden et al., 1984; Trump et al., 1984; Short et al., 1986, 1987, 1989a; Dietrich & Swenberg, 1991b; Umemura et al., 1992; Lehman-McKeeman, 1995). Dramatic reduction in cell proliferation occurs within days of stopping exposure (Short et al., 1987), and typically recovery can occur, and normal renal architecture is restored, if treatment is stopped at this time (Mattie et al., 1991). However, if treatment continues, linear papillary mineralization, caused

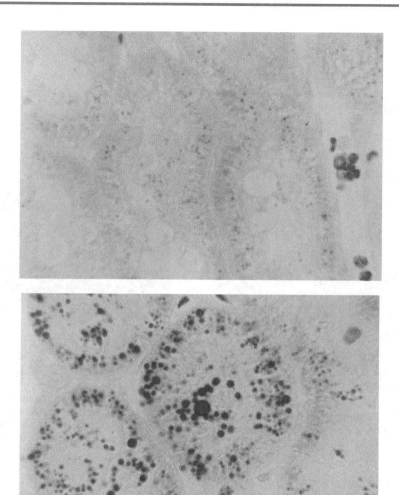

Figure 1. Histopathological characterization of the spontaneous and exacerbated formation of hyaline droplets, the hallmark of α_{2u}-globulin nephropathy, in male rat kidneys (× 320). When stained with Mallory-Heidenhain stain, small, lightly-stained eosinophilic droplets are observed in the proximal tubule epithelium of untreated male rats (top). No similar spontaneous droplet formation is observed in the kidneys of any other species. Following a single oral dosage of d-limonene to male rats (150 mg/kg), the number, size and staining intensity of the droplets is markedly increased within 24 hours (bottom).

by accumulation of calcium hydroxyapatite in the thin limbs of Henle, is noted after several months of treatment (Figure 5) and there is an accelerated onset of the cortical changes typical of chronic progressive nephropathy typically seen in older male rats (Alden *et al.*, 1984; Trump *et al.*, 1984; Short *et al.*, 1987). With chronic exposure, sporadic foci of atypical hyperplasia, defined as a focal aggregation of morphologically abnormal cells (Dietrich & Swenberg, 1993), can be observed in the proximal tubules, and the atypical foci progress to renal adenomas and carcinomas on prolonged exposure. Again, these changes are observed only in male rats. No similar renal changes have been observed in female rats or in any other species including mice, dogs or monkeys (US National Toxicology Program, 1983, 1986a, b, 1987a, b, 1990; Kitchen, 1984; Webb *et al.*, 1990).

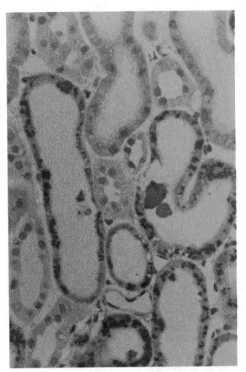

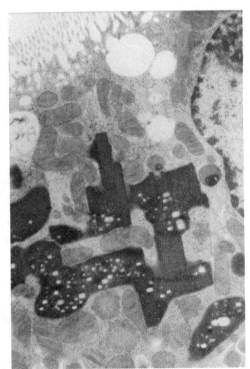

Figure 2. Immunohistochemical localization of α_{2u}-globulin in the proximal tubule cells. A polyclonal antibody to α_{2u}-globulin was used to detect the presence of α_{2u}-globulin within the protein droplets induced following *d*-limonene treatment.

Figure 3. Electron micrograph of a renal proximal tubule cell showing the appearance of crystalloid inclusions in the cell following the development of α_{2u}-globulin nephropathy.

A major factor that determines the pathophysiological progression of this syndrome and the carcinogenic outcome is the duration of exposure. For example, if exposures are limited, such as in the 90-day stop study on decalin (Gaworski *et al.*, 1985), the hallmark hyaline droplet response is observed, but the renal changes do not progress to include the chronic sequelae and no tumours are seen. As discussed below, the increased cell turnover and sustained cell proliferation are prerequisites for, and ultimately involved in, the tumour development associated with this syndrome.

The protein droplet nephropathy described above is specific for male rats. If a protein droplet nephropathy is also produced in female rats (exception would be an androgen) or mice of either sex, it cannot be called α_{2u}-globulin nephropathy. If other dose-related degenerative renal lesions are produced by a chemical in female rats or in mice, establishment of a causal relationship between α_{2u}-globulin and the nephropathy and/or carcinogenicity in male rats will require more extensive research. This distinction should not pertain to minor exacerbations of common spontaneous renal disease.

α_{2u}-Globulin

The histological characteristics of this syndrome were determined well before the role of α_{2u}-globulin in renal toxicity and tumorigenesis was defined. Given that the droplets observed histologically appeared to contain protein, initial biochemical experiments focused on identifying what protein or proteins had accumulated in the droplets following exposure. Using two-dimensional electrophoresis, Alden *et al.* (1984) demonstrated that only one protein had accumulated in the kidney after chemical treatment, and this protein was subsequently identified as α_{2u}-globulin. Moreover, immunohistochemical studies have localized the

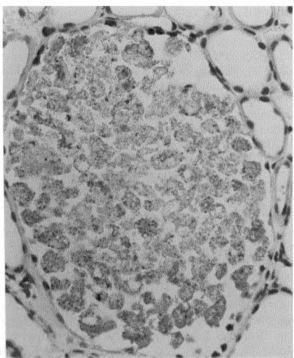

Figure 4. Immunohistochemical localization of α_{2u}-globulin within the granular casts which appear at the cortico-medullary junction following repeated administration of a compound (TMP) that induces acute α_{2u}-globulin nephropathy.

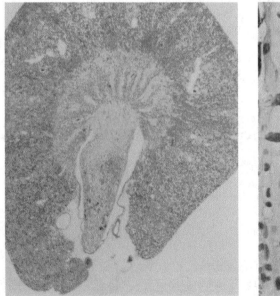
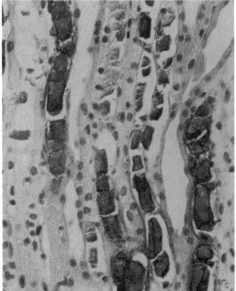

Figure 5. Chronic exposure to chemicals which cause α_{2u}-globulin nephropathy leads to the development of papillary mineralization resulting from the accumulation of calcium hydroxyapatite in the thin limbs of the loops of Henle. The mineralization is readily apparent in cross sections (left) of the kidney, and upon microscopic evaluation of the medullary region (right).

accumulation of α_{2u}-globulin to the protein droplets (Figure 2; Burnett et al., 1989; Dietrich & Swenberg, 1991a).

The identification of α_{2u}-globulin immediately put into perspective the male rat specificity of this syndrome. α_{2u}-Globulin is an unusual protein synthesized exclusively by adult male rats (Table 2). It was originally isolated from male rat urine by Roy et al. (1966). It is synthesized predominantly in liver (Roy & Neuhaus, 1966; Kurtz, 1981) but extrahepatic sites of synthesis, including the salivary, lachrymal, preputial, meibomian and perianal glands, have been identified (MacInnes et al., 1986; Murty et al., 1987; Mancini et al., 1989). However, α_{2u}-globulin purified from these accessory glands is electrophoretically distinct from the hepatic form of the protein, and is not male-specific as the protein has been detected in the salivary, lachrymal and preputial glands of female rats (MacInnes et al., 1986; Murty et al., 1987).

α_{2u}-Globulin is encoded by a multi-gene family clustered on chromosome 5 (Kurtz, 1981) and its expression is regulated by a complex hormonal interaction, requiring testosterone, glucocorticoids, insulin, thyroid hormone and growth hormone (Kurtz et al., 1976a,b, 1978a,b; Kurtz & Feigelson, 1978; Roy et al., 1980). It is generally recognized that gene expression is maximal in a hormonally intact, sexually mature male rat, and expression cannot be induced further (Kurtz & Feigelson, 1978). α_{2u}-Globulin mRNA is very abundant in liver, accounting for the second highest mRNA levels in the male rat liver. Only albumin is more

abundant (Sippel et al., 1976; Kurtz et al., 1978a). Although female rats possess the entire complement of hepatic α_{2u}-globulin genes, oestrogen is a very effective repressor of their expression (Roy et al., 1975). Masculinization of female rats stimulates expression of α_{2u}-globulin, but not to the levels seen in males (Roy & Neuhaus, 1967; Chatterjee et al., 1989).

The α_{2u}-globulin detected in the kidney is considered to be hepatic in origin (Roy et al., 1966; MacInnes et al., 1986). Once synthesized, the protein is rapidly secreted from the liver and hepatic levels are very low at steady state (Roy et al., 1966). The molecular weight of α_{2u}-globulin is approximately 18.5 kDa, and the protein is freely filtered across the glomerulus (Roy et al., 1966; Neuhaus, 1986). In fact, renal clearance of the protein is so effective that plasma concentrations of α_{2u}-globulin are low, typically no higher than 3 mg/100 ml (Roy & Neuhaus, 1966). It is estimated that adult male rats synthesize about 50 mg α_{2u}-globulin per day, and the entire amount synthesized is filtered by the kidney (Roy et al., 1966; Neuhaus et al., 1981; Lehman-McKeeman & Caudill, 1992a). Only about 60% of the filtered α_{2u}-globulin (or approximately 30 mg/day) is reabsorbed by the kidney (Neuhaus, 1986; Lehman-McKeeman & Caudill, 1992a), in contrast to the complete reabsorption of most other proteins by the proximal tubule cells (Maack et al., 1979). Because it is so abundant, the large amount of α_{2u}-globulin which is reabsorbed is thought to contribute to the spontaneous formation of protein droplets in the

---

Table 2. Characteristics of α_{2u}-globulin

Synthesized primarily in the liver of adult male rats; not synthesized by any other species

Complex hormonal regulation of hepatic gene expression

Required for expression: testosterone, glucocorticoids, insulin, thyroid hormone, growth hormone

Inhibits expression: oestrogen

Low molecular weight (18.5 kDa) allows for glomerular filtration

Major urinary protein excreted by adult male rats

Member of the α_{2u}-globulin protein superfamily, also referred to as lipocalins

Unlike other lipocalins, no endogenous ligand is detected, and its function is unknown

Binds hyaline droplet inducing agents in a reversible manner and with a molar ratio of 1

Ligand binding cavity is spherical and has a molecular volume of about 85 Å^3

male rat kidney. The remaining, non-absorbed protein (15–20 mg/day) is excreted in the urine, where, as the most abundant urinary protein, it accounts for about 35% of the total urinary protein (Roy *et al.*, 1966; Neuhaus *et al.*, 1981; Lehman-McKeeman & Caudill, 1991).

Although male rats synthesize a large quantity of α_{2u}-globulin, the function of this protein remains unknown. The detection of α_{2u}-globulin in pheromone-producing glands (preputial, meibomian and perianal glands) suggests a function relating to the transport of pheromones. However, no endogenous ligand for α_{2u}-globulin has been identified (Roy *et al.*, 1966; Lehman-McKeeman & Caudill, 1992b; Lehman-McKeeman *et al.*, 1998). Other functions which have been suggested for the protein include roles in renal fatty acid binding (Kimura *et al.*, 1989) or in the regulation or modulation of spermatogenesis (Roy *et al.*, 1976).

Whereas no physiological function for α_{2u}-globulin is known, its role in the pathophysiology of male-rat-specific protein droplet nephropathy and renal carcinogenesis is unequivocal. Only α_{2u}-globulin accumulates in the protein droplets, only male rats synthesize α_{2u}-globulin, and only male rats develop this syndrome. The nephropathy is not seen in female rats or any other species (Alden *et al.*, 1984; Swenberg *et al.*, 1989; Borghoff *et al.*, 1990; Hard *et al.*, 1993). Furthermore, the nephropathy does not develop in juvenile male rats (Alden *et al.*, 1984), since synthesis of the protein is not detected until puberty (Roy *et al.*, 1983), nor is it observed in the male NCI-Black Reiter (NBR) rat (Dietrich & Swenberg, 1991a), an unusual strain which does not synthesize α_{2u}-globulin (Chatterjee *et al.*, 1989). Finally, although mice are refractory to this toxicity, the nephropathy can be produced in transgenic mice engineered to express α_{2u}-globulin (Lehman-McKeeman & Caudill, 1994).

Biochemical mechanisms of α_{2u}-globulin nephropathy

A common characteristic of all chemicals that produce α_{2u}-globulin nephropathy is the ability to bind to the protein, which appears to be the rate-limiting step in the development of the nephropathy (Swenberg *et al.*, 1989; Borghoff *et al.*, 1990;

Lehman-McKeeman, 1993, 1997). In the kidney there is a sex-dependent retention of chemical, with more compound distributing to and being retained by the kidney in male rats than in female rats (Charbonneau *et al.*, 1987; Lehman-McKeeman *et al.*, 1989, 1991), and in the male rat kidney, 20–40% of the chemical is bound specifically to α_{2u}-globulin (Lock *et al.*, 1987; Charbonneau *et al.*, 1989; Lehman-McKeeman *et al.*, 1989, 1991). The bound chemical can be dissociated by protein denaturation, indicating that the binding is reversible, but the ligand–protein complex survives tissue homogenization, centrifugation and lyophilization, suggesting that the complex is stable and does not dissociate *in vivo* (Lock *et al.*, 1987; Lehman-McKeeman *et al.*, 1989, 1991). The stability of the protein–chemical complex is also suggested by time course studies which show that as the chemical is cleared from the kidney, the percentage of chemical that is protein-bound increases (Lock *et al.*, 1987). Data on equilibrium saturation binding *in vitro* indicate that the dissociation constant for xenobiotic binding to α_{2u}-globulin is approximately 10^{-7} M (Borghoff *et al.*, 1991; Lehman-McKeeman & Caudill, 1992a,b).

For several chemicals, the moieties that bind to α_{2u}-globulin have been identified (Table 1). These ligands are as structurally diverse as the class of compounds which produce the syndrome. In some cases, parent compound will bind directly to the protein (isophorone), while in others, oxidative metabolites, including epoxides (*d*-limonene-1,2-epoxide), ketones (γ-lactone of 3,5,5-trimethylhexanoic acid) and hydroxylated metabolites of aliphatic (2,4,4-trimethyl-2-pentanol) or aromatic compounds (2,5-dichlorophenol) have been isolated from α_{2u}-globulin. It is clear that the ligand-binding site of α_{2u}-globulin must accommodate very diverse chemical structures. More information on the nature of the binding site in α_{2u}-globulin and the orientation of the chemical in the binding site is becoming available as the X-ray crystal structure of the protein is solved (see below). However, it is clear that ligands must be hydrophobic in nature and have a molecular volume of no greater than 100 Å^3 to fit into the protein binding site (Borghoff *et al.*, 1991; Bocskei *et al.*, 1992; Lehman-McKeeman, 1997).

Although the ligand–protein complex can be isolated from the kidney *in vivo*, it is not known where the interaction between the xenobiotic and α_{2u}-globulin occurs. The complex appears to be localized in the phagolysosomal compartment, suggesting that binding does not take place in the kidney. Rather, the interaction probably occurs outside the kidney (in liver or blood), and following glomerular filtration, the complex enters the proximal tubule cells by endocytosis, accumulating in the phagolysosomes after lysosomal fusion.

Following binding of a ligand to α_{2u}-globulin, the rate of lysosomal degradation of the protein is reduced relative to the native protein. In experiments with renal cortical lysosomal lysates as enzyme source, the rate of degradation *in vitro* of α_{2u}-globulin to which *d*-limonene-1,2-epoxide, isophorone or 2,5-dichlorophenol was bound decreased by about 30% (Lehman-McKeeman *et al.*, 1990). In contrast, lysosomal degradation of other proteins such as albumin was not altered by the presence of any of these chemicals, and there was no change in lysosomal cathepsin activity towards model substrates in the presence of the chemicals or the α_{2u}-globulin complexes (Lehman-McKeeman *et al.*, 1990). Using immunoblotting techniques, it has been found that α_{2u}-globulin exists in two forms in the kidney. One form is the native protein (18.5 kDa), whereas the second is a smaller form (about 16 kDa) representing the native protein from which the first nine amino acids have been cleaved. In general, the quantities of both forms of the protein increase after chemical treatment (Saito *et al.*, 1991; Kurata *et al.*, 1994). Therefore, the increase in amounts of protein droplets seen following chemical treatment occurs because the rate of degradation of α_{2u}-globulin is reduced by ligand binding, and with chemical binding, protein begins to accumulate in the phagolysosomes.

As chemical treatment continues, the lysosomes become enlarged, engorged with protein and polyangular (Figure 3). Although the mechanisms of cell death are not understood for this syndrome, cytotoxicity is evidenced by single cell necrosis in the P_2 segment of the proximal tubule (Short *et al.*, 1986; Swenberg *et al.*, 1989); loss of renal function is dose- and time-dependent. Renal functional perturbations include reduced uptake of organic anions, cations and amino acids and a mild proteinuria resulting from a large increase in the amount of α_{2u}-globulin excreted in urine (Lehman-

McKeeman, 1995). These functional changes occur only in male rats and only at dosages which exacerbate the protein droplet formation (Figure 6). In response to the cell death and functional changes, there is a compensatory increase in cell proliferation in the kidney, most notably in the P_2 segment of the proximal tubules, the site of protein accumulation (Short *et al.*, 1989a; Umemura *et al.*, 1992; Lehman-McKeeman, 1995). With continued treatment, the cell proliferation persists for as long as exposure continues, but it does not restore renal function. The increase in renal cell proliferation is believed to exert a promotional influence on the kidney, such that sustained cell turnover is mechanistically linked to the development of renal tubule tumours via tumour promotion (Short *et al.*, 1989a,b; Dietrich & Swenberg, 1991b, Kurata *et al.*, 1994). Thus, α_{2u}-globulin nephropathy begins acutely as protein accumulation, but represents a continuum of changes that ultimately progress to renal tumours (Swenberg *et al.*, 1989; Flamm & Lehman-McKeeman, 1991; Hard *et al.*, 1993; Hard & Whysner, 1994).

Renal tubule tumour formation in α_{2u}-globulin nephropathy

In bioassays conducted by the National Toxicology Program, renal tubule tumours are uncommon in rats, occurring spontaneously at incidences of 0.96 and 0.07% for male and female Fischer 344 rats, respectively (US National Institute of Environmental Health Sciences, 1996). As noted in Table 1, several chemicals causing renal tubule tumours exclusively in male rats have been identified, and the highest tumour rate (seen with *d*-limonene) was approximately 25% (US National Toxicology Program, 1990). In this respect, these chemicals differ from classical renal carcinogens such as the nitrosamines, for which tumour incidences approach 100%. The renal tumours associated with α_{2u}-globulin nephropathy are also distinguished from classical renal carcinogens in that they show a much longer latency period, requiring at least 18 months of continued dosing, and the chemicals that cause the male rat-specific renal tumours are not genotoxic (Hard, 1984, 1987; Dietrich & Swenberg, 1993; Hard *et al.*, 1993). For the renal carcinogens listed in Table 1, there is generally no evidence of mutagenicity in *Salmonella*

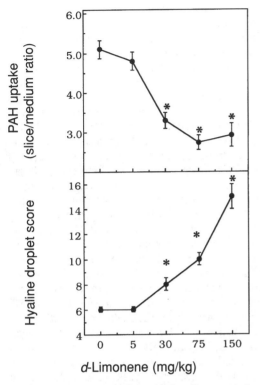

Figure 6. Dose-response relationship for *d*-limonene-induced acute (single exposure) exacerbation of hyaline droplet formation and subchronic changes (91 days of repeat dosing) in renal function. Exacerbation of hyaline droplets was evaluated histologically 24 hours after a single oral dosage of *d*-limonene (150 mg/kg). Droplets were graded on a scale from 0-16 (with a maximum score of 16) after staining with Mallory-Heidenhain stain. In this example, renal function was assessed as the in vitro uptake of *p*-aminohippurate (PAH) in cortical slices prepared from rats dosed daily with *d*-limonene for 91 days. Asterisks indicate dosages for which both hyaline droplet scores and PAH uptake were statistically different from control ($p < 0.05$). A dosage of 5 mg/kg did not exacerbate hyaline droplet formation and did not change PAH uptake. At dosages of 30 mg/kg and higher, dose-dependent increases in hyaline droplet severity were observed along with a dose-dependent decrease in PAH uptake.

typhimurium (with or without metabolic activation) or mouse lymphoma cells, or clastogenicity in Chinese hamster ovary cells (US National Toxicology Program, 1983, 1986a,b, 1987a,b, 1990). The identification of a potentially reactive epoxide intermediate of *d*-limonene that binds to α₂ᵤ-globulin might raise some concern that the epoxide was directly involved in the carcinogenicity of *d*-limonene. However, this epoxide, an unusually

stable chemical, also shows negative results in a battery of mutagenicity tests (Watabe *et al.*, 1980, 1981; Burnett *et al.*, 1989; von der Hude *et al.*, 1989).

The lack of genotoxicity among the chemicals causing α₂ᵤ-globulin nephropathy and male-rat-specific renal tumours supports the concept that nongenotoxic mechanisms are involved in the carcinogenic response. The cell proliferation seen with subchronic and chronic exposure to these chemicals is necessary for the tumour formation associated with this syndrome (Short *et al.*, 1989a,b; Swenberg *et al.*, 1989; Dietrich & Swenberg, 1991b; Umemura *et al.*, 1992). Sustained cell proliferation is believed to be a primary mechanism underlying the tumour response to many nongenotoxic chemicals, as accelerated cell turnover can promote clonal expansion of spontaneously initiated cells (Grasso, 1987; Swenberg *et al.*, 1989; Cohen & Ellwein, 1990; Williams & Whysner, 1996). Dose-related and male-rat-specific increases in cell proliferation have been demonstrated with all of the chemicals evaluated, and the dose–response relationships for cell proliferation parallel those for hyaline droplet formation and the induction of renal tumours (Figure 7; Short *et al.*, 1987, 1989a,b). As mentioned earlier, the increased cell proliferation is dependent on continued exposure to the agent inducing the nephropathy. When male and female rats were exposed to unleaded gasoline or TMP in the same inhalation chambers, cell proliferation did not increase in females, but there were clear, concentration-dependent increases in male rats (Short *et al.*, 1989a). Furthermore, the link between the nephropathy and cell proliferation was established in experiments comparing NBR and Fischer 344 rats exposed to *d*-limonene (Dietrich & Swenberg, 1991a,b). Cell proliferation was increased in Fischer 344 rats, but not in NBR rats which lack α₂ᵤ-globulin and do not develop α₂ᵤ-globulin nephropathy following 4 or 31 weeks of exposure to *d*-limonene (Figure 8). Thus, the increase in cell proliferation was shown to be totally dependent on the presence of α₂ᵤ-globulin.

The concept that chemicals inducing α₂ᵤ-globulin nephropathy cause renal tubule tumours by secondary, non-genotoxic mechanisms is further supported by the results of several initiation–promotion studies. After unleaded gasoline and *d*-limonene were identified as causing α₂ᵤ-globulin

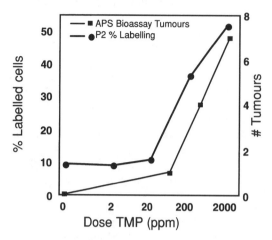

Figure 7. Dose-response relationship for TMP -induced proximal tubule cell proliferation and the development of renal tubule tumours.

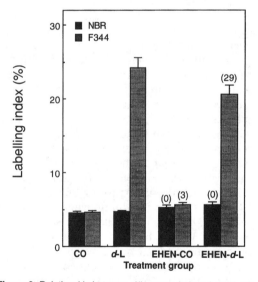

Figure 8. Relationship between *d*-limonene induced renal cell proliferation and kidney tumour promotion in male Fischer 344 and NBR rats. No increase in cell proliferation was observed in the NBR rat, which does not synthesize α_{2u} -globulin, whereas increased cell proliferation and promotion of EHEN-initiated renal tumours was observed in the Fischer 344 rat.

nephropathy, two large initiation-promotion experiments were conducted. The first was a classical initiation–promotion experiment on unleaded gasoline and TMP that included all of the sequence controls and was conducted on male and female rats (Short *et al.*, 1989b). In this study, *N*-nitroso-ethylhydroxyethylamine (EHEN) was used as the initiator and three concentrations of unleaded gasoline or 50 ppm TMP were evaluated for their ability to promote atypical renal foci and renal tumour formation. Parallel studies on cell proliferation were conducted (Short *et al.*, 1989a). Evidence of tumour promotion was present only in male rats, demonstrating that promotion parallel-led the findings in the carcinogenicity bioassay on unleaded gasoline (Kitchen, 1984). Promotion was concentration-dependent, with significant increases in renal foci and tumours in nitrosamine-initiated rats exposed to 300 ppm unleaded gasoline, paralleling the results of the carcinogenicity bioassay. Promotion (nitrosamine followed by TMP or unleaded gasoline) was much more effective than administration of the same substances in the reverse sequence, i.e., animals were exposed to TMP or unleaded gasoline for 24 weeks, then given nitrosamine for two weeks and held for an additional 35 weeks (Short *et al.*, 1989b).

A second initiation–promotion study, conducted with EHEN and *d*-limonene, compared the response of NBR and Fischer 344 male rats (Dietrich & Swenberg, 1991b) in order to evaluate the requirement for α_{2u}-globulin in formation of renal foci and tumours. In this study, cell proliferation, atypical tubules, atypical hyperplasia and renal adenomas were evaluated. EHEN was an effective initiator when administered alone to either strain of rat, causing increases in atypical tubules, the earliest preneoplastic lesion (Dietrich & Swenberg, 1993). When EHEN treatment was followed by *d*-limonene, marked increases in atypical tubules (Figure 9) and atypical hyperplasia (Figure 10) were induced in male Fischer 344 rats, but no increase was seen in NBR rats. Likewise, incidence of renal adenomas (Figure 11) was significantly increased in Fischer 344 rats, but none occurred in NBR rats. Increased cell proliferation was present at 7 and 32 weeks of promotion in Fischer 344, but never in NBR rats.

The initiation–promotion studies conducted with unleaded gasoline and *d*-limonene were performed after the ability of these chemicals to cause α_{2u}-globulin nephropathy had been characterized. In contrast, the renal tumour-promoting activity of sodium barbital and a major hydrolysis product, diethylacetylurea, was established well before these two chemicals were shown to cause α_{2u}-globulin nephropathy in male rats. Briefly, in standard initiation–promotion protocols, both sodium barbital and diethylacetylurea have been shown to promote renal tumour formation in male Fischer 344 rats following initiation by N-nitrosodiethylamine (Diwan et al., 1985, 1989a,b). Both agents also produced nephrotoxicity and increased renal cell proliferation (Ward et al., 1991), but only after kidneys were evaluated by Mallory– Heidenhain staining and immunohistochemical analysis was their ability to induce α_{2u}-globulin nephropathy recognized (Kurata et al., 1994).

Collectively, the initiation–promotion studies provide compelling evidence that unleaded gasoline, TMP, d-limonene and sodium barbital act as renal tubule tumour promoters and that this

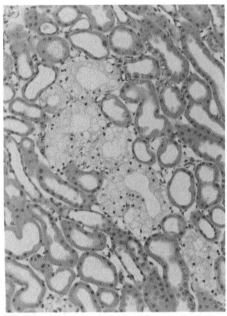

Figure 10. Microscopic appearance of atypical renal cell hyperplasia in a male Fischer 344 rat initiated with EHEN and promoted with d-limonene.

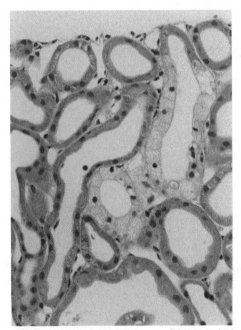

Figure 9. Microscopic appearance of an atypical tubule in a male Fischer 344 rat initiated with EHEN and promoted with d-limonene.

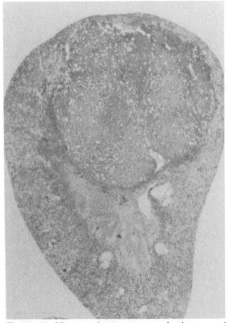

Figure 11. Microscopic appearance of a large renal adenoma in a male Fischer 344 rat initiated with EHEN and promoted with d-limonene.

promoting effect requires α_{2u}-globulin. The requirement for α_{2u}-globulin also explains why the renal tumour induction by these agents is a male-rat-specific effect. The link between the acute development of α_{2u}-globulin nephropathy and the chronic development of renal tubule tumours is the renal cell injury which stimulates sustained cell proliferation. In this manner, the biochemical and pathophysiological data support the conclusion that α_{2u}-globulin nephropathy begins as an acute protein overload but represents a continuum of changes that ultimately progress to renal tumours. The major mechanistic events in this continuum are summarized in Figure 12.

Human relevance of α_{2u}-globulin nephropathy

Given the compelling and comprehensive evidence that α_{2u}-globulin is necessary for the development of this syndrome and that the protein is synthesized exclusively by adult male rats, it seems reasonable to conclude that α_{2u}-globulin nephropathy is unique to the male rat. However, α_{2u}-globulin is a member of a large protein superfamily (Brooks, 1987; Flower et al., 1993; Flower, 1994) characterized by a very unusual tertiary structure. The proteins in this family, described as lipocalins and often referred to as the α_{2u}-globulin protein superfamily, are synthesized in many species, including humans. The primary function of the lipocalins is

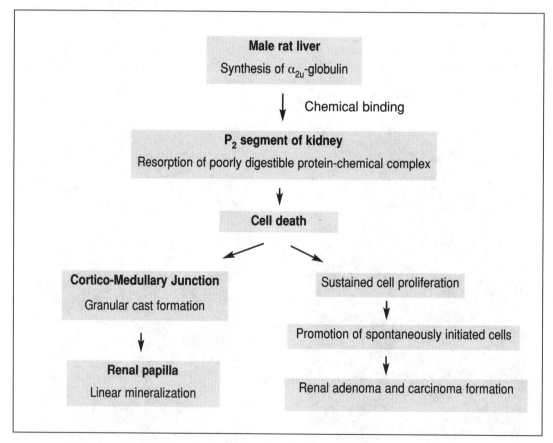

Figure 12. Schematic representation of the continuum of changes initiated by the binding of a xenobiotic to α_{2u}-globulin. Small droplets form spontaneously in male rat kidneys due to the large amount of α_{2u}-globulin in the kidney. When a chemical binds to α_{2u}-globulin, the acute, pathognomonic response is the rapid exacerbation of hyaline droplet formation, and with repeated exposure, the syndrome progresses from protein overload to renal cell injury, cell death and compensatory sustained hyperplasia prior to the development of renal tubule tumours.

to bind and transport small hydrophobic molecules, and for many of them, endogenous ligands have been identified (Table 3). The unique structural motif is a β-barrel with eight anti-parallel β-strands that fold into an orthogonal calyx, or cup-like structure. Ligands are bound within the β-barrel cavity which is lined almost exclusively by hydrophobic amino acids and which form the shape of the pocket and contribute to ligand specificity (Papiz et al., 1986; Brooks, 1987; Godovac-Zimmerman, 1988; Cowan et al., 1990).

The superfamily protein that is most similar to α_{2u}-globulin is mouse urinary protein (MUP). MUP is the mouse homologue of α_{2u}-globulin, sharing nearly 90% sequence homology and hormonally controlled in a manner similar to that described previously for α_{2u}-globulin (Hastie et al., 1979; Shaw et al., 1983). MUP is also the major urinary protein excreted by mice (Finlayson et al., 1963; Lehman-McKeeman & Caudill, 1992a) and represents the most abundant mRNA species in the mouse liver (Hastie et al., 1979). However, unlike α_{2u}-globulin, MUP expression is not fully repressed by oestrogen, so that female mice synthesize and excrete MUP, albeit at levels that are much lower than in males (Rumke & Thung, 1964; Hastie et al., 1979; Knopf et al., 1983;). It is estimated that male mice excrete about 15 mg of MUP daily (Lehman-McKeeman & Caudill, 1992a).

If similarities in molecular structure are sufficient for the superfamily proteins to bind to chemicals that cause α_{2u}-globulin nephropathy, then, because of the very high homology between

α_{2u}-globulin and MUP, mice should be sensitive to developing a similar renal syndrome. However, studies conducted in mice have clearly indicated that no renal changes, including renal tumours, occur following exposure to any of the chemicals known to cause renal tumours in male rats (US National Toxicology Program, 1983, 1986a,b, 1987a,b, 1990; Bomhard et al., 1988; Lehman-McKeeman et al., 1991; Lake et al., 1997). The lack of toxicity in mice treated with agents that induce hyaline droplets is attributed to several major differences between MUP and α_{2u}-globulin. Specifically, MUP does not bind any of the chemicals known to bind to α_{2u}-globulin (Lehman-McKeeman & Caudill, 1992a) and MUP is not reabsorbed into the kidney to any significant extent (Larsen et al., 1990; Lehman-McKeeman & Caudill, 1992a). In direct contrast, α_{2u}-globulin transgenic mice are sensitive to d-limonene-induced α_{2u}-globulin nephropathy although the renal handling of MUP is not affected in any way (Lehman-McKeeman & Caudill, 1994).

There are two other major differences between α_{2u}-globulin and the lipocalin superfamily proteins that distinguish α_{2u}-globulin from all of these proteins. The first difference is that for most of the proteins in the superfamily, important endogenous ligands have been identified. In direct contrast, no endogenous ligand has been detected for α_{2u}-globulin (Table 3; Lehman-McKeeman et al., 1998). For example, it is well established that retinol-binding protein (RBP) binds and transports retinol (Blaner, 1989) and apolipoprotein D transports cholesterol in the circulation (Drayna et al., 1987). Similarly, a variety of ligands have been identified for odorant-binding protein (Pevnser et al., 1990) and α1-acid glycoprotein (Ganguly et al., 1967; Urien et al., 1982). For MUP, 2-sec-butyl-4,5-dihydrothiazole, a compound with established pheromonal properties, has been isolated from the purified protein (Liebich et al., 1977; Bocskei et al., 1992; Lehman-McKeeman et al., 1998). The presence of endogenous ligands not only indicates a function for these proteins, but is also likely to prevent the binding of hyaline droplet-inducing agents to the superfamily proteins. In this regard, it has been shown empirically that other superfamily proteins, particularly those synthesized by humans, do not bind to agents that induce α_{2u}-globulin nephropathy (Lehman-McKeeman & Caudill, 1992b). In the

Table 3. Members of the lipocalin or α_{2u}-globulin superfamily[a]	
Protein	**Endogenous ligand**
α_{2u}-Globulin	Unknown
Mouse urinary protein	2-(sec-butyl)-4,5-Dihydrothiazole
Retinol binding protein	Retinol
α1-Acid glycoprotein	Drugs, steroids
β-LactoGlobulin	Retinol
Odorant-binding protein	Odorants
Apolipoprotein D	Cholesterol

[a] Abridged from Lehman-McKeeman, 1997

absence of an endogenous ligand for α_{2u}-globulin, the empty binding pocket allows chemicals to bind to the protein. Furthermore, it also appears that the binding of ligands to other superfamily proteins does not affect the renal handling of the protein, whereas for α_{2u}-globulin, binding of a chemical clearly alters the renal degradation of the protein (Urien et al., 1982; Blaner, 1989; Lehman-McKeeman et al., 1990). Therefore, although the other superfamily proteins are reabsorbed by the proximal tubule, they do not accumulate in the kidney either spontaneously or following chemical treatment (Alden et al., 1984). This observation also holds true for humans, as no α_{2u}-globulin-like protein has been detected in human kidney tissue (Borghoff & Lagarde, 1993).

The last and most important difference between α_{2u}-globulin and the other members of the lipocalin superfamily concerns the nature of the binding cavity in α_{2u}-globulin. X-ray crystallographic data for α_{2u}-globulin show that the binding pocket (1) is closed off to water; (2) is lined by extremely hydrophobic amino acid residues, and (3) has a probe-accessible volume of 84.0 ± 0.9 Å^3, which is very similar to that (75 Å^3) of the (also hydrophobic) binding pocket in MUP (Bocskei et al., 1992; Lehman-McKeeman, 1997). However, subtle differences in the amino acids that line the binding pocket markedly affect the shape of the cavities, which differs greatly between MUP and α_{2u}-globulin (Figure 13). Specifically, two phenylalanine residues in α_{2u}-globulin (Phe-54 and Phe-103) serve to close off the back of the binding cavity, creating a pocket that is spherical in shape (Lehman-McKeeman, 1997). The large spherical shape of this pocket does not restrict binding, supporting the fact that a diverse array of chemical structures can bind to α_{2u}-globulin. In contrast, the amino acid residues at positions 54 and 103 in MUP are leucine and alanine, respectively. These amino acids do not close off the pocket, yielding a cavity that is flattened and elongated (Bocskei et a., 1992). In this manner, the MUP cavity is restricted by its elongated shape, and cannot accommodate bulky chemicals such as d-limonene-1,2-epoxide (Lehman-McKeeman & Caudill, 1992a; Lehman-McKeeman et al. , 1998). Other lipocalins, such as retinol-binding protein also have flattened, elongated binding cavities that overlap only by about 20 Å^3 with that of α_{2u}-globulin when the

protein structures are superimposed (Cowan et al., 1990). Thus, the specific binding of chemicals to α_{2u}-globulin is ultimately attributable to the unique nature and shape of its ligand binding site, which does not restrict chemical binding.

Collectively, the present data support the conclusions that only α_{2u}-globulin contributes to this renal syndrome and that structurally-similar α_{2u}-globulin superfamily proteins synthesized by humans are not predictive of any risk for humans to develop renal cancer when exposed to agents that induce α_{2u}-globulin nephropathy. At the same time, however, there is the possibility, albeit remote, that other, unrelated proteins which bind xenobiotics might serve as a surrogate for α_{2u}-globulin in humans. To directly address this issue, Borghoff and Lagarde (1993) characterized the protein composition of human (male) kidneys and determined whether agents known to bind to α_{2u}-globulin could bind to human kidney proteins. The results of this work demonstrated that the protein composition of human kidney was very different from that of male rat kidneys and there was no specific binding of α_{2u}-globulin ligands to human renal proteins. These results provide convincing evidence that there is no protein in humans that can contribute to a renal syndrome like α_{2u}-globulin nephropathy.

Alternative hypotheses

During the past 15 years, a significant body of data, including biochemical, cellular and molecular evidence, has been assembled by a number of research groups to support the conclusion that α_{2u}-globulin plays a central role in the continuum described for the development of male-rat-specific renal tubule tumours (Figure 12). Furthermore, extensive data support the conclusion that the properties of α_{2u}-globulin are so unique that no other protein can contribute to such a syndrome. Most importantly, even in cases of potentially high human exposure to agents that induce the syndrome in male rats (as in the case of therapeutic uses), there are no data implicating these chemicals as human nephrotoxins or carcinogens. Despite the thorough evaluation of the mechanisms underlying this syndrome, the possibility that other mechanisms may contribute to the toxicity has been suggested.

One alternative proposal is that the chemicals themselves are nephrotoxic and that binding to

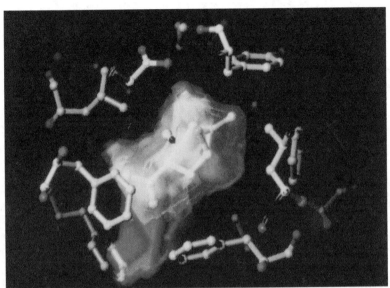

Figure 13. Depiction of the ligand-binding cavities in α_{2u}-globulin (blue cloud) and mouse urinary protein (MUP) (red cloud) as determined by X-ray crystallography. For α_{2u}-globulin, the shape of the binding cavity is essentially spherical, resulting from the orientation of two phenylalanine residues which close off the back of the cavity. The two phenylalanine residues in α_{2u}-globulin are replaced by leucine and alanine, respectively in MUP, resulting in a binding cavity that is elongated and flattened (red cloud) relative to the binding pocket in α_{2u}-globulin. Although the binding cavities of the two proteins are similar in volume, the actual overlap in shape (the highlighted, pink region) is very small. The spherical binding cavity in α_{2u}-globulin is far less restrictive, thereby allowing for a broad spectrum of chemicals to bind to the protein.

α_{2u}-globulin simply serves to concentrate them in the male rat kidney (Melnick, 1992; Melnick & Kohn, this volume). In this manner, toxicity is observed because the delivered dose to the target organ is increased. Accordingly, this proposal is still dependent on the presence of α_{2u}-globulin, and given the unique properties of the protein, the lack of human relevance still holds. At the same time, however, existing data do not support the contention that direct toxicity of the chemicals themselves is involved in renal toxicity and carcinogenicity. First, as noted earlier, the α_{2u}-globulin–ligand complex is quite stable, arguing against the notion that the chemical can be released from the kidney without protein denaturation. Second, direct evaluation of TMP metabolites has indicated that they are not nephrotoxic (Borghoff & Lagarde, 1993). Finally, the most compelling data supporting the non-toxic effects of these chemicals exists for d-limonene, an agent currently being developed as a cancer chemotherapeutic agent (Crowell & Gould, 1994). In early animal studies to address its

anti-carcinogenic activity, d-limonene was fed in the diet to female rats at levels up to 100 000 ppm (10% of diet), and no toxicity was observed (Elegbede *et al.*, 1986; Elson *et al.*, 1988). Furthermore, in a 13-week study conducted by the US National Toxicology Program before the bioassay for d-limonene, female rats were given doses ranging from 150 to 2400 mg/kg by gavage and no renal toxicity was detected, whereas in male rats, renal lesions were observed at all dosages (US National Toxicology Program, 1990). Although there are no accompanying toxicokinetic data for these studies, it is reasonable to assume that the renal concentrations of d-limonene achieved at the extremely high dosages tolerated by female rats are at least equal to the renal concentrations achieved in male rats at much lower dosages.

It is also important to emphasize that the syndrome characterized by α_{2u}-globulin nephropathy is specific to male rats and involves non-genotoxic mechanisms. Therefore, if a chemical is deemed to be genotoxic or causes renal injury and tumours in female rats or other species, mechanisms other than or in addition to α_{2u}-globulin nephropathy must be contributing. It is possible that for certain chemicals, particularly halogenated hydrocarbons, α_{2u}-globulin may contribute to nephrotoxic and nephrocarcinogenic responses in male rats, but other mechanisms, including metabolic activation by glutathione conjugation (Dekant et al., 1989; Lock, 1989) may also be involved in the development of toxicity and carcinogenicity.

Another argument put forward as providing evidence in conflict with the existing mechanism of α_{2u}-globulin nephropathy is that, for several chemicals, there is a discontinuity between the acute nephropathy and the development of renal tumours (Huff, 1996). As discussed earlier, there is a critical level of sustained cell proliferation that is necessary to promote renal tubule tumour formation. If the severity of the acute nephropathy and subsequent regenerative hyperplasia is below that critical level, a chemical (e.g., gabapentin) may not produce renal tumours. The concept of a non-linear dose–response relationship for this syndrome is entirely consistent with the hypothesis that non-genotoxic mechanisms are involved in the development of the renal tubule tumours in male rats (Grasso, 1987; Short et al., 1987; Williams & Whysner, 1996). Furthermore, as emphasized earlier, the cell proliferation that links renal injury to renal foci and tumours must be sustained chronically. Consequently, it is inappropriate to infer carcinogenic outcome based on subchronic regimens such as a 90-day stop study (Gaworski et al., 1985).

Overall, although alternative hypotheses have been suggested, they are not supported by the existing data, and no effort has been made to generate new data in support of these hypotheses.

Risk assessment for species-specific carcinogenicity caused by α_{2u}-globulin nephropathy

If sufficient data are generated to demonstrate that a chemical causes renal tubule tumours in male rats via a mechanism involving α_{2u}-globulin nephropathy, the existing evidence implies that the renal tumours are not predictive of a similar risk to humans. Thus, any evaluation of risk is based on a qualitative, rather than a quantitative analysis. However, this is not a determination to be made lightly, and it is critical that the appropriate

scientific evidence is developed to support the conclusion that a chemical does not pose a cancer risk to humans. The US Environmental Protection Agency Risk Assessment Forum has developed criteria which must be met in order to establish that a chemical causes renal tubule tumours via a mechanism involving α_{2u}-globulin. These criteria, and their impact on risk evaluation are presented here to summarize the extensive review incorporated into the human risk assessment for male rat-specific renal tumours (US Environmental Protection Agency, 1991).

Given some of the current misconceptions that have led to the development of alternative hypotheses, it is important that the criteria used to establish that an agent causes renal tumours in male rats by a mechanism involving α_{2u}-globulin nephropathy be stringent, clearly communicated and strictly adhered to. The essential criteria which need to be satisfied to conclude that an agent causes kidney tumours in male rats through a response associated with α_{2u}-globulin are listed in Table 4. The first criterion is that an agent causing renal tumours should be negative in a battery of genetic toxicity tests, thereby supporting a non-genotoxic mechanism of tumour formation. Both the acute renal effects as well as the renal tubule

---

Table 4. Criteria for establishing the role of α_{2u}-globulin nephropathy in male rat renal carcinogenesis

Essential evidence
- Renal tumours occur only in male rats
- Acute exposure exacerbates hyaline droplet formation
- α_{2u}-Globulin accumulates in hyaline droplets
- Subchronic histopathological changes including granular cast formation and linear papillary mineralization
- Absence of hyaline droplets and characteristic histopathological changes in female rats and mice
- Negative for genotoxicity in a battery of tests

Additional supporting evidence
- Reversible binding of chemical (or metabolites) to α_{2u}-globulin
- Increased and sustained cell proliferation in P_2 segment of proximal tubules in male rat kidneys
- Dose response relationship between hyaline droplet severity and renal tumour incidence

tumours must be male rat-specific. If clear evidence of renal toxicity or an increased incidence of renal tumours are observed in female rats or in other species, these criteria do not apply. Thirdly, the chemical should present with the common histological and biochemical features of α_{2u}-globulin nephropathy, namely the exacerbated formation of hyaline droplets in proximal tubule cells, the development of subchronic renal changes including granular cast formation and linear papillary mineralization, and the absence of similar histological changes in female rats or in other species. It is also essential to show that α_{2u}-globulin accumulates in the kidney and that the chemical (or metabolites) can bind reversibly to α_{2u}-globulin. Data showing that chemical treatment causes sustained increases in renal cell proliferation in the P_2 segment of the proximal tubule are important to link the acute toxicity with tumour development. Lastly, dose-response relationships which characterize toxicity and the carcinogenic outcome should be similar.

In reviewing chemicals listed in Table 1, it is obvious that only a few of the compounds studied meet all these criteria. Those agents for which all criteria have been fulfilled include *d*-limonene, unleaded gasoline, sodium barbital (and its metabolite, diethylacetylurea), 1,4-dichlorobenzene and isophorone. The fact that only a few chemicals meet the described criteria underscores the stringency of the criteria and the breadth of mechanistic evidence that is required to prove this mechanism. Collectively, however, the data supporting these criteria demonstrate a mechanism that is unique to the male rat, a mechanism that is predicated on the unusual features of α_{2u}-globulin, and a mechanism that has no correlate in humans.

References

Alden, C.L., Kanerva, R.L., Ridder, G. & Stone, L.C. (1984) The pathogenesis of the nephrotoxicity of volatile hydrocarbons in the male. In: *Renal Effects of Petroleum Hydrocarbons*. Mehlman, M. A., Hemstreet, C.P., Thorpe, J.J. & Weaver, N.K., eds, *Advances in Modern Environmental Toxicology*, Vol. 7, Princeton Sci. Pub., Princeton, New Jersey, pp. 107–120

Basler, A., von der Hude, W. & Seelbach, A. (1989) Genotoxicity of epoxides. I. Investigations with the SOS Chromotest and the Salmonella/mammalian microsome test. *Mutagenesis*, **4**, 313–314

Blaner, W.S. (1989) Retinol-binding protein: The serum transport protein for vitamin A. *Endocrine Rev.*, **10**, 308–316

Bocskei, Z., Groom, C.R., Flower, D.R., Wright, C.E., Phillips, S.E.V., Cavaggioni, A., Findlay, J.B.C. & North, A.C.T. (1992) Pheromone binding to two rodent urinary proteins revealed by X-ray crystallography. *Nature*, **360**, 186–188

Bomhard, E., Luckhaus, G., Voigt, W.-H. & Loeser, E. (1988) Induction of light hydrocarbon nephropathy by *p*-dichlorobenzene. *Arch. Toxicol.*, **61**, 433–439

Borghoff, S.J. & Lagarde, W.H. (1993) Assessment of binding of 2,4,4-trimethyl-2-pentanol to low molecular weight proteins isolated from kidneys of male rats and humans. *Toxicol. Appl. Pharmacol.*, **119**, 228–235

Borghoff, S.J., Short, B.G. & Swenberg, J.A. (1990) Biochemical mechanisms and pathobiology of α_{2u}-globulin nephropathy. *Annu. Rev. Pharmacol. Toxicol.*, **30**, 349–367

Borghoff, S.J., Miller, A.B., Bowen, J.P. & Swenberg, J.A. (1991) Characteristics of chemical binding to α_{2u}-globulin *in vitro*–evaluating structure activity relationships. *Toxicol. Appl. Pharmacol.*, **107**, 228–238

Brooks, D.E. (1987) The major androgen-regulated secretory proteins of the rat epididymis bear sequence homology with members of the α_{2u}-globulin superfamily. *Biochem. Int.*, **14**, 235–240

Burnett, V.L., Short, B.G. & Swenberg, J.A. (1989) Localization of α_{2u}-globulin within protein droplets of male rat kidney: Immunohistochemistry using perfusion-fixed, GMA-embedded tissue sections. *J. Histochem. Cytochem.*, **37**, 813–818

Carpenter, C.P., Kinkead, E.R., Geary, D.L., Jr, Sullivan, L.J. & King, J.M. (1975) Petroleum hydrocarbon toxicity studies. II. Animal and human response to vapors of varnish makers' and painters' naphtha. *Toxicol. Appl. Pharmacol.*, **32**, 263–281

Charbonneau, M., Lock, E.A., Strasser, J, Cox, M.G., Turner, M.J. & Bus, J.S. (1987) 2,2,4-Trimethylpentane-induced nephrotoxicity. I. Metabolic disposition of TMP in male and female Fischer 344 rats. *Toxicol. Appl. Pharmacol.*, **97**, 171–181

Charbonneau, M., Strasser, J., Lock, E.A., Turner, M.J. & Swenberg, J.A. (1989) Involvement of reversible binding for α_{2u}-globulin in 1,4-dichlorobenzene-induced nephrotoxicity. *Toxicol. Appl. Pharmacol.*, **99**, 122–132

Chatterjee, B., Demyan, W.F., Song, C.S., Garg, B.D. & Roy, A.K. (1989) Loss of androgenic induction of α_{2u}-globulin gene family in the liver of NIH Black rats. *Endocrinology*, **125**, 1385–1388

Cohen, S.M. & Ellwein, L.B. (1990) Cell proliferation in carcinogenesis. *Science*, **249**, 1007–1011

Cowan, S.W., Newcomer, M.E. & Jones, T.A. (1990) Crystallographic refinement of human serum retinol binding protein at 2 Å resolution. *Proteins*, **8**, 44–61

Crowell, P.L. & Gould, M.N. (1994) Chemoprevention and therapy of cancer by *d*-limonene. *Crit. Rev. Oncog.*, **5**, 1–22

Dekant, W., Vamvakas, S. & Anders, M.W. (1989) Bioactivation of nephrotoxic haloalkenes by glutathione conjugation: Formation of toxic and mutagenic intermediates by cysteine conjugate β-lyase. *Drug Metab. Rev.*, **20**, 43–83

Dietrich, D.R. & Swenberg, J.A. (1991a) NCI-Black-Reiter (NBR) male rats fail to develop renal disease following exposure to agents that induce alpha-$_{2u}$-globulin (α_{2u}) nephropathy. *Fund. Appl. Toxicol.*, **16**, 749–762

Dietrich, D.R. & Swenberg, J.A. (1991b) The presence of α_{2u}-globulin is necessary for d-limonene promotion of male rat kidney tumors. *Cancer Res.*, **51**, 3512–3521

Dietrich, D.R. & Swenberg, J.A. (1993) Renal carcinogenesis. In: *Toxicology of the Kidney*, 2nd ed., Hook, J.B. & Goldstein, R.S., eds, *Target Organ Toxicology Series*, Raven Press, Ltd., New York, pp. 495–537

Diwan, B.A., Rice, J.M., Ohshima, M., Ward, J.M. & Dove, L.F. (1985) Comparative tumor promoting activities of phenobarbital, amobarbital, barbital sodium, and barbituric acid on livers and other organs of male F344/NCr rats following initiation with N-nitrosodiethylamine. *J. Natl Cancer Inst.*, **74**, 509–516

Diwan, B. A., Ohshima, M. & Rice, J.M. (1989a) Promotion by sodium barbital of renal cortical and transitional cell tumors, but not intestinal tumors, in F344 rats given methyl (acetoxymethyl)nitrosamine, and lack of effect of phenobarbital, amobarbital, or barbituric acid on development of either renal or intestinal tumors. *Carcinogenesis*, **10**, 183–188

Diwan, B.A., Nims, R.W., Ward, J.M., Hu, H., Lubet, R.A. & Rice, J. M. (1989b) Tumor promoting activities of ethylphenylacetylurea and diethylacetylurea, the ring hydrolysis products of barbiturate tumor promoters phenobarbital and barbital, in rat liver and kidney initiated by N-nitrosodiethylamine. *Carcinogenesis*, **10**, 189–194

Dominick, M.A., Robertson, D.G., Bleavins, M.R., Sigler, R.E., Bobrowski, W.F. & Gough, A.W. (1991) α_{2u}-Globulin nephropathy without nephrocarcinogenesis in male Wistar rats administered 1-(aminomethyl)cyclohexaneacetic acid. *Toxicol. Appl. Pharmacol.*, **111**, 375–387

Drayna, D.T., McLean, J.W., Wion, K.L., Trent, J.M., Drabkin, H.A. & Lawn, R.M. (1987) Human apolipoprotein D gene: Gene sequence, chromosome localization, and homology to the α_{2u}-globulin superfamily. *DNA*, **6**, 199–204

Elegbede, J.A., Elson, C.E., Tanner, M.A., Qureshi, A. & Gould, M.N. (1986) Regression of rat primary mammary tumors following dietary d-limonene exposure. *J. Natl Cancer Inst.*, **76**, 323–325

Elson, C.E., Maltzman, T.H., Boston, J.L., Tanner, M.A. & Gould, M.N. (1988) Anti-carcinogenic activity of *d*-limonene during inititation and promotion/progression stages of DMBA-induced rat mammary carcinogenesis. *Carcinogenesis*, **9**, 331–332

Finlayson, J.S., Potter, M. & Runner, C.R. (1963) Electrophoretic variation and sex dimorphism of the major urinary protein complex in inbred mice: A new genetic marker. *J. Natl Cancer Inst.*, **31**, 91–107

Flamm, W.G. & Lehman-McKeeman, L.D. (1991) The human relevance of the renal tumor-inducing potential of *d*-limonene in male rats: Implications for risk assessment. *Reg. Toxicol. Pharmacol.*, **13**, 70–86

Flower, D. R. (1994) The lipocalin protein family: A role in cell regulation. *FEBS Lett.*, **354**, 7–11

Flower, D.R., North, A.C. & Attwood, T.K. (1993) Structure and sequence relationships in the lipocalins and related proteins. *Protein Sci.*, **2**, 753–761

Ganguly, M., Carnighan, R.H. & Westphal, U. (1967) Steroid protein interactions. XIV. Interaction between human α1-acid glycoprotein and progesterone. *Biochemistry*, **6**, 2803–2814

Garg, B.D., Olson, M.J., Li, L.C. & Roy, A.K. (1989) Phagolysosomal alterations induced by unleaded gasoline in epithelial cells of the proximal convoluted tubules of male rats: Effect of dose and treatment duration. *J. Toxicol Environ. Health*, **26**, 101–118

Gaworski, C.L., Haun, C.C., MacEwen, J.D., Vernot, E.H., Bruner, R.H., Amster, R.L. & Cowan, M.J., Jr (1985) A 90-day vapor inhalation toxicity study of decalin. *Fund. Appl. Toxicol.*, **5**, 785–793

Godovac-Zimmerman, J. (1988) The structural motif of β-lactoglobulin and retinol-binding protein: A basic framework for binding and transport of small hydrophobic molecules? *Trends Biochem. Sci.*, **13**, 64–66

Grasso, P. (1987) Persistent organ damage and cancer production in rats and mice. *Arch. Toxicol.*, Suppl. 11, 75–83

Hard, G.C. (1984) High frequency, single-dose model of renal adenoma/carcinoma induction using dimethylnitrosamine in Crl: (W)BR rats. *Carcinogenesis*, **5**, 1047–1050

Hard, G. C. (1987) Chemically induced epithelial tumours and carcinogenesis of the renal parenchyma. In: *Nephrotoxicity in the Experimental and Clinical Situation. Part 1*, Bach, P.H. & Lock, E.A., eds, *Developments in Nephrology*, Martinus Nighoff Publishers, Boston, MA, pp. 211–250

Hard, G.C. & Whysner, J. (1994) Risk assessment of *d*-limonene: An example of male rat-specific renal tumorigens. *Crit. Rev. Toxicol.*, **24**, 231–254

Hard, G.C., Rodgers, I.S., Baetcke, K.P., Richards, W.L., McGaughy, R.E. & Valcovic, L.R. (1993) Hazard evaluation of chemicals that cause α_{2u}-globulin, hyaline droplet nephropathy, and tubule neoplasia in the kidneys of male rats. *Environ. Health Perspect.*, **99**, 313–349

Hastie, N.D., Held, W.A. & Toole, J.J. (1979) Multiple genes coding for the androgen-regulated major urinary proteins of the mouse. *Cell*, **17**, 449–457

von der Hude, W., Basler, A., Mateblowski, R. & Obe, G. (1989) Genotoxicity of epoxides. II. *In vitro* investigations with the sister-chromatid exchange (SCE) test and the unscheduled DNA synthesis (UDS) test. *Mutagenesis*, **4**, 323–324

Huff, J. (1996) Response: α_{2u}-globulin nephropathy, posed mechanisms and white ravens. *Environ. Health Perspect.*, **104**, 1264–1267

Kimura, H., Odani, S., Suzuki, J.-I., Arakawa, M. & Ono, T. (1989) Kidney fatty acid-binding protein: Identification as α_{2u}-globulin. *FEBS Lett.*, **246**, 101–104

Kitchen, D.N. (1984) Neoplastic renal effects of unleaded gasoline in Fischer 344 rats. In: *Renal Effects of Petroleum Hydrocarbons*, Mehlman, M.A., Hemstreet, C.P., Thorpe, J.J. & Weaver, N.K., eds, *Advances in Modern Environmental Toxicology*, Vol. 7, Princeton Scientific Publishers, Inc., Princeton, New Jersey, pp. 65–71

Knopf, J.L., Gallagher, J.F. & Held, W.A. (1983) Differential, multihormonal regulation of the mouse major urinary protein gene family in the liver. *Mol. Cell Biol.*, **3**, 2232–2240

Kretchmer, N. & Bernstein, J. (1974) The dynamic morphology of the nephron: Morphogenesis of the 'protein droplet'. *Kidney Int.*, **5**, 96–105

Kurata, Y., Diwan, B.A., Lehman-McKeeman, L.D., Rice, J.M. & Ward, J.M. (1994) Comparative hyaline droplet nephropathy in male F344/NCr rats induced by sodium barbital and diacetylurea, a breakdown product of sodium barbital. *Toxicol. Appl. Pharmacol.*, **126**, 224–232

Kurtz, D.T. (1981) Rat α_{2u}-globulin is encoded by a multigene family. *J. Mol. Appl. Gen.*, **1**, 29–38

Kurtz, D.T. & Feigelson, P. (1978) Multihormonal control of the messenger RNA for the hepatic protein globulin. In: *Biochemical Actions of Hormones*, Vol. V, Litwack, G., ed., Academic Press, New York, pp. 433–455

Kurtz, D.T., Sippel, A.E. & Feigelson, P. (1976a) Effect of thyroid hormones on the level of the hepatic mRNA for α_{2u}-globulin. *Biochemistry*, **15**, 1031–1036

Kurtz, D.T., Sippel, A.E., Ansah-Yiadom, R. & Feigelson, P. (1976b) Effects of sex hormones on the level of messenger RNA for the rat hepatic protein α_{2u}-globulin. *J. Biol. Chem.*, **251**, 3594–3598

Kurtz, D., Chan, K.-M. & Feigelson, P. (1978a) Translational control of hepatic α_{2u}-globulin synthesis by growth hormone. *Cell*, **15**, 743–750

Kurtz, D.T., Chan, K.-M. & Fiegelson, P. (1978b) Glucocorticoid induction of hepatic α_{2u}-globulin synthesis and messenger RNA level in castrated male rats *in vivo*. *J. Biol. Chem.*, **253**, 7886–7890

Lake, B.G., Cunninghame, M.E. & Price, R.J. (1997) Comparison of the hepatic and renal effects of 1,4-dichlorobenzene in the rat and mouse. *Fund. Appl. Toxicol.*, **39**, 67–75

Larsen, G.L., Bergman, A. & Klasson-Wehler, A. (1990) A methylsulphonyl metabolite of a polychlorinated biphenyl can serve as a ligand for α_{2u}-globulin in rat and major urinary protein in mice. *Xenobiotica*, **20**, 1343–1352

Lehman-McKeeman, L.D. (1993) Light hydrocarbon nephropathy. In: *Toxicology of the Kidney*, Hook, J.B. & Goldstein, R.S., eds, Raven Press, Ltd., New York, pp. 477–494

Lehman-McKeeman, L.D. (1995) Dose-response relationships for male rat specific α_{2u}-globulin nephropathy and renal carcinogenesis. In: *Monograph of the Cancer Dose Response Working Group*, ILSI Press, Lyons, France, pp. 175–183

Lehman-McKeeman, L.D. (1997) α_{2u}-Globulin nephropathy. In: *Renal Toxicology*, Sipes, I.G., McQueen, C.A. & Gandolfi, A.J., eds, *Comprehensive Toxicology*, Vol. 7, Pergamon Press, New York, pp. 677–692

Lehman-McKeeman, L.D. & Caudill, D. (1991) Quantitation of urinary α_{2u}-globulin and albumin by reverse-phase high performance liquid chromatography. *J. Pharmacol. Meth.*, **26**, 239–247

Lehman-McKeeman, L.D. & Caudill, D. (1992a) Biochemical basis for mouse resistance to hyaline droplet nephropathy: Lack of relevance of the α_{2u}-globulin protein superfamily in this male rat-specific syndrome. *Toxicol. Appl. Pharmacol.*, **112**, 214–221

Lehman-McKeeman, L.D. & Caudill, D. (1992b) α_{2u}-Globulin is the only member of the lipocalin protein superfamily that binds to hyaline droplet inducing agents. *Toxicol. Appl. Pharmacol.*, **116**, 170–176

Lehman-McKeeman, L.D. & Caudill, D. (1994) *d*-Limonene-induced hyaline droplet nephropathy in α_{2u}-globulin transgenic mice. *Fund. Appl. Toxicol.*, **23**, 562–568

Lehman-McKeeman, L.D., Rodriguez, P.A., Takigiku, R., Caudill, D. & Fey, M.L. (1989) *d*-Limonene-induced male rat-specific nephrotoxicity: Evaluation of the association between *d*-Limonene and α_{2u}-globulin. *Toxicol. Appl. Pharmacol.*, 99, 250–259

Lehman-McKeeman, L.D., Rivera-Torres, M.I. & Caudill, D. (1990) Lysosomal degradation of α_{2u}-globulin and α_{2u}-globulin-xenobiotic conjugates. *Toxicol. Appl. Pharmacol.*, 103, 539–548

Lehman-McKeeman, L.D., Rodriguez, P.A., Caudill, D., Fey, M.L., Eddy, C.L. & Asquith, T.N. (1991) Hyaline droplet nephropathy resulting from exposure to 3,5,5-trimethyl hexanoyloxybenzene sulfonate. *Toxicol. Appl. Pharmacol.*, 107, 429–438

Lehman-McKeeman, L.D., Caudill, D., Rodriguez, P.A. & Eddy, C. (1998) 2-sec-Butyl-4,5-dihydrothiazole is a ligand for mouse urinary protein and rat α_{2u}-globulin: Physiological and toxicological relevance. *Toxicol. Appl. Pharmacol.*, 149, 32–40

Liebich, H.M., Zlatkis, A., Bertsch, W., Van Dahm, R. & Whitten,W.K. (1977) Identification of dihydrothiazoles in urine of male mice. *Biomed. Mass Spectrom.*, 4, 69–72

Lock, E.A. (1989) Mechanism of nephrotoxic action due to organohalogenated compounds. *Toxicol. Lett.*, 49, 93–106

Lock, E.A., Charbonneau, M., Strasser, J., Swenberg, J.A. & Bus, J.S. (1987) 2,2,4-Trimethylpentane-induced nephrotoxicity. II. The reversible binding of a TMP metabolite to a renal protein fraction containing α_{2u}-globulin. *Toxicol. Appl. Pharmacol.*, 91, 182–192

Maack, T., Johnson, V., Kau, S.T., Figueiredo, J. & Sigulem, D. (1979) Renal filtration, transport and metabolism of low-molecular-weight proteins: A review. *Kidney Int.*, 16, 251–270

MacInnes, J.I., Nozik, E.S. & Kurtz, D.T. (1986) Tissue-specific expression of the rat α_{2u}-globulin gene family. *Mol. Cell. Biol.*, 6, 3563–3567

Mancini, M.A., Majumdar, D., Chartterjee, B. & Roy, A.K. (1989) α_{2u}-Globulin in modified sebaceous glands with pheromonal functions: Localization of the protein and its mRNA in preputial, meibomian and perianal glands. *J. Histochem. Cytochem.*, 37, 149–157

Mattie, D.R., Alden, C.L., Newell, T.K., Gaworski, C.L. & Flemming, C.D. (1991) A 90-day continuous vapor inhalation toxicity study of JP-8 jet fuel followed by 20 or 21 months of recovery in Fischer 344 rats and C57BL/6 mice. *Toxicol. Pathol.*, 19, 77–87

Maunsbach, A.B. (1966) Electron microscopic observations of cytoplasmic bodies with crystalline patterns in rat kidney proximal tubule cells. *J. Ultrastruct. Res.*, 14, 167–196

Melnick, R.L. (1992) An alternative hypothesis on the role of chemically induced protein droplet (α_{2u}-globulin) nephropathy in renal carcinogenesis. *Reg. Toxicol. Pharmacol.*, 16, 111–125

Murty, C.V.R., Sarkar, F.H., Mancini, M.A. & Roy, A.K. (1987) Sex-independent synthesis of α_{2u}-globulin and its messenger ribonucleic acid in the rat preputial gland: Biochemical and immunocytochemical analyses. *Endocrinology*, 121, 1000–1005

Neuhaus, O.W. (1986) Renal reabsorption of low molecular weight proteins in adult male rats: α_{2u}-Globulin. *Proc. Soc. Exp. Biol. Med.*, 182, 531–539

Neuhaus, O., Flory, W., Biswas, N. & Hollerman, C.E. (1981) Urinary excretion of α_{2u}-globulin and albumin by adult male rats following treatment with nephrotoxic agents. *Nephron*, 28, 133–140

Papiz, M.Z., Sawyer, L., Eliopoulos, E.E., North, A.C.T., Findlay, J.B.C., Sivaprasadarao, R., Jones, T.A., Newcomer, M.E. & Kraulis, P.J. (1986) The structure of β-lactoglobulin and its similarity to plasma retinol-binding protein. *Nature*, 324, 383–385

Pevsner, J., Hou, V., Snowman, A.M. & Snyder, S.H. (1990) Odorant-binding protein: Characterization of ligand binding. *J. Biol. Chem.*, 265, 6118–6125

Roy, A.K. & Neuhaus, O.W. (1966) Proof of the hepatic synthesis of a sex-dependent protein in the rat. *Biochim. Biophys. Acta*, 127, 82–87

Roy, A.K. & Neuhaus, O.W. (1967) Androgenic control of a sex-dependent protein in the rat. *Nature*, 214, 618–620

Roy, A.K., Neuhaus, O.W. & Harmison, C.R. (1966) Preparation and characterization of a sex-dependent rat urinary protein. *Biochim. Biophys. Acta*, 127, 72–81

Roy, A.K., McMinn, D.M. & Biswas, N.M. (1975) Estrogenic inhibition of the hepatic synthesis of α_{2u}-globulin in the rat. *Endocrinology*, 97, 1501–1508

Roy, A.K., Byrd, J.G., Biswas, N.M. & Chowdhury, A.K. (1976) Protection of spermatogenesis by α_{2u}-globulin in rats treated with oestrogen. *Nature*, 260, 719–721

Roy, A.K., Chatterjee, B., Prasad, M.S.K. & Unakar, N. (1980) Role of insulin in the regulation of the hepatic messenger RNA for α_{2u}-globulin in diabetic rats. *J. Biol. Chem.*, 255, 11614–11618

Roy, A.K., Nath, T.S., Motwani, N.M. & Chatterjee, B. (1983) Age-dependent regulation of the polymorphic forms of α_{2u}-globulin. *J. Biol. Chem.*, 258, 10123–10127

Rumke, P.H. & Thung, P.J. (1964) Immunological studies on the sex-dependent prealbumin in mouse urine and its occurrence in the serum. *Acta. Endocrinol.*, 47, 156–164

Saito, K., Uwagawa, S., Kaneko, H. & Yoshitake, A. (1991) Behavior of α_{2u}-globulin accumulating in kidneys of male rats treated with *d*-limonene: Kidney-type α_{2u}-globulin in the urine as a marker of *d*-limonene nephropathy. *Toxicology*, **70**, 173–183

Shaw, P.H., Held, W.A. & Hastie, N.D. (1983) The gene family for major urinary proteins: Expresson in several secretory tissues of the mouse. *Cell*, **32**, 755–761

Short, B.G., Burnett, V.L. & Swenberg, J.A. (1986) Histopathology and cell proliferation induced by 2,2,4-trimethylpentane in the male rat kidney. *Toxicol. Pathol.*, **14**, 194–203

Short, B.G., Burnett, V.L., Cox, M.G., Bus, J.S. & Swenberg, J.A. (1987) Site-specific renal cytotoxicity and cell proliferation in male rats exposed to petroleum hydrocarbons. *Lab. Invest.*, **57**, 564–577

Short, B.G., Burnett, V.L. & Swenberg, J.A. (1989a) Elevated proliferation of proximal tubule cells and localization of accumulated α_{2u}-globulin in F344 rats during chronic exposure to unleaded gasoline or 2,2,4-trimethylpentane. *Toxicol. Appl. Pharmacol.*, **101**, 414–431

Short, B.G., Steinhagen, W.H. & Swenberg, J.A. (1989b) Promoting effects of unleaded gasoline and 2,4,4-trimethylpentane on the development of atypical cell foci and renal tubular cell tumors in rats exposed to *N*-ethyl-*N*-hydroxyethylnitrosamine. *Cancer Res.*, **49**, 6369–6378

Sippel, A.E., Kurtz, D.T., Morris, H.P. & Feigelson, P. (1976) Comparison of *in vivo* translational rates and messenger RNA levels of α_{2u}-globulin in rat liver and Morris hepatoma 5123D. *Cancer Res.*, **36**, 3588–3593

Stone, L.C., Kanerva, R.L., Burns, J.L. & Alden, C.L. (1987) Decalin-induced nephrotoxicity: Light and electron microscopic examination of the effects of oral dosing on the development of kidney lesions in the rat. *Food. Chem. Toxicol.*, **25**, 43–52

Swenberg, J.A. (1993) α_{2u}-Globulin nephropathy: Review of the cellular and molecular mechanisms involved and their implications for human risk assessment. *Environ. Health Perspect.*, **101** (Suppl. 6), 39–44

Swenberg, J.A., Short, B.G., Borghoff, S.J., Strasser, J. & Charbonneau, M. (1989) The comparative pathobiology of α_{2u}-globulin nephropathy. *Toxicol. Appl. Pharmacol.*, **97**, 35–46

Trump, B.F., Lipsky, M.M., Jones, T.W., Heatfield, B.M., Higgonson, J., Endicott, K. & Hess, H.B. (1984) An evaluation of the significance of experimental hydrocarbon toxicity to man. In: *Renal Effects of Petroleum Hydrocarbons*. Vol. 7, Mehlman, M.A., Hemstreet, C.P., Thorpe, J.J. & Weaver, N.K., eds, *Advances in Modern Environmental Toxicology*, Princeton Scientific, Princeton, New Jersey, pp. 273–288

Umemura, T., Tokumo, K. & Williams, G.M. (1992) Cell proliferation induced in the kidneys and livers of rats and mice by short term exposure to the carcinogen p-dichlorobenzene. *Arch. Toxicol.*, **66**, 503–507

Urien, S., Albengres, E., Zini, R. & Tillement, J.-P. (1982) Evidence for binding of certain acidic drugs to α1-acid glycoprotein. *Biochem. Pharmacol.*, **31**, 3687–3689

US Environmental Protection Agency (1991) α_{2u}-Globulin: Association with chemically induced renal toxicity and neoplasia in the male rat. *Risk Assessment Forum*. EPA/625/3-91/019F

US National Institute of Environmental Health Sciences (1996) Tumor incidence in control animals by route and vehicle of administration. F344/N rats. Contract #N01-ES-65401, Analytical Sciences, Inc., Durham, NC

US National Toxicology Program (NTP) (1983) *Carcinogenesis Bioassay of Pentachloroethane in F-344/N Rats and B6C3F1 Mice (Gavage Study)* (NTP Technical Report No. 232), U.S. Department of Health and Human Services, Public Health Service, National Institutes of Health, Bethesda, MD

US National Toxicology Program (1986a) *Toxicology and Carcinogenesis Studies of Isophorone in F344/N rats and B6C3F1 Mice (Gavage Study)* (NTP Technical Report No. 291), US Department of Health and Human Services, Public Health Service, National Institutes of Health, Research Triangle Park, NC

US National Toxicology Program (1986b) *Carcinogenesis Bioassay of Tetrachloroethylene (Perchloroethylene) in F344/N rats and B6C3F1 Mice (Inhalation Study)* (NTP Technical Report No. 311), U.S. Department of Health and Human Services, Public Health Service, National Institutes of Health, Bethesda, MD

US National Toxicology Program (NTP) (1987a) *Toxicology and Carcinogenesis Studies of 1,4-Dichlorobenzene in F344/N Rats and B6C3F1 Mice* (NTP Technical Report No. 319), U.S. Department of Health and Human Services, Public Health Service, National Institutes of Health, Bethesda, MD

US National Toxicology Program (NTP) (1987b) *Carcinogenesis Studies of Dimethyl Methylphosphonate in F344/N Rats and B6C3F1 Mice (Gavage Study)* (NTP Technical Report No. 323), U.S. Department of Health and Human Services, Public Health Service, National Institutes of Health, Bethesda, MD

US National Toxicology Program (1990) *Toxicology and Carcinogenesis Studies of d-Limonene in F344/N Rats and B6C3F1 Mice (Gavage Studies)* (NTP Technical Report No. 347), U.S. Department of Health and Human Services, Public Health Service, National Institutes of Health, Bethesda, MD

Ward, J.M., Weghorst, C.W., Diwan, B.A., Konishi, N., Lubet, R.A., Henneman, J.R. & Devor, D.E. (1991) Evaluation of cell proliferation in the kidneys of rodents with bromodeoxyuridine immunohisto-chemistry or tritiated thymidine autoradiography after exposure to renal toxins, tumor promoters and carcinogens. Butterworth, B.E., Slaga, T.J., Farland, W. and McClain, M., eds, *Chemically Induced Cell Proliferation: Implications for Risk Assessment*, Wiley-Liss, New York, pp. 369–388

Watabe, T., Hiratsuka, A., Isobe, M. & Ozawa, N. (1980) Metabolism of d-limonene by hepatic microsomes to non-mutagenic epoxides toward Salmonella typhi-murium. *Biochem. Pharmacol.*, **29**, 1068–1071

Watabe, T., Hiratsuka, A., Ozawa, N. & Isobe, M. (1981) A comparative study on the metabolism of *d*-limonene and 4-vinylcyclohex-1-ene by hepatic microsomes. *Xenobiotica*, **11**, 333–344

Webb, D.R., Kanerva, R.L., Hysell, D.K., Alden, C.L. & Lehman-McKeeman, L.D. (1990) Assessment of the sub-chronic oral toxicity of *d*-limonene in dogs. *Food. Chem. Toxicol.*, **28**, 669–675

Williams, G.M. & Whysner, J. (1996) Epigenetic carcino-gens: Evaluation and risk assessment. *Exp. Toxicol. Pathol.*, **48**, 189–195

Corresponding authors

J.A. Swenberg
Department of Environmental Sciences and Engineering and Pathology, University of North Carolina, Chapel Hill, NC, USA

L.D. Lehman-McKeeman
Human and Environmental Safety Division Miami Valley Laboratories, Procter and Gamble Co., Cincinnati, OH, USA

Species Differences in Thyroid, Kidney and Urinary Bladder Carcinogenesis
C. C. Capen, E. Dybing, J.M. Rice and J.D Wilbourn, eds
IARC Scientific Publications No. 147
International Agency for Research on Cancer, Lyon, 1999

Possible mechanisms of induction of renal tubule cell neoplasms in rats associated with α_{2u}-globulin: role of protein accumulation versus ligand delivery to the kidney

R. L. Melnick and M. C. Kohn

Introduction

In 1991, the US Environmental Protection Agency (EPA) adopted the view that when kidney tumours are induced in male rats, but not in female rats, and α_{2u}-globulin accumulation is also observed in the kidney, the kidney tumour response may not be applicable to human risk assessment (USEPA, 1991). Three criteria were established by EPA for examining evidence linking α_{2u}-globulin accumulation with the tumour response, namely:

(1) increased number and size of hyaline droplets in renal proximal tubule cells of treated male rats,
(2) identification of the accumulating protein in the hyaline droplets as α_{2u}-globulin, and
(3) presence of additional aspects of the pathological sequence of lesions associated with α_{2u}-globulin nephropathy (single cell necrosis, exfoliation of epithelial cell into the proximal tubule lumen, formation of granular casts, linear mineralization of papillary tubules, and tubule hyperplasia).

Additional information to be considered includes reversible binding of ligand to α_{2u}-globulin, decreased lysosomal degradation of α_{2u}-globulin, and sustained cell proliferation in the P_2 segment of the proximal tubule of male rats at doses that induce renal neoplasms. However, demonstration of the latter factors was not necessary, even though they are more mechanistically linked to the α_{2u}-globulin hypothesis. The EPA specifies that if experimental data do not meet the criteria in any one of the three categories listed above, the α_{2u}-globulin process alone is not considered to be responsible and the kidney tumour response may be used for both hazard identification and quantitative risk estimation. If experimental data reasonably fulfil these criteria but some tumours are attributable to other carcinogenic processes, the EPA's cancer risk assessment policy is to include the tumour response for hazard identification but to engage in quantitative risk estimation only if the non-α_{2u}-globulin potency can be estimated. If the tumour response is *solely* attributable to α_{2u}-globulin nephropathy, the EPA does not use that response in human hazard identification or quantitative risk estimation. In several cases, much debate has ensued on the applicability of these criteria and about the α_{2u}-globulin hypothesis for evaluation of human cancer risk (Huff, 1996; Dietrich, 1997; Melnick *et al.*, 1997).

A previous review of this topic (Melnick, 1992) identified several inconsistencies and important data gaps in the hypothesis linking α_{2u}-globulin nephropathy to the induction of kidney tumours in male rats and demonstrated how alternative hypotheses based on the same available information are plausible. Thus the mechanisms of chemically induced α_{2u}-globulin nephropathy and chemically induced renal cancer remain at the level of operational hypotheses.

When generalized classification schemes cannot accommodate wide variations in response to various toxicants or when quantitative relationships between the supposed early-stage carcinogenic events and cancer outcome cannot be established, then use of hypothetical schemes may result in excessive reliance on preconceived notions rather than on data from definitive experiments.

The purpose of the previous review (Melnick, 1992) was to stimulate further research that would lead to a better understanding of the mechanisms involved in chemically induced renal carcinogenesis. Research findings that address assumptions in mechanistic hypotheses of chemical carcinogenesis can be valuable in reducing uncertainties in predictions of human risk and lead to improved scientifically based public health decisions. Unfortunately, little progress has been made on some of the fundamental issues that were previously raised. It seems that the creation of imprecisely formulated classification systems based on mechanistic assumptions and qualitative correlations of response stifles the advancement of basic science. Thus in several studies of chemical induction of kidney tumours in male rats, research goals appear to have been focused more on showing that criteria for dismissing positive animal findings had been reached than on improving our understanding of the quantitative relationships in the biological processes leading to the carcinogenic effect.

The development of public health policies for judging the relevance of animal findings in evaluations of human hazard potential demands rigorous and objective scrutiny of the strengths and weaknesses of hypotheses, especially when decisions based on such hypothesis may contribute to widespread exposure to chemicals that would otherwise be restricted. This is particularly important for kidney carcinogens, since the incidence of human kidney cancer (in the USA) has increased by 30% between 1973 and 1989 (Miller et al., 1992), and the incidence is higher in males than in females, both in humans (Miller et al., 1992) and in animals (Barrett & Huff, 1991). Instructive in this respect are reports of increased kidney cancer risk associated with human exposure to gasoline vapours (Siemiatycki et al., 1987; Partanen et al., 1991; Lynge et al., 1997), while animal exposure to totally vaporized unleaded gasoline is associated with the induction of α_{2u}-globulin nephropathy and kidney tumours in male rats (MacFarland et al., 1984; Short et al., 1987, 1989a, 1989b; Gérin et al., 1991). Because of changes in the composition of hydrocarbons and additives in gasoline over the past 50 years (e.g.,

benzene, tetraethyl lead) and differences in the composition of gasoline vapour exposures and totally vaporized gasoline (Halder et al., 1986), it is likely that the animal and human exposures differed significantly; however, the results of these studies indicate that some constituents of gasoline increase the incidence of kidney cancer in animals and in humans.

The extent and quality of data for individual chemicals that induce α_{2u}-globulin nephropathy and kidney cancer varies greatly. Consequently, Swenberg (1993) cautioned that "this necessitates a case-by-case analysis of the available data when determining the relevance for humans of this chemically induced renal disease in male rats." This paper examines reported relationships between exposure to chemicals that cause α_{2u}-globulin accumulation in the kidneys of male rats and the induction of renal tubule cell neoplasms.

The α_{2u}-globulin hypothesis

The hypothesis on the role of α_{2u}-globulin in chemical induction of kidney cancer was developed based on the observation that protein droplets containing α_{2u}-globulin accumulate in epithelial cells of the proximal convoluted tubules of male rats exposed to hydrocarbons that had been reported to cause kidney cancer in male rats after long-term exposure. α_{2u}-Globulin is a protein of low molecular weight (18.7 kDa) synthesized in the liver of mature male rats under androgenic control (Roy & Neuhaus, 1967). It is not synthesized by hepatocytes of female rats, mice of either sex, or several other species including humans. Hydrocarbons or their metabolites that bind reversibly to α_{2u}-globulin do not appear to cause an increase in the hepatic concentration of this protein (Viau et al., 1986; Olson et al., 1987; Murty et al., 1988).

α_{2u}-Globulin is secreted into the blood, filtered through the glomerulus, and partially reabsorbed (~60%) by endocytosis into renal tubule epithelial cells of the P_2 segment (Neuhaus et al., 1981). The unabsorbed fraction is excreted in the urine, while the reabsorbed portion is presumably hydrolysed to amino acids after fusion of endocytotic vesicles with epithelial cell lysosomes. The accumulation of protein droplets containing α_{2u}-globulin was suggested to be due to reversible binding of xenobiotic ligands to this protein, rendering it more resistant to proteolytic degradation by lysosomal enzymes (Swenberg et al., 1989; Lehman-McKeeman et al., 1990). Binding is considered to be critical for α_{2u}-globulin accumulation; however, since binding affinities for various ligands have been reported to vary by more than three orders of magnitude (1.8 x 10^{-7} to 5.2 x 10^{-4} M), other factors were suggested to be involved in α_{2u}-globulin accumulation (Borghoff et al., 1991). In vitro studies of lysosomal degradation of α_{2u}-globulin purified from the urine of control male rats showed a 24–33% decrease in the rate of degradation when the protein was incubated with excess amounts of ligands that cause α_{2u}-globulin accumulation in the male rat kidney (Lehman-McKeeman et al., 1990).

Proteolytic processing of α_{2u}-globulin during its resorption into renal proximal tubules results in the accumulation of a kidney-type α_{2u}-globulin (α_{2u}-K; 17 kDa), which was identified as a kidney fatty acid-binding protein (Kimura et al., 1989; Uchida et al., 1995). Proteolytic processing at the brush border membrane appears to precede the endocytotic uptake of this protein. Treatment of male rats with agents that cause α_{2u}-globulin accumulation results in large increases in α_{2u}-K in the male rat kidney (Saito et al., 1992). The major form of the protein excreted in the urine of control rats is the native type (18.7 kDa), whereas in the urine of rats treated with chemicals that induce α_{2u}-globulin accumulation, dose-dependent increases in α_{2u}-K excretion have been observed (Saito et al., 1996).

The excessive accumulation of α_{2u}-globulin is hypothesized to cause lysosomal dysfunction, resulting in cell killing (Swenberg et al., 1989). The actual cause of cell death is not known. Sloughing of necrotic epithelial cells into the tubule lumen has been observed and intratubular granular casts of necrotic cellular debris accumulate at the junction of the P_3 segment of the proximal tubule and the thin loop of Henle. Regenerative proliferation of epithelial cells in the P_2 segment occurs in response to the cell loss (Short et al., 1987, 1989a; Dietrich & Swenberg, 1991a).

Although the mechanistic link between cell proliferation and kidney cancer is unknown, it has been suggested that regenerative hyperplasia causes the tumorigenic response in the male rat kidney by increasing the likelihood of fixing presumed spontaneous cancer-initiating DNA damage into heritable mutations or by promoting the clonal expansion of spontaneously initiated cells (Short et al., 1989b; Dietrich & Swenberg, 1991a). In support of this hypothesis, neither protein droplet nephropathy nor increases in renal tumours have been observed in female rats or in mice of either sex exposed to chemicals that induce α_{2u}-globulin accumulation in the kidneys of male rats. Further, protein droplet nephropathy was not induced in NIH-Black-Reiter (NBR) rats (Dietrich & Swenberg, 1991b), a strain that is deficient in hepatic α_{2u}-globulin synthesis. However, no two-year carcinogenicity study in NBR rats has been reported and renal tumours induced by these chemicals in male rats have not been analysed for genetic alterations.

Changes in renal α_{2u}-globulin levels and relationships to kidney cancer
Unleaded gasoline
Two-year inhalation studies of unleaded gasoline, at exposure concentrations of 0, 67, 292 and 2056 ppm, resulted in dose-related increased incidences of kidney tumours in male Fischer 344 rats (0, 2, 9 and 16%, respectively) and liver tumours in female B6C3F$_1$ mice (MacFarland et al., 1984). The kidney findings are particularly noteworthy, because renal tubule cell neoplasms are uncommon in untreated male Fischer 344 rats, occurring at a rate of approximately 0.6% (Solleveld et al., 1984).

Halder et al. (1985) examined the toxicity of 15 hydrocarbon compounds found in unleaded gasoline, and concluded that the nephrotoxicity of gasoline was due primarily to the alkane components, and that the nephrotoxic potency of these compounds increased with the degree of alkane branching. Consequently, 2,2,4-trimethylpentane (TMP), one of the most active nephrotoxic components in this mixture, has been used as a model compound to study the mechanism of renal toxicity induced by unleaded gasoline. In male Fischer 344 rats treated with TMP for three weeks, the dose–response curve for renal protein droplet accumulation correlated with that for increased replication of epithelial cells in the P_2 segment of renal proximal tubules (Short et al., 1987).

A similar dose-dependence was observed for the kidney tumour response in male Fischer 344 rats exposed to unleaded gasoline for two years and for the increased replication rates of P_2 epithelial cells after three weeks of inhalation exposure to unleaded gasoline (Short *et al.*, 1987). An enhanced rate of cell proliferation (4–11-fold) in the P_2 segment has been observed through 48 weeks of exposure of male Fischer 344 rats to 300 ppm unleaded gasoline (Short *et al.*, 1989a). Enhanced cell proliferation (4–8-fold) was also observed in P_3 epithelial cells through 22 weeks of exposure to 300 ppm unleaded gasoline. Because no increase in cell replication was seen in the kidney of female rats at any time point, it was hypothesized that chronic cell proliferation associated with α_{2u}-globulin nephropathy may be responsible for the apparent sex- and species-specificity of the kidney carcinogenic effects of unleaded gasoline in laboratory animals. However, as noted above, elevated risk of kidney cancer associated with human exposure to gasoline vapours has been reported, so it cannot be stated that the carcinogenic effects of complex gasoline mixtures are entirely species-specific.

Selected intermediates of TMP metabolism were administered to male Fischer 344 rats, and kidney sections were examined for evidence of α_{2u}-globulin accumulation (Charbonneau *et al.*, 1987a). All chemicals studied, including the carboxylic acid metabolites of TMP (Charbonneau *et al.*, 1987b), which do not bind to α_{2u}-globulin, caused accumulation of α_{2u}-globulin. This observation suggests that binding to α_{2u}-globulin may not be the only process associated with TMP-induced renal accumulation of this protein.

2,4,4-Trimethyl-2-pentanol (TMP-2-OH) was the major metabolite of TMP detected in the male rat kidney and was associated with an increase in the renal concentration of α_{2u}-globulin; this metabolite was not detected in the female rat kidney (Charbonneau *et al.*, 1987b). TMP-2-OH has a high binding affinity for α_{2u}-globulin ($K_d = 0.2 \mu M$; Borghoff *et al.*, 1991). The reason for the sex differences in urinary metabolite profiles and in the renal distribution of TMP-2-OH may be important in understanding sex or species differences in the induction of renal nephropathy by TMP. Charbonneau *et al.* (1987b) also presented data on the kidney concentrations of α_{2u}-globulin and of TMP-equivalents in male Fischer 344 rats at 24 hours after treatment with [^{14}C]TMP by gavage. At doses of TMP that elicited accumulation of α_{2u}-globulin, the renal molar concentrations of α_{2u}-globulin were substantially higher than the renal molar concentrations of radiolabelled TMP equivalents. For example, as the dose of TMP was increased from 5 to 50 mg/kg body weight, the increase in renal α_{2u}-globulin was 3.5 times greater than the increase in TMP equivalents. Thus, at a dose of TMP (50 mg/kg) that has been shown to induce severe protein droplet nephropathy and high levels of regenerative hyperplasia (Short *et al.*, 1987), a large percentage (~70%) of the α_{2u}-globulin present in the kidney of male rats is unbound. This point is also illustrated in studies with TMP-2-OH (Table 1). Twenty-four hours after administration of a single oral dose of 600 mg/kg, the renal concentration of α_{2u}-globulin in male rats was approximately 3100 μM whereas the renal concentration of TMP-2-OH was only about 800

Table 1. Renal stoichiometry of α_{2u}-globulin and TMP-2-OH in male Fischer 344 rats 24 hours after an oral dose of TMP-2-OH[a]			
Dose (mg/kg)	α_{2u}-globulin (μM)	TMP-2-OH (μM)	α_{2u}-globulin: TMP-2-OH (molar ratio)
6	950	400	2.4
60	1900	800	2.4
600	3100	800	3.9

[a] Adapted from Borghoff *et al.* (1995)

μM (Borghoff *et al.*, 1995). This study shows that as the dose of TMP-2-OH was increased, the concentration of α_{2u}-globulin increased to a greater extent than that of the ligand. Because of the large excess of α_{2u}-globulin compared to TMP-2-OH and the 1:1 stoichiometry of ligand binding to α_{2u}-globulin (Lehman-McKeeman & Caudill, 1992), accumulation of α_{2u}-globulin in the male rat kidney is unlikely to be due simply to ligand binding and inhibited degradation of the ligand-bound protein.

Borghoff *et al.* (1992) compared the accumulation of α_{2u}-globulin and the level of cell proliferation in the kidney of male Fischer 344 rats administered European high test (EHT) gasoline or unleaded gasoline for 10 days. Unleaded gasoline has a higher concentration of branched hydrocarbons than EHT and produced a greater increase in α_{2u}-globulin accumulation. At doses containing approximately equivalent amounts of TMP (500 mg/kg body weight of EHT and 16 mg/kg body weight of unleaded gasoline), protein droplet scores and renal concentrations of α_{2u}-globulin were similar, while the level of cell proliferation in the renal proximal tubules was nearly two times greater with the EHT dose than with the unleaded gasoline dose. Evidently, stimulation of renal cell proliferation in rats administered EHT must have involved mechanisms unrelated to α_{2u}-globulin accumulation, possibly induced by other components in this complex mixture. Hence, the observation of both α_{2u}-globulin accumulation and cell proliferation in kidney tubules of male rats does not necessarily indicate that the proliferative response was due solely to α_{2u}-globulin nephropathy.

Short *et al.* (1989b) observed a dose-related increase in the incidence of atypical cell foci (considered by the authors to be preneoplastic lesions) in the kidneys of male Fischer 344 rats, but not in female rats, initiated with N-nitroso-ethyl(hydroxyethyl)amine (EHEN) and then exposed for 59 weeks to unleaded gasoline at exposures ranging from 10 to 300 ppm. An increase was similarly observed in EHEN-initiated male rats that were exposed to 50 ppm TMP. Renal lesions were not increased significantly in male rats treated with unleaded gasoline or TMP alone. These studies indicate that unleaded gasoline and TMP can promote the development of chemically induced preneoplastic lesions in the kidney of male rats.

Methyl t-butyl ether (MTBE) and t-butyl alcohol (TBA)

Inhalation exposure of Fischer 344 rats to 0, 400, 3000 or 8000 ppm MTBE (6 hours/day, 5 days/week, for up to two years) produced increased incidences of renal tubule adenomas and carcinomas and of interstitial cell adenomas of the testes in male rats (Chun *et al.*, 1992). The severity of chronic nephropathy was increased in exposed male and female rats, though no carcinogenic response was observed in females. The severity of nephropathy in male rats was greater than that typically seen with chemicals that induce α_{2u}-globulin accumulation. The same exposures in CD-1 mice, but for only 18 months, produced increased incidences of hepatocellular carcinomas in males and hepatocellular adenomas and carcinomas in females (Burleigh-Flayer *et al.*, 1992).

Administration of the MTBE metabolite t-butyl alcohol in drinking water to Fischer 344 rats for two years produced increased incidences of renal tubule hyperplasias and renal tubule adenomas or carcinomas in male rats but not in female rats. As with MTBE, t-butyl alcohol treatment increased the severity of nephropathy in both male and female rats (Cirvello *et al.*, 1995; National Toxicology Program, 1995). Interestingly, a treatment-related increase in hyaline droplet accumulation was observed in the renal proximal tubules of male rats but not in female rats given t-butyl alcohol in drinking water for 13 weeks. In addition, an increase in renal tubule cell replication was observed in male rats, but only at exposures that exceeded the carcinogenic doses used in the two-year study (Takahashi *et al.*, 1993).

Immunohistochemical studies of α_{2u}-globulin in kidney sections from male rats exposed to MTBE for 13 weeks did not show an exposure-related increase in staining for this protein (Swenberg & Dietrich, 1991). Because staining was equivalent after exposure to 400, 3000 or 8000 ppm MTBE, yet only the two higher concentrations produced kidney tumours, a clear relationship between α_{2u}-globulin accumulation and kidney carcinogenesis could not be established. Furthermore, proteinaceous casts localized at the junction of the proximal tubules and the thin loop of Henle did not stain positively for α_{2u}-globulin. Thus, classical effects of α_{2u}-globulin nephropathy-inducing agents are not evident in rats exposed to MTBE

(Swenberg & Dietrich, 1991), suggesting that other factors are involved in MTBE-induced nephropathy and renal carcinogenicity in male rats.

Ten-day exposures to MTBE vapours, at 0, 400, 1500 or 3000 ppm, produced exposure-related increases in protein droplet accumulation and renal epithelial cell proliferation in proximal tubules of male Fischer 344 rats but not in female rats (Prescott-Mathews *et al.*, 1997). Unlike other chemicals that induce α_{2u}-globulin nephropathy, a very mild exposure-related increase in the kidney concentration of α_{2u}-globulin was observed in male rats (by the enzyme-linked immunosorbent assay, which is more quantitative than α_{2u}-globulin immunohistochemical staining), with a significant increase seen only at 3000 ppm.

A comparison between the renal effects of unleaded gasoline and MTBE evaluated in the same laboratory is worth noting (Figures 1 and 2). Exposure of male Fischer 344 rats to unleaded gasoline for 10 days produced dose-related

increases in protein droplets, α_{2u}-globulin accumulation and renal epithelial cell proliferation (Borghoff *et al.*, 1992). At exposures to unleaded gasoline and MTBE that produced comparable increases in protein droplets and cell proliferation, male rats treated with unleaded gasoline had much greater increases in α_{2u}-globulin (300%) than those treated with MTBE (40%). Further, the slope of plots of protein droplet score (Figure 1) or elevated cell proliferation (Figure 2) versus concentration of α_{2u}-globulin in the kidneys of exposed male rats is much steeper for MTBE than it is for unleaded gasoline. These slopes should be invariant with the identity of the α_{2u}-globulin-inducing chemical if α_{2u}-globulin accumulation alone is the cause of these effects. The divergence between increases in protein droplets or cell proliferation and α_{2u}-globulin accumulation suggests that other factors than α_{2u}-globulin are largely responsible for the protein droplet and cell proliferation responses in the kidneys of male rats exposed to MTBE.

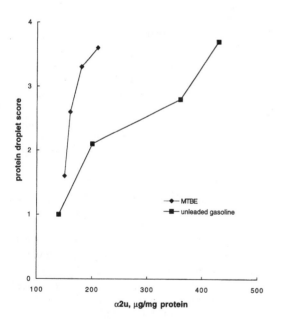

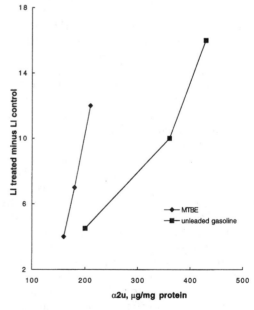

Figure 1. Relationship between α_{2u}-globulin(α2u) concentration and protein droplet score in the proximal tubules of male Fischer 344 rats exposed to methyl *t*-butyl ether by inhalation (Prescott-Mathews *et al.*, 1997) or to unleaded gasoline (Borghoff *et al.*, 1992) by gavage for 10 consecutive days.

Figure 2. Relationship between α_{2u}-globulin (α2u) concentration and increases in labelling index (LI) in the proximal tubules of male Fischer 344 rats exposed to methyl *t*-butyl ether by inhalation (Prescott-Mathews *et al.*, 1997) or to unleaded gasoline (Borghoff *et al.*, 1992) by gavage for 10 consecutive days.

Poet *et al.* (1996) found that the interaction between kidney proteins and MTBE did not withstand dialysis in buffer or anion exchange chromatography and suggested that binding between MTBE and kidney proteins was either very weak or nonspecific. For other chemicals that induce α_{2u}-globulin accumulation in the male rat kidney, approximately 20–40% of the ligand remains bound after dialysis in buffer. This finding is true even for chemicals such as 1,4-dichlorobenzene and its metabolite 2,5-dichlorophenol (Charbonneau *et al.*, 1989), which also have weak binding affinities for α_{2u}-globulin ($\sim 5 \times 10^{-4}$ M; Borghoff *et al.*, 1991). Thus, interactions between MTBE and α_{2u}-globulin appear to be different from those of other chemicals that induce the accumulation of this protein.

In spite of the differences in behaviour between MTBE and other chemicals that induce α_{2u}-globulin nephropathy, a review panel assembled by the US National Research Council (NRC) concluded that results of the 10-day study of MTBE in rats showed that α_{2u}-globulin was involved in the causation of the kidney tumours observed in the two-year inhalation study and that the kidney cancer findings should not be used for human risk assessment (National Research Council, 1996). The evaluation by the NRC panel shows how reliance on simplistic classification systems applied to renal carcinogenesis can lead to less than rigorous scrutiny of the strengths and weaknesses of available data in the decision-making process.

d-Limonene

A two-year study of *d*-limonene administered by gavage in corn oil showed increased incidences of renal tubule neoplasms in male rats (0/50 control; 8/50 at 75 mg/kg; 11/50 at 150 mg/kg), but not in female rats that received 300 or 600 mg/kg or mice that received up to 1000 mg/kg (National Toxicology Program, 1990).

Most chemicals that have been shown to induce protein droplet nephropathy and renal carcinogenesis also increased tumour incidence at other organ sites; mouse liver was the site of the most common tumour response. *d*-Limonene is an exception to this common occurrence. Although *d*-limonene has a weak binding affinity for α_{2u}-globulin, its metabolite, *d*-limonene oxide has

a strong binding affinity (5.6×10^{-7} M) for α_{2u}-globulin (Borghoff *et al.*, 1991; Lehman-McKeeman & Caudill, 1992). In rats dosed with *d*-[^{14}C]-limonene, the renal concentration of *d*-limonene equivalents was 2.5 times higher in male rats than in female rats, and *d*-limonene oxide was identified associated with α_{2u}-globulin in the male rat kidney (Lehman-McKeeman *et al.*, 1989).

Dietrich and Swenberg (1991a) reported that administration of *d*-limonene by gavage at 150 mg/kg for 30 weeks promoted renal tumour development in male Fischer 344 rats, but not in male NBR rats, after EHEN initiation. This species difference was attributed to hepatic synthesis and renal accumulation of α_{2u}-globulin in the Fischer rats and the associated increase in renal tubule cell proliferation. Other differences between these strains of rats might have had an effect on the results. For example, EHEN produced a much higher incidence of atypical hyperplasias in renal tubules and a higher incidence of liver tumours in Fischer 344 rats than in NBR rats. Because no two-year carcinogenicity study has been performed with NBR rats, it is not known whether this strain of rat responds to initiators and promoters of renal carcinogenesis similarly as do Fischer 344 rats.

Gabapentin

The anticonvulsant drug gabapentin (1-(aminomethyl)cyclohexaneacetic acid) caused α_{2u}-globulin nephropathy, including a moderate to marked increase in hyaline droplets, in male Wistar rats given 2000 mg/kg for 104 weeks, without producing kidney tumours (Dominick *et al.*, 1991). In a 13-week study, this dose of gabapentin caused hyaline droplet accumulation in proximal tubules, granular cast formation in the renal cortex and outer medulla, and tubule epithelial regeneration. Thus, the accumulation of hyaline droplets containing α_{2u}-globulin and the degenerative/regenerative changes in the proximal tubule epithelium (P_2 segment) that occurred in male rats exposed to gabapentin were not predictive of renal carcinogenesis with chronic exposure. Renal tubule cell proliferation data are not available for rats exposed to this drug.

Lindane

Administration of lindane by gavage to male Fischer 344 rats (4 days) at 10 mg/kg per day induced α_{2u}-globulin nephropathy (Dietrich & Swenberg, 1990); this dose is similar to the doses of lindane used in a long-term feeding study (up to 470 ppm) that did not increase the incidence of renal tumours in male rats (National Cancer Institute, 1977). Thus, this study, like the one above, shows that renal changes associated with α_{2u}-globulin nephropathy are not always predictive of renal carcinogenicity.

1,4-Dichlorobenzene (1,4-DCB)

Administration of 1,4-dichlorobenzene by gavage for two years led to increased incidences of renal tubule cell neoplasms in male rats (1/50 control, 3/50 at 150 mg/kg, and 8/50 at 300 mg/kg) and hepatocellular neoplasms in mice of both sexes (National Toxicology Program, 1987); no neoplastic effects were observed in female rats. The severity of nephropathy was greater in dosed male rats than in controls, while dose-related increases in the incidence of nephropathy were observed in female rats and in mice of both sexes.

1,4-DCB and its major metabolite, 2,5-dichlorophenol, bind reversibly to α_{2u}-globulin (Charbonneau et al., 1989) but with affinities three orders of magnitude lower than TMP-2-OH or d-limonene oxide (Borghoff et al., 1991). Cell proliferation studies in rats administered 1,4-DCB by gavage for 4 days showed increases in proliferating cells in the proximal tubule of males at the high dose (300 mg/kg), but not at 150 mg/kg or in female rats at either dose level (Umemura et al., 1992). Increases in cell proliferation were also observed in the livers of rats of both sexes, even though this was not a target site of 1,4-DCB carcinogenesis. Evidently, increases in cell proliferation after short-term exposures are not reliably predictive of carcinogenesis due to long-term exposure.

Species differences in the biotransformation of 1,4-DCB may be important in the organ-specific carcinogenic effects of this chemical. Glutathione conjugates of 2,5-dichlorohydroquinone, a metabolite of 1,4-DCB, have been suggested to contribute to the nephrotoxic effects of 1,4-DCB in the male rat (Klos & Dekant, 1994), while 2,5-dichlorobenzoquinone may be more important in the hepatocarcinogenicity of 1,4-DCB in mice (Hissink et al., 1997).

Relevant to the consideration of a possible role of dichlorohydroquinone in the renal carcino-genicity of 1,4-DCB are results of studies on its congener, hydroquinone. Hydroquinone is a clastogenic agent that produced kidney tumours in male rats at gavage doses of 25 or 50 mg/kg body weight but no kidney tumours in female rats. The kidney tumour response in male rats was not associated with hyaline droplet accumulation (National Toxicology Program, 1989a). The severity of spontaneous nephropathy commonly seen in aged Fischer 344 rats was increased in high-dose males; however, in comparison to controls, the severity of this lesion was not increased in the low-dose group of male rats. The incidence of liver tumours was also increased in treated female mice. This pattern of tumour response (kidney tumours in male rats but not in female rats and liver tumours in mice) was seen with 1,4-DCB and several other chemicals that induce α_{2u}-globulin accumulation in the kidney of male rats. Hence, it is evident that factors in addition to α_{2u}-globulin contribute to the greater susceptibility of male Fischer 344 rats compared with female rats or mice to the development of renal tumours. Because nephrotoxic metabolites of 1,4-DCB are congeners of hydroquinone, these chemicals may produce kidney tumours in male rats by similar mechanisms. In that case, the male rat kidney tumour response to 1,4-DCB would not simply be a consequence of weak binding to α_{2u}-globulin and subsequent accumulation of this protein.

Tetrachloroethylene

Tetrachloroethylene, a dry-cleaning agent and industrial degreaser, induced renal tubule cell neoplasms in male rats in a two-year inhalation study at exposure concentrations of 200 and 400 ppm (National Toxicology Program, 1986a). Protein droplets, α_{2u}-globulin accumulation, and increased cell replication rates were observed in the proximal tubules of male rats dosed with 1000 mg/kg tetrachloroethylene by gavage for 10 days (Goldsworthy et al., 1988); however, hyaline droplets containing α_{2u}-globulin were not increased in proximal tubules of male rats exposed to 400 ppm tetrachloroethylene by inhalation for four weeks (Green et al., 1990). The latter finding indicates that α_{2u}-globulin nephropathy was not involved in the induction of the renal tubule cell neoplasms that were observed in the NTP inhalation study of tetrachloroethylene. A glutathione/-β-lyase activation pathway producing a mutagenic intermediate may be involved in the renal carcinogenicity of tetrachloroethylene (Green *et al.*, 1990).

Potassium bromate (KBrO₃)

$KBrO_3$, an oxidizing agent used as a food additive for treatment of wheat flour, was administered to male and female Fischer 344 rats in drinking water for 110 weeks at concentrations of 250 and 500 ppm. This treatment produced high incidences of renal cell tumours in both sexes (males: 6% controls, 60% low-dose, 88% high-dose; females: 0% controls, 56% low-dose, 80% high-dose; Kurokawa *et al.*, 1990). The renal carcinogenicity of $KBrO_3$ has been attributed to oxidative DNA damage (Sai *et al.*, 1994; Umemura *et al.*, 1995). Levels of 8-hydroxydeoxyguanosine, a product of oxidative DNA damage formed by oxygen-radical-generating agents, were increased in kidney DNA but not in liver DNA of rats given oral doses of $KBrO_3$.

The finding that hyaline droplets containing α_{2u}-globulin accumulated in male rats treated with $KBrO_3$ led to the suggestion that α_{2u}-globulin nephropathy may contribute an additive effect in the renal carcinogenicity of $KBrO_3$ in male rats (Umemura *et al.*, 1993). However, in the absence of data on binding of bromate to α_{2u}-globulin and demonstration of consequent reduced proteolytic degradation of the bound protein, it is not possible to determine whether α_{2u}-globulin accumulation resulted from the α_{2u}-globulin mechanism described above or perhaps resulted from oxidative damage associated with $KBrO_3$ treatment. Because the incidences of renal cell tumours were similarly elevated in male and female rats given equivalent concentrations of $KBrO_3$ in their drinking water and because treatment with $KBrO_3$ caused increased cell proliferation in the female rat kidney (Umemura *et al.*, 1995), it is likely that α_{2u}-globulin accumulation was irrelevant to the carcinogenic effects of $KBrO_3$ in the kidney.

Ferric nitrilotriacetate (Fe-NTA)

A single administration of Fe-NTA to male rats suppresses proteolytic processing of α_{2u}-globulin in renal proximal tubules, resulting in an increase in native α_{2u}-globulin in the kidney and a decrease in α_{2u}-K levels (Uchida *et al.*, 1995). Repeated administration of Fe-NTA caused renal tubule

necrosis as a consequence of membrane lipid peroxidation and produced a high incidence of renal adenocarcinomas in male rats and mice (Ebina *et al.*, 1986). Interestingly, the corresponding aluminium salt (Al-NTA) produced renal tubule necrosis and regenerative hyperplasia similar to that induced by Fe-NTA, but did not elicit a renal tumour response. $KBrO_3$ and Fe-NTA induce poly(ADP-ribosyl)ation and DNA double-strand breaks in renal cortical nuclei of exposed male rats (McLaren *et al.*, 1994). Poly(ADP-ribosyl)ation is thought to represent a post-translational modification of nuclear proteins involved in DNA repair. The above findings show that kidney changes unrelated to ligand binding to α_{2u}-globulin can also affect α_{2u}-globulin accumulation in the male rat and that nephrotoxicity and renal carcinogenicity can occur as independent phenomena. Hence, renal accumulation of α_{2u}-globulin may be a consequence rather than a cause of nephrotoxicity.

Hexachlorobenzene (HCB)

Dietary administration of HCB (75 and 150 ppm), a polychlorinated aromatic fungicide, produced high incidences of liver and kidney neoplasms in rats of both sexes (Ertürk *et al.*, 1986). At equivalent doses, female rats had higher incidences of liver neoplasms and male rats had higher incidences of kidney neoplasms. Administration of HCB (50 or 100 mg/kg) by gavage produced α_{2u}-globulin nephropathy in male rats but no renal changes in female rats (Bouthillier *et al.*, 1991). HCB was also found to bind reversibly to α_{2u}-globulin. Because kidney tumours were also induced in female rats treated with HCB, the tumour response in males cannot be attributed simply to the associated increase in renal α_{2u}-globulin levels.

Modelling α_{2u}-globulin accumulation and ligand dosimetry in the male rat kidney

The studies described above indicate that renal accumulation of α_{2u}-globulin in male rats may result from inhibition of renal lysosomal proteinases or from certain degenerative changes (e.g., oxidative damage). Because the relationship between α_{2u}-globulin accumulation and nephrotoxicity has not been elucidated, the possibility that observed increases in renal α_{2u}-globulin levels may be a consequence rather than a cause of renal toxicity cannot be excluded. Integrating data on the relationships between xenobiotic exposure, α_{2u}-globulin accumulation, and tumour outcome in a comprehensive mathematical model of the involved processes, rather than simply relying on qualitative correlations, would help to distinguish between several possible explanations for the observations.

One attempt to evaluate the toxicokinetics of a specific α_{2u}-globulin-inducing chemical (2,4,4-trimethyl-2-pentanol, TMP-2-OH) in the male rat kidney has been described (Borghoff et al., 1995). This mechanism-based dosimetry model includes ligand interaction with α_{2u}-globulin, reduced lysosomal degradation of α_{2u}-globulin as a result of ligand binding, and renal accumulation of α_{2u}-globulin. The model was developed using literature values for secretion of α_{2u}-globulin from the liver, the fraction of α_{2u}-globulin excreted in urine, the fraction cleared from plasma by glomerular filtration, and the rate of α_{2u}-globulin degradation. In trying to reproduce experimental data on α_{2u}-globulin and TMP-2-OH levels in the blood and kidneys, several parameter values were altered but without any clear justifications. The authors found that their model underpredicted the measured renal concentrations of α_{2u}-globulin and overpredicted renal TMP-2-OH concentrations in treated male rats, even when they tripled the reported rate of α_{2u}-globulin synthesis in the liver. Furthermore, to simulate the increased level of renal α_{2u}-globulin following oral administration of TMP-2-OH, the rate of renal degradation of the α_{2u}-globulin-TMP-2-OH complex had to be reduced to zero; however, this tactic prevented the model from reproducing the observed later decline in renal α_{2u}-globulin after an oral dose of 600 mg TMP-2-OH/kg body weight. This large decrease in the degradation rate of the ligand–protein complex is not consistent with reported data (as indicated above, the rate of α_{2u}-globulin degradation in vitro was decreased by about 30% in the presence of excess ligand; Lehman-McKeeman et al., 1990).

The lack of correspondence between this model's predictions and the experimental data indicates that the model's structure does not adequately describe the quantitative relationships among the processes involved in α_{2u}-globulin accumulation in the male rat kidney and/or that parameter values may be incorrect. This

modelling effort, which is the first quantitative test of the α_{2u}-globulin hypothesis, demonstrates that a 30% reduction in the degradation rate of α_{2u}-globulin resulting from ligand binding is inadequate to explain the observed accumulation of α_{2u}-globulin in the male rat kidney. Clearly, processes not included in the α_{2u}-globulin hypothesis must be involved.

The α_{2u}-globulin hypothesis is based on several qualitative observations; however, quantitative linkages between the critical biological processes in the hypothesis not only remain unproved, but have not even been tested. Two critical steps in the α_{2u}-globulin hypothesis are the reversible binding of the xenobiotic ligand to α_{2u}-globulin and subsequent reduction in the proteolytic degradation of the bound protein. Any model of α_{2u}-globulin accumulation in the male rat kidney must be consistent with the effects of strong and weak binding ligands. The α_{2u}-globulin hypothesis focuses largely on effects of the ligand on α_{2u}-globulin without adequate consideration of the effects of α_{2u}-globulin on the ligand. The presence of a binding protein such as α_{2u}-globulin in the male rat can have important consequences on the disposition of the binding ligand. Hence, evaluations of the α_{2u}-globulin hypothesis must address the mutual effects of the protein and ligand on each other in the male rat; these issues were included in the TMP-2-OH/α_{2u}-globulin model developed by Borghoff et al. (1995).

In male rats exposed to a chemical that binds to α_{2u}-globulin or that is metabolized to an α_{2u}-globulin–binding ligand, retention of the ligand in tissues will be affected by the presence and amount of α_{2u}-globulin, as well as the binding affinity of the ligand for α_{2u}-globulin. A realistic model of these processes must include descriptions of the absorption, distribution and metabolism of the parent compound, as well as the hepatic secretion, resorption and renal degradation of α_{2u}-globulin (e.g., Figure 3). If the binding ligand is the parent compound, the kinetics of its metabolism and elimination must be included in the model; if one or more metabolites bind to α_{2u}-globulin, the kinetics of their formation and elimination must be included.

The presence of α_{2u}-globulin in the liver, blood and kidney will affect the distribution of α_{2u}-globulin–binding ligands. Estimations of tissue partition coefficients must account for ligand binding to

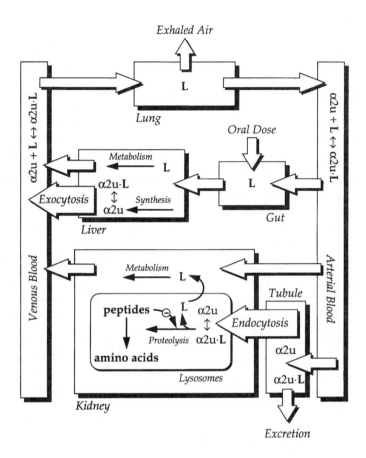

Figure 3. Partial block diagram of the physiologically based pharmacokinetic model of the disposition of an α_{2u}-globulin ($\alpha 2u$) ligand (L) and its effect on the renal accumulation of α_{2u}-globulin.

α_{2u}-globulin in homogenates of these tissues. Binding of ligand to α_{2u}-globulin in the liver may occur if the ligand can cross the secretory vesicle membrane. In that case, the rate of hepatic metabolism of the ligand would be affected by both its rate of transport across the membrane and its binding affinity for α_{2u}-globulin. If the ligand can cross the lysosomal membrane, it may appear in the cytosol of the renal proximal tubule cells following resorption and partial degradation of bound α_{2u}-globulin.

A related issue to be considered is whether the presence of ligand affects hepatic secretion of α_{2u}-globulin. Exposure of mature male rats to unleaded gasoline by gavage with doses that resulted in large increases in the concentration of

α_{2u}-globulin in the kidney did not alter significantly the hepatic concentrations of α_{2u}-globulin or its mRNA when measured 18 to 24 hours after the last exposure (Olson *et al.*, 1987; Murty *et al.*, 1988). Inhalation exposure of male rats to an isoparaffinic solvent did not significantly increase hepatic levels of α_{2u}-globulin, but doubled the plasma α_{2u}-globulin concentration (Viau *et al.*, 1986), suggesting that exposure to isoparaffinic solvents may result in a coordinated elevation in the hepatic synthesis and secretion of α_{2u}-globulin. The issue of hepatic response to an α_{2u}-globulin-binding ligand has been only partially addressed for relatively few chemicals. Because potential effects of binding ligands on hepatic synthesis of α_{2u}-globulin may be largely resolved within 18 hours after exposure, studies are needed that include evaluations at times much closer to the last exposure. Regardless of whether hepatic α_{2u}-globulin is secreted as the free or ligand-bound form, in the blood the equilibrium between these forms would be established as determined by the binding affinity of the ligand for this protein.

An adequate toxicokinetic model also must reflect the glomerular filtration and resorption of α_{2u}-globulin followed by its degradation. The filtered fraction that is not reabsorbed (~40%) (Neuhaus et al., 1981) is excreted in the urine. The assumption that free and bound α_{2u}-globulin are equally resorbed has not been examined, but the data of Saito et al. (1996) are consistent with this assumption. Finally, the model must accurately represent the degradation of α_{2u}-globulin in proximal tubule cells. Lehman-McKeeman et al. (1990) reported that degradation of α_{2u}-globulin by lysosomal proteinases was reduced by about 30% in the presence of excess xenobiotic ligand. Accumulation of α_{2u}-globulin in the male rat kidney may not be due only to ligand binding; Olson et al. (1988) found that treatment of male rats with leupeptin, an inhibitor of lysosomal proteolysis, resulted in renal accumulation of hyaline droplets containing α_{2u}-globulin. Furthermore, consideration of potential changes in renal lysosomal proteinase activities in vivo in response to protein accumulation need additional investigation, because increases of 60% in renal cortical cathepsin B and D activities were seen in male rats four days after administration of unleaded gasoline (Murty et al., 1988).

Because the model by Borghoff et al. (1995) was not able to simulate the renal accumulation of α_{2u}-globulin in male rats dosed with TMP-2-OH, we suggest that several assumptions in the α_{2u}-globulin hypothesis are incorrect. First, ligand binding to α_{2u}-globulin may increase the rate of hepatic secretion of this protein. Second, degradation of unbound α_{2u}-globulin may also be reduced as a consequence of accumulation of the ligand in proximal tubule cells (Lehman-McKeeman et al., 1990). Release of ligand, perhaps early during the degradation of α_{2u}-globulin, and subsequent binding to formerly free α_{2u}-globulin may reduce proteolytic degradation of both bound and free α_{2u}-globulin. Third, increased uptake of protein (e.g., α_{2u}-globulin) induces lysosomal cathepsins

(Olbricht et al., 1993; Eisenberger et al., 1995) and would be expected to stimulate proteolysis of α_{2u}-globulin (Murty et al., 1988). Fourth, liver and kidney are known to possess cytoplasmic fatty acid-binding proteins with a broad range of lipophilic ligands (Maatman et al., 1991). Binding of TMP-2-OH to such proteins would significantly affect the concentration of free ligand. We are testing these hypotheses by comparing a new model's predictions with the published data.

Relationships between α_{2u}-globulin accumulation, cell proliferation, and kidney cancer

Foci of chronic progressive nephrosis, characterized by degeneration/regeneration of the proximal tubule epithelium, are common in ageing male and female rats and are even seen to a minimal degree in renal proximal tubules of control Fischer 344 rats by 20 weeks of age. The frequency of these lesions and their severity increase with age. Short et al. (1989a) reported that the rates of regenerative cell replication in these lesions in control rats are higher than the cell replication rates of proximal tubule segments affected by chemicals that induce α_{2u}-globulin accumulation. Konishi and Ward (1989) also observed high levels of cell proliferation associated with chronic progressive nephrosis in control female Fischer 344 rats. In spite of the high frequency of these spontaneous proliferative lesions, the incidence of kidney tumours in untreated male rats is low (<1.0 %), even when they are maintained for up to 146 weeks of age (Solleveld et al., 1984).

High rates of renal tubule cell proliferation in rats are not reliable predictors of kidney cancer. For example, in the bioassay of chloroform in rats, renal tumours were significantly increased in males but not in females (National Cancer Institute, 1976). In contrast to these findings, the labelling index in renal proximal tubules was not increased in male rats given bioassay doses of chloroform by gavage for three weeks (Larson et al., 1995a) but was increased 17-fold and 26-fold in female rats given bioassay doses of this nephrotoxic agent (Larson et al., 1995b).

Although cell proliferation is a basic component of multistage carcinogenesis, there are no data demonstrating that cell division is the limiting factor in kidney cancer (Barrett & Huff, 1991). Cell proliferation data for exposures longer than three weeks are available for only two chemicals (unleaded gasoline and *d*-limonene) that form α_{2u}-globulin ligands and induce renal tumours in long-term studies. Cell proliferation data for 48 weeks of exposure to TMP are also available; however, a carcinogenicity study of this chemical has not been reported. Thus, quantitative dose-response relationships between sustained cell proliferation and renal carcinogenesis in male rats have not been established for most chemicals that induce α_{2u}-globulin nephropathy.

Alternatively, the unbound ligand (e.g., TMP-2-OH) that accumulates in the kidney cytosol by one of the mechanisms suggested above may be subsequently converted to the proximate nephrotoxicant or carcinogen (e.g., the aldehyde or carboxylic acid metabolites). In this case, α_{2u}-globulin may simply serve as a vector affecting the levels of the renal toxicant/carcinogen or its precursor in the male rat kidney.

Summary and conclusions

The α_{2u}-globulin hypothesis is supported by the findings that :

(1) Several nongenotoxic chemicals that cause α_{2u}-globulin accumulation and renal carcinogenesis in male rats do not induce kidney tumours in animals that lack the ability to synthesize α_{2u}-globulin in the liver (e.g., female rats or mice of either sex).

(2) Chemicals that cause α_{2u}-globulin accumulation in the kidney of male Fischer 344 or Sprague-Dawley rats do not induce protein droplet nephropathy in male NBR rats (Dietrich & Swenberg, 1991b), a strain deficient in hepatic α_{2u}-globulin synthesis.

(3) Chemicals (or their metabolites) that bind reversibly to α_{2u}-globulin cause α_{2u}-globulin accumulation in the male rat kidney (Borghoff *et al.*, 1991).

(4) *In vitro* degradation of ligand-bound α_{2u}-globulin by lysosomal extracts was decreased in the presence of excess α_{2u}-globulin ligand (Lehman-McKeeman *et al.*, 1990).

(5) S-phase labelling index in the P_2 segment of renal proximal tubules was increased in male rats exposed to several chemicals or chemical mixtures that induce α_{2u}-globulin accumulation, and for unleaded gasoline, the dose-

dependence for the renal epithelial cell labelling index is similar to that of the kidney tumour response (Short *et al.*, 1987, 1989a).

(6) Unleaded gasoline and *d*-limonene elicited tumour-promoting activity in the kidney of male Fischer 344 rats initiated with EHEN (Short *et al.*, 1989b; Dietrich & Swenberg, 1991a), whereas *d*-limonene did not promote renal carcinogenesis in EHEN-initiated male NBR rats (Dietrich & Swenberg, 1991a).

This review has identified several inconsistencies and critical gaps in the data claimed to prove the α_{2u}-globulin hypothesis. These deficiencies reveal how limited is our understanding of the proposed linkage between the reversible binding of xenobiotic ligands to α_{2u}-globulin, the accumulation of α_{2u}-globulin in the male rat kidney, and male rat-specific kidney carcinogenesis.

(1) Several contradictory observations have been reported; for example, gabapentin and lindane induce α_{2u}-globulin accumulation and nephropathy in male rats at doses that did not increase kidney tumour incidence.

(2) α_{2u}-globulin accumulation may arise by mechanisms unrelated to ligand binding to this protein; for example, 2,2,4-trimethylpentanoic acid, a metabolite of TMP (Charbonneau *et al.*, 1987a), and leupeptin, an inhibitor of lysosomal proteolysis (Olson *et al.*, 1988), cause α_{2u}-globulin accumulation without binding. In addition, increases in α_{2u}-globulin accumulation in male rats treated with potassium bromate or Fe-NTA may occur secondary to oxidative damage rather than protein binding (Sai *et al.*, 1994; Uchida *et al.*, 1995).

(3) A 30% reduction in the lysosomal degradation rate of α_{2u}-globulin resulting from ligand binding was inadequate to explain the observed accumulation of α_{2u}-globulin in the male rat kidney (Borghoff *et al.*, 1995).

(4) α_{2u}-globulin accumulation in the male rat kidney has been observed under conditions in which ~70% of the protein was unbound (Charbonneau *et al.*, 1987b; Borghoff *et al.*, 1995).

(5) Some compounds with weak binding affinity for α_{2u}-globulin (e.g., MTBE) cause hyaline droplet accumulation and induce kidney

tumours in male rats but give rise to very small increases in renal concentrations of α_{2u}-globulin (Chun et al., 1992; Prescott-Mathews et al., 1997).

(6) Except for d-limonene, the chemicals that induce both α_{2u}-globulin accumulation and kidney carcinogenesis also induce cancer at other sites (see Table 2); mouse liver neoplasms were the most common (Melnick, 1992). This finding suggests that other mechanisms are involved in the carcinogenicity of these chemicals.

(7) Several compounds that cause α_{2u}-globulin nephropathy and induce kidney tumours in male rats also induce renal toxicity and/or renal carcinogenesis in female rats or in mice (e.g., 1,4-DCB, MTBE, HCB, potassium bromate). Kidney toxicity and carcinogenicity induced by these chemicals can certainly not be attributed simply to the presence of α_{2u}-globulin.

(8) The potential contributions of alternative metabolites in the toxic and carcinogenic processes have not been adequately investigated (e.g., 2,5-dichlorohydroquinone or a subsequent metabolite from 1,4-DCB, the glutathione conjugate of tetrachloroethylene, and the acid and aldehyde metabolites of TMP).

(9) Foci of chronic progressive nephrosis, which are renal tubule lesions appearing in control Fischer 344 rats by 20 weeks of age, have cellular replication rates that are higher than those of P_2 proximal tubule cells in male rats exposed to chemicals that induce α_{2u}-globulin accumulation (Short et al., 1989a); however, the incidence of spontaneous kidney tumours in untreated male rats is low (<1.0%) even at 146 weeks of age (Solleveld et al.,1984).

(10) Although cell proliferation is a basic component of multistage carcinogenesis, there are no data demonstrating that the carcinogenic outcome in the kidney is determined by the cell division rate (Barrett & Huff, 1991). Furthermore, there is no adequate database

Table 2. Sites of tumour induction in rats or mice exposed to chemicals that induce α_{2u}-globulin accumulation, in addition to kidney tumours in male rats

Chemical	Rats	Mice	Reference
Unleaded gasoline	–	Liver	MacFarland et al., 1984
Methyl t-butyl ether/-t-butyl alcohol	Testis, haematopoietic system	Liver, thyroid	Chun et al., 1992; Burleigh-Flayer et al., 1992; Belpoggi et al., 1995; Cirvello et al., 1995
d-Limonene	–	–	NTP, 1990
1,4-Dichlorobenzene	–	Liver	NTP, 1987
Tetrachloroethylene	Haematopoietic system	Liver	NTP, 1986a
Hexachlorobenzene	Kidney (females) liver	Liver	Ertürk et al., 1986; Cabral et al., 1979
Potassium bromate	Kidney (females) mesothelium thyroid	Kidney	Kurokawa et al., 1990
Ferric nitriloacetate	Kidney (females)	Kidney	Ebina et al., 1986; Li et al., 1987
Hexachloroethane	–	Liver	NTP, 1989b
Isophorone	Preputial gland	Liver	NTP, 1986b

relating cell proliferation rate to renal tumour response in male rats (Melnick, 1992).

(11) Dose–response studies do not support a relationship between the increase in hyaline droplets containing α_{2u}-globulin and kidney carcinogenicity in male rats (e.g., tetrachloroethylene).

(12) Human exposure to gasoline vapours has been associated with increased kidney cancer risk, indicating that the renal tumorigenicity of gasoline may not be species–specific.

These findings suggest that among the chemicals reviewed in this paper, only *d*-limonene meets the criteria presented in the consensus report in this volume for agents causing kidney tumours through an α_{2u}-globulin-associated response in male rats.

The hypothesis that kidney tumours in the male rat are caused by promotion of initiated cells by regenerative hyperplasia consequent to cytotoxicity due to α_{2u}-globulin accumulation is consistent with some observations and inconsistent with others. Therefore, the hypothesis is unproved and, at best, represents only one element in a complex etiology of kidney cancer. To embrace this hypothesis as an adequate explanation of the renal carcinogenic effects of α_{2u}-globulin ligands would be to elevate hypothesis to the level of data and liable to result in a failure to perform definitive experiments that are needed to identify mechanistic details.

Mechanisms of hydrocarbon-induced nephropathy and renal carcinogenesis are not well understood. Correlative studies do not prove causal relationships, and hypotheses that are styled to influence public health policies need strong scientific support. The "widely accepted hypothesis" links the kidney tumour response in male rats to α_{2u}-globulin accumulation resulting from reversible binding of a xenobiotic ligand to this protein, which renders α_{2u}-globulin less susceptible to proteolytic degradation. However, exceptions have been identified and a test of this hypothesis failed to demonstrate critical quantitative relationships that would be expected between exposure to an α_{2u}-globulin-binding ligand and α_{2u}-globulin accumulation in the male rat kidney. Further, the α_{2u}-globulin hypothesis ignores the fact that the presence of α_{2u}-globulin in the male rat affects the concentration of the binding ligand in the kidney, as well as the potential impact of this alteration on target organ dosimetry. Alternative hypotheses based on the same information are plausible. For example, α_{2u}-globulin accumulation may be a consequence of renal toxicity rather than its cause. Two chemicals that cause α_{2u}-globulin accumulation (TMP-2-OH and 2,5-dichlorophenol) were toxic to proximal tubule epithelial fragments *in vitro* (Wilke et al., 1994).

We hypothesize that α_{2u}-globulin may serve to increase the concentration of the carcinogenic agent or its precursor in the male rat kidney. In this case, α_{2u}-globulin may cause a left-shift in the kidney cancer dose–response curve for α_{2u}-globulin-binding ligands in male rats relative to responses in female rats or mice. If the effect of α_{2u}-globulin is largely on the renal concentration of toxicant, then extrapolations across species should adjust for differences in target dose rather than consider the effects in male rats to be irrelevant to humans.

It should be recognized that the mechanisms of chemically induced α_{2u}-globulin nephropathy and chemically induced renal cancer have yet to become more than operational hypotheses and that the alternative view advanced here must also be considered an unproved hypothesis. It would be inappropriate to accept or reject either hypothesis before the mechanisms of renal carcinogenesis are more fully understood and these or any other reasonable hypotheses have been adequately tested. Further experimental studies and mathematical models that address assumptions in the hypotheses relating exposure to α_{2u}-globulin-binding chemicals with α_{2u}-globulin accumulation and kidney cancer in the male rat are needed to better understand the processes involved and to strengthen the scientific basis for any public health decisions.

References

Barrett, J.C. & Huff, J.E. (1991) Cellular and molecular mechanisms of chemically induced renal carcinogenesis. *Renal Failure*, 13, 211–225

Belpoggi, F., Soffritti, M. & Maltoni, C. (1995) Methyl-tertiary-butyl ether (MTBE)–a gasoline additive–causes testicular and lymphohaematopoietic cancers in rats. *Toxicol. Ind. Health*, 11, 119–149

Borghoff, S.J., Miller, A.B., Bowen, J.P. & Swenberg, J.A. (1991) Characteristics of chemical binding to α_{2u}-globulin in vitro – evaluating structure-activity relationships. Toxicol. Appl. Pharmacol., 107, 228–238

Borghoff, S.J., Youtsey, N.L. & Swenberg, J.A. (1992) A comparison of European High Test gasoline and PS-6 unleaded gasoline in their abilities to induce α_{2u}-globulin nephropathy and renal cell proliferation. Toxicol. Lett., 63, 21–33

Borghoff, S.J., Gargas, M.L., Andersen, M.E. & Conolly, R.B. (1995) Development of a mechanism-based dosimetry model for 2,4,4-trimethyl-2-pentanol-induced α_{2u}-globulin nephropathy in male Fischer 344 rats. Fundam. Appl. Toxicol., 25, 124–137

Bouthillier, L., Greselin, E., Brodeur, J., Viau, C. & Charbonneau, M. (1991) Male rat specific nephrotoxicity resulting from subchronic administration of hexachlorobenzene. Toxicol. Appl. Pharmacol., 110, 315–326

Burleigh-Flayer, H.D., Chun, J.S. & Kintigh, W.J. (1992) Methyl tertiary butyl ether: vapor inhalation oncogenicity study in CD-1 mice. Export, PA: Bushy Run Research Center; OPTS-42098

Cabral, J.R.P., Mollner, T., Raitano, F. & Shubik, P. (1979) Carcinogenesis of hexachlorobenzene in mice. Int. J. Cancer, 23, 47–51

Charbonneau, M., Lock, E.A., Strasser, J., Short, B.G. & Bus, J.S. (1987a) Nephrotoxicity of 2,2,4-trimethylpentane (TMP) metabolites in male Fischer 344 rats. Toxicologist, 7, 89

Charbonneau, M., Lock, E.A., Strasser, J., Cox, M.G., Turner, M.J. & Bus, J.S. (1987b) 2,2,4-Trimethylpentane-induced nephrotoxicity. I. Metabolic disposition of TMP in male and female Fischer 344 rats. Toxicol. Appl. Pharmacol., 91, 171–181

Charbonneau, M., Strasser, J., Jr, Lock, E.A., Turner, M.J., Jr & Swenberg, J.A. (1989) Involvement of reversible binding to α_{2u}-globulin in 1,4-dichlorobenzene-induced nephrotoxicity. Toxicol. Appl. Pharmacol., 99, 122–132

Chun, J.S., Burleigh-Flayer, H.D. & Kintigh, W.J. (1992) Methyl tertiary butyl ether: vapor inhalation oncogenicity study in Fischer 344 rats. Export, PA: Bushy Run Research Center; Report 91N0013B

Cirvello, J.D., Radovsky A., Heath, J.E., Farnell, D.R. & Lindamood, C. (1995) Toxicity and carcinogenicity of t-butyl alcohol in rats and mice following chronic exposure in drinking water. Toxicol. Ind. Health, 11, 151–165

Dietrich, D.R. (1997) Doubting nongenotoxic mechanisms of renal cancer: comparing apples and oranges in the α_{2u}-globulin hypothesis. Environ. Health Perspect., 105, 898–902

Dietrich, D.R. & Swenberg, J.A. (1990) Lindane induces nephropathy and renal accumulation of α_{2u}-globulin in male but not female Fischer 344 rats or male NBR rats. Toxicol. Lett., 53, 179–181

Dietrich, D.R. & Swenberg, J.A. (1991a) The presence of α_{2u}-globulin is necessary for d-limonene promotion of male rat kidney tumors. Cancer Res., 51, 3512–3521

Dietrich, D.R. & Swenberg, J.A. (1991b) NCI-Black-Reiter (NBR) male rats fail to develop renal disease following exposure to agents that induce α_{2u}-globulin (α_{2u}) nephropathy. Fundam. Appl. Toxicol., 16, 749–762

Dominick, M.A., Robertson, D.G., Bleavins, M.R., Sigler, R.E., Bobrowski, W.F. & Gough, A.W. (1991) α_{2u}-Glo- bulin nephropathy without nephrocarcinogenesis in male Wistar rats administered 1-(aminomethyl)cyclohexaneacetic acid. Toxicol. Appl. Pharmacol., 111, 375–387

Ebina, Y., Okada, S., Hamazaki, S., Ogino, F., Li, J.L. & Midorikawa, O. (1986) Nephrotoxicity and renal cell carcinoma after use of iron- and aluminum-nitrilotriacetate complexes in rats. J. Natl Cancer Inst., 76, 107–113

Eisenberger, U., Fels, L.M., Olbricht, C.J. & Stolte, H. (1995) Cathepsin B and L in isolated proximal tubular segments during acute and chronic proteinuria. Ren. Physiol. Biochem., 18, 89–96

Ertürk, E., Lambrecht, R.W., Peters, H.A., Cripps, D.J., Gocmen, A., Morris, C.R. & Bryan, G.T. (1986) Oncogenicity of hexachlorobenzene. In: Morris, C.R. & Cabral, J.R.P., eds, Hexachlorobenzene: Proceedings of an International Symposium, (IARC Scientific Publications No. 77), Lyon, International Agency for Research on Cancer, pp. 417–423

Gérin, M., Viau, C., Talbot, D. & Greselin, E. (1991) Nephrotoxicity of aviation gasoline in the rat. In: Bach, P.H., Gregg, N.J., Wilks, M.F. & Delacruz, L., eds, Nephrotoxicity: Mechanisms, Early Diagnosis, and Therapeutic Management, New York, Dekker, pp. 267–272

Goldsworthy, T.L., Lyght, O., Burnett, V.L. & Popp, J.A. (1988) Potential role of α_{2u}-globulin, protein droplet accumulation, and cell replication in the renal carcinogenicity of rats exposed to trichloroethylene, perchloroethylene, and pentachloroethane. Toxicol. Appl. Pharmacol., 96, 367–379

Green, T., Odum, J., Nash, J.A. & Foster, J.R. (1990) Perchloroethylene-induced rat kidney tumors: an investigation of the mechanisms involved and their relevance to humans. Toxicol. Appl. Pharmacol., 103, 77–89

Halder, C.A., Holdsworth, C.E., Cockrell, B.Y. & Piccirillo, V.J. (1985) Hydrocarbon nephropathy in male rats:

identification of the nephrotoxic components of unleaded gasoline. *Toxicol. Ind. Health*, 1, 67–87

Halder, C.A., Van Gorp, G.S., Hatoum, N.S. & Warne, T.M. (1986) Gasoline vapor exposures. Part I. Characterization of workplace exposures. *Am. Ind. Hyg. Assoc. J.*, 47, 164–172

Hissink, A.M., Oudshoorn, M.J., Van Ommen, B. & Van Bladeren, P.J. (1997) Species and strain differences in the hepatic cytochrome P450-mediated biotransformation of 1,4-dichlorobenzene. *Toxicol. Appl. Pharmacol.*, 145, 1–9

Huff, J. (1996) Response: α_{2u}-globulin nephropathy, posed mechanisms, and white ravens [letter]. *Environ. Health Perspect.*, 104, 1264-1267

Kimura, H., Odani, S., Suzuki, J., Arakawa, M. & Ono, T. (1989) Kidney fatty acid-binding protein: identification as α_{2u}-globulin. *FEBS Lett.*, 246, 101–104

Klos, C. & Dekant, W. (1994) Comparative metabolism of the renal carcinogen 1,4-dichlorobenzene in the rat: identification and quantitation of novel metabolites. *Xenobiotica*, 24, 965–976

Konishi, N. & Ward, J.M. (1989) Increased levels of DNA synthesis in hyperplastic renal tubules of aging nephropathy in female F344/NCr rats. *Vet. Pathol.*, 26, 6–10

Kurokawa, Y., Maekawa, A., Takahashi, M. & Hayashi, Y. (1990) Toxicity and carcinogenicity of potassium bromate – a new renal carcinogen. *Environ. Health Perspect.*, 87, 309–335

Larson, J.L., Wolf, D.C. & Butterworth, B.E. (1995a) Induced regenerative cell proliferation in livers and kidney of male F-344 rats given chloroform in corn oil by gavage or *ad libitum* in drinking water. *Toxicology*, 95, 73–86

Larson, J.L., Wolf, D.C., Méry, S., Morgan, K.T. & Butterworth, B.E. (1995b) Toxicity and cell proliferation in the liver, kidneys and nasal passages of female F-344 rats induced by chloroform administered by gavage. *Food. Chem. Toxicol.*, 33, 443–456

Lehman-McKeeman, L.D. & Caudill, D. (1992) α_{2u}-Globulin is the only member of the lipocalin protein superfamily that binds to hyaline droplet inducing agents. *Toxicol. Appl. Pharmacol.*, 116, 170–176

Lehman-McKeeman, L.D., Rodriguez, P.A., Takigiku, R., Caudill, D. & Fey, M.L. (1989) *d*-Limonene-induced male rat-specific nephrotoxicity: evaluation of the association between *d*-limonene and α_{2u}-globulin. *Toxicol. Appl. Pharmacol.*, 99, 250–259

Lehman-McKeeman, L.D., Rivera-Torres, M.I. & Caudill, D. (1990) Lysosomal degradation of α_{2u}-globulin and α_{2u}-globulin-xenobiotic conjugates. *Toxicol. Appl. Pharmacol.*, 103, 539–548

Li, J.L., Okada, S., Hamazaki, S., Ebina, Y. & Midorikawa, O. (1987) Subacute nephrotoxicity and induction of renal cell carcinoma in mice treated with ferric nitriloacetate. *Cancer Res.*, 47, 1867–1869

Lynge, E., Andersen, A., Nilsson, R., Barlow, L., Pukkala, E., Nordlinder, R., Boffetta, P., Grandjean, P., Heikkilä, P., Hörte, L.G., Jakobsson, R., Lundberg, I., Moen, B., Partanen, T. & Riise, T. (1997) Risk of cancer and exposure to gasoline vapors. *Am. J. Epidemiol.*, 145, 449–458

Maatman, R.G.H.J., Van Kuppevelt, T.H.M.S.M. & Veerkamp, J.H. (1991) Two types of fatty acid-binding protein in human kidney. Isolation, characterization and localization. *Biochem. J.*, 273, 759–766

MacFarland, H.N., Ulrich, C.E., Holdsworth, C.E., Kitchen, D.N., Haliwell, W.H. & Blum, S.C. (1984) A chronic inhalation study with unleaded gasoline vapor. *J. Am. Coll. Toxicol.*, 3, 231–248

McLaren, J., Boulikas, T. & Vamvakas, S. (1994) Induction of poly(ADP-ribosyl)ation in the kidney after in vivo application of renal carcinogens. *Toxicology*, 88, 101–112

Melnick, R.L. (1992) An alternative hypothesis on the role of chemically induced protein droplet (α_{2u}-globulin) nephropathy in renal carcinogenesis. *Reg. Toxicol. Pharmacol.*, 16, 111–125

Melnick, R.L., Kohn, M.C. & Huff, J. (1997) Weight of evidence versus weight of speculation to evaluate the α_{2u}-globulin hypothesis. *Environ. Health Perspect.*, 105, 904–906

Miller, B.A., Ries, L.A.G., Hankey, B.F., Kosary, C.L. & Edwards, B.K., eds (1992) *Cancer Statistics Review: 1973-1989, National Cancer Institute* (NIH Publication No. 92-2789), Bethesda, MD, National Institutes of Health

Murty, C.V.R., Olson, M.J., Garg, B.D. & Roy, A.K. (1988) Hydrocarbon-induced hyaline droplet nephropathy in male rats during senescence. *Toxicol. Appl. Pharmacol.*, 96, 380–392

National Cancer Institute (NCI) (1976) *Report on Carcinogenesis Bioassay of Chloroform* NCI, National Tech. Inform. Service No. PB264018/AS) Bethesda, MD

National Cancer Institute (NCI) (1977) *Bioassay of Lindane for Possible Carcinogenicity (CAS No. 58-89-9)* (NCI Carcinogenesis Technical Report No. 14) Bethesda, MD, National Institutes of Health

National Research Council (NRC) (1996) *Toxicological and Performance Aspects of Oxygenated Motor Vehicle Fuels*, Washington DC, National Academy Press

National Toxicology Program (NTP) (1986a) *Toxicology and Carcinogenesis Studies of Tetrachloroethylene (perchloroethylene) (CAS No. 127-18-4) in F344/N Rats and B6C3F$_1$ Mice (Inhalation Studies)* (NTP Technical Report No. 311), Bethesda, MD, National Institutes of Health

National Toxicology Program (NTP) (1986b) *Toxicology and Carcinogenesis Studies of Isophorone (CAS No. 78-59-1) in F344/N Rats and B6C3F₁ Mice (Gavage Studies)*. (NTP Technical Report No. 291), Bethesda, MD, National Institutes of Health

National Toxicology Program (NTP) (1987) *Toxicology and Carcinogenesis Studies of 1,4-Dichlorobenzene (CAS No. 106-46-7) in F344/N Rats and B6C3F1 Mice (Gavage Studies)*. (NTP Technical Report No. 319), Bethesda, MD, National Institutes of Health

National Toxicology Program (NTP) (1989a) *Toxicology and Carcinogenesis Studies of Hydroquinone (CAS No. 123-31-9) in F344/N Rats and B6C3F₁ Mice (Gavage Studies)* (NTP Technical Report No. 366), Bethesda, MD, National Institutes of Health

National Toxicology Program (NTP) (1989b) *Toxicology and Carcinogenesis Studies of Hexachloroethane (CAS No. 67-72-1) in F344/N Rats (Gavage Studies)* (NTP Technical Report No. 361), Bethesda, MD, National Institutes of Health

National Toxicology Program (NTP) (1990) *Toxicology and Carcinogenesis Studies of d-Limonene (CAS No. 5989-27-5) in F344/N Rats and B6C3F1 Mice (Gavage Studies)* (NTP Technical Report No. 347), Bethesda, MD, National Institutes of Health

National Toxicology Program (NTP) (1995) *Toxicology and Carcinogenesis Studies of t-Butyl Alcohol (CAS No. 76-65-0) in F344/N Rats and B6C3F1 Mice (Drinking Water Studies)* (Technical Report Series No. 436, NIH Publication No. 94-3167), Research Triangle Park, NC; National Institutes of Health

Neuhaus, O.W., Flory, W., Biswas, N. & Hollerman, C.E. (1981) Urinary excretion of α_{2u}-globulin and albumin by adult male rats following treatment with nephrotoxic agents. *Nephron, 28*, 133–140

Olbricht, C.J., Irmler, H., Gutjahr, E. & Koch, K.M. (1993) Effect of low-molecular-weight dextran on proteolytic and nonproteolytic lysosomal enzymes in isolated segments of rat proximal tubule. *Nephron, 64*, 262–267

Olson, M.J., Garg, B.D., Murty, C.V.R. & Roy, A.K. (1987) Accumulation of α_{2u}-globulin in the renal proximal tubules of male rats exposed to unleaded gasoline. *Toxicol. Appl. Pharmacol., 90*, 43–51

Olson, M.J., Mancini, M.A., Garg, B.D. & Roy, A.K. (1988) Leupeptin-mediated alteration of renal phagolysosomes: similarity to hyaline droplet nephropathy of male rats exposed to unleaded gasoline. *Toxicol. Lett., 41*, 245–254

Partanen, T., Heikkila, P., Hernberg, S., Kauppinen, T., Moneta, G. & Ojajarvi, A. (1991) Renal cancer and occupational exposure to chemical agents. *Scand. J. Work Environ. Health, 17*, 231–239

Poet, T.S., Murphy, J.E. & Borghoff, S.J. (1996) In vitro uptake of methyl *t*-butyl ether (MTBE) in male and female rat kidney homogenate: solubility and protein interactions. *Toxicologist, 30*, 305

Prescott-Mathews, J.S., Wolf, D.C., Wong, B.A. & Borghoff, S.J. (1997) Methyl *tert*-butyl ether causes α_{2u}-globulin nephropathy and enhanced renal cell proliferation in male Fischer-344 rats. *Toxicol. Appl. Pharmacol., 143*, 301–314

Roy, A.K. & Neuhaus, O.W. (1967) Androgenic control of a sex-dependent protein in the rat. *Nature, 214*, 618–620

Sai, K., Tyson, C.A., Thomas, D.W., Dabbs, J.E., Hasegawa, R. & Kurokawa, Y. (1994) Oxidative DNA damage induced by potassium bromate in isolated rat renal proximal tubules and renal nuclei. *Cancer Lett., 87*, 1–7

Saito, K., Kaneko, H., Isobe, N., Nakatsuka, I., Yoshitake, A. & Yamada, H.(1992) Differences in α_{2u}-globulins increased in male rat kidneys following treatment with several α_{2u}-globulin accumulating agents: cystein protease(s) play(s) an important role in production of kidney-type-α_{2u}-globulin. *Toxicology, 76*, 177–186

Saito, K., Uwagawa, S., Kaneko, H., Shiba, K., Tomigahara, Y. & Nakatsuka, I. (1996) α_{2u}-Globulins in the urine of male rats: a reliable indicator of α_{2u}-globulin accumulation in the kidney. *Toxicology, 106*, 149–157

Short, B.G., Burnett, V.L., Cox, M.G., Bus, J.S. & Swenberg, J.A. (1987) Site-specific renal cytotoxicity and cell proliferation in male rats exposed to petroleum hydrocarbons. *Lab. Invest., 57*, 564–577

Short, B.G., Burnett, V.L. & Swenberg, J.A. (1989a) Elevated proliferation of proximal tubule cells and localization of accumulated α_{2u}-globulin in F344 rats during chronic exposure to unleaded gasoline or 2,2,4-trimethylpentane. *Toxicol. Appl. Pharmacol., 101*, 414–431

Short, B.G., Steinhagen, W.H. & Swenberg, J.A. (1989b) Promoting effects of unleaded gasoline and 2,2,4-trimethylpentane on the development of atypical cell foci and renal tubular cell tumors in rats exposed to N-ethyl-N-hydroxyethylnitrosamine. *Cancer Res., 49*, 6369–6378

Siemiatycki, J., Dewar, R., Nadon, L., Gérin, M., Richardson, L. & Wacholder, S. (1987) Associations between several sites of cancer and twelve petroleum-derived liquids. Results from a case study in Montreal. *Scand. J. Work Environ. Health, 13*, 493–504

Solleveld, H.A., Haseman, J.K. & McConnell, E.E. (1984) Natural history of body weight gain, survival, and neoplasia in the F344 rat. *J. Natl Cancer Inst., 72*, 929–940

Swenberg, J.A. (1993) α_{2u}-Globulin nephropathy: review of the cellular and molecular mechanisms involved and their implications for human risk assessment. *Environ. Health Perspect.,* **101** (Suppl. 6), 39–44

Swenberg, J.A. & Dietrich, D.R. (1991) Immuno-histochemical localization of α_{2u}-globulin in kidneys of treated and control rats of a 13-week vapor inhalation study undertaken with methyl tertiary butyl ether (MTBE). Report to the MTBE Health Effects Testing Task Force

Swenberg, J.A., Short, B., Borghoff, S., Strasser, J. & Charbonneau, M. (1989) The comparative pathobiology of α_{2u}-globulin nephropathy. *Toxicol. Appl. Pharmacol.,* **97**, 35–46

Takahashi, K., Lindamood, C., III & Maronpot, R.R. (1993) Retrospective study of possible α_{2u}-globulin nephropathy and associated cell proliferation in male Fischer 344 rats dosed with *t*-butyl alcohol. *Environ. Health Perspect.,* **101** (Suppl. 5), 281–285

Uchida, K., Fukuda, A., Kawakishi, S., Toyokuni, S., Hiai, H., Ikeda, S. & Horio, F. (1995) Acute nephrotoxicity of a carcinogenic iron chelate. Selective inhibition of a pro-teolytic conversion of α_{2u}-globulin to the kidney fatty acid-binding protein. *FEBS Lett.,* **357**, 165–167

Umemura, T., Tokumo, K. & Williams, G.M. (1992) Cell proliferation induced in the kidneys and livers of rats and mice by short term exposure to the carcinogen *p*-dichlorobenzene. *Arch. Toxicol.,* **66**, 503–507

Umemura, T., Sai, K., Takagi, A., Hasegawa, R. & Kurokawa, Y. (1993) A possible role for cell proliferation in potassium bromate ($KBrO_3$) carcinogenesis. *J. Cancer Res. Clin. Oncol.,* **119**, 463–469

Umemura, T., Sai, K., Takagi, A., Hasegawa, R. & Kurokawa, Y. (1995) A possible role for oxidative stress in potassium bromate ($KBrO_3$) carcinogenesis. *Carcinogenesis,* **16**, 593–597

USEPA (United States Environmental Protection Agency) (1991) *Alpha-2U-Globulin: Association with Chemically-Induced Renal Toxicity and Neoplasia in the Male Rat* (EPA/625/3-91/019F), Washington, DC, US Environmental Protection Agency

Viau, C., Bernard, A., Gueret, F., Maldague, P., Gengoux, P. & Lauwerys, R. (1986) Isoparaffinic solvent-induced nephrotoxicity in the rat. *Toxicology,* **38**, 227–240

Wilke, A.V., Dorman, D.C. & Borghoff, S.J. (1994) Use of primary rat proximal tubule fragments for study of α_{2u}-globulin, 2,5-dichlorophenol, and 2,4,4-trimethyl-2-pentanol toxicity. *In Vitro Toxicol.,* **7**, 357–368

Corresponding author

R.L. Melnick
National Institute of Environmental Health Sciences
P.O. box 12233
Research Triangle Park,
NC 27709, USA

Species Differences in Thyroid, Kidney and Urinary Bladder Carcinogenesis
C.C. Capen, E. Dybing, J.M. Rice and J.D. Wilbourn, eds
IARC Scientific Publications No. 147
International Agency for Research on Cancer, Lyon, 1999

Human bladder cancer: epidemiological, pathological and mechanistic aspects

C. La Vecchia and L. Airoldi

Introduction

Among risk factors that have been associated with bladder carcinoma in humans are cigarette smoking, occupational exposure to various chemicals including aromatic amines, bladder infections by *Schistosoma haematobium* and the use of some drugs such as phenacetin-containing analgesics, chlornaphazine and cyclophosphamide. Associations with coffee drinking and artificial sweeteners, saccharin and cyclamates, have also been suspected, but the epidemiological evidence is now reassuring (Matanoski & Elliott, 1981; La Vecchia & Decarli, 1996; Ross *et al.*, 1996; Silverman *et al.*, 1996).

The possibility that bladder cancer is associated with many different chemical agents is not surprising, since most metabolites and carcinogens are excreted through the urinary tract. For example, tobacco smoking contains various mutagenic substances that, after being absorbed into the circulation, pass into the urine. Consequently, the urine of smokers is mutagenic in the Ames test (Doll & Peto, 1981; Silverman *et al.*, 1996).

The present paper reviews major aspects of the descriptive and analytical epidemiology of bladder cancer. Most data refer to transitional-cell carcinoma of the bladder, which accounts for about 95% of bladder cancer in white populations — but only about 85% in American blacks and even less in Middle East populations (Bedwani *et al.*, 1993). In the latter region, squamous-cell cancers are frequent and have considerably worse prognoses than transitional-cell types.

Descriptive epidemiology

Between 1973 and 1994 in the United States, bladder cancer incidence increased moderately in both sexes and various races, whereas mortality tended to decline, most noticeably in men (Kosary

et al., 1996). In Europe, high incidence rates for bladder carcinoma have been recorded in areas with a high concentration of chemical industries (northern Italy, Saarland and Bas-Rhin). Death rates also tend to be high in heavily industrialized countries (Figure 1), as well as in Egypt where bladder schistosomiasis is endemic (Bedwani *et al.*, 1993; Levi *et al.*, 1993, 1994).

Problems of case ascertainment and death certification may affect bladder cancer mortality data. In several countries rates in men have shown increases in the elderly, but stable or declining rates in middle age. Some of these patterns, however, are probably real, and reflect cohort effects in tobacco exposure, since this is one of the smoking-related neoplasms (US Office of Smoking and Health, 1982; IARC, 1985). Within Europe, there are in fact several similarities with the pattern of rates observed for lung cancer, with downward trends over the last one or two decades in several northern European countries, but persistent rises in southern and eastern Europe (La Vecchia *et al.*, 1992; Figure 2). Changes in occupational exposure to carcinogens (which are another major cause of bladder cancer (Matanoski & Elliott, 1981; La Vecchia & Decarli, 1996) in subsequent generations of European men may also have caused earlier rises and subsequent declines in rates, which are particularly large at younger ages.

In the late 1980s, most of the age-adjusted mortality rates for men within Europe fell in the rather narrow range of 5 to 8 per 100 000. Only Denmark (9.5) and Italy (9.1) had rates above 8. Low rates were registered in Sweden and a few southern European countries. Rates for women were between 1 and 3 per 100 000 in most countries, and showed no appreciable trend over time.

When an age, period and cohort model (Osmond & Gardner, 1982; Decarli & La Vecchia,

Figure 1. Bladder cancer mortality (age-standardized, world standard) in countries providing data to the World Health Organization database (from Levi *et al.*, 1994).

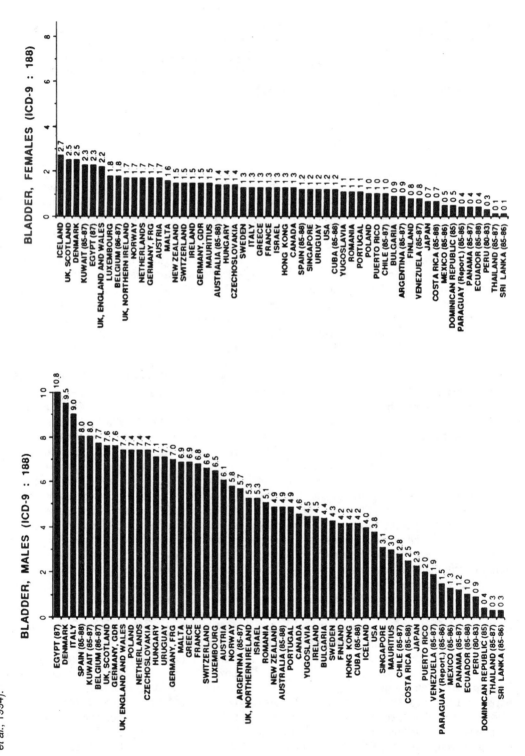

Figure 2. Trends in age-standardized mortality rates from bladder cancer in selected European countries (La Vecchia *et al.*, 1992). Males, +; females, ❑. Solid line: all ages; broken line, ages 35–64.

Deaths from bladder cancer

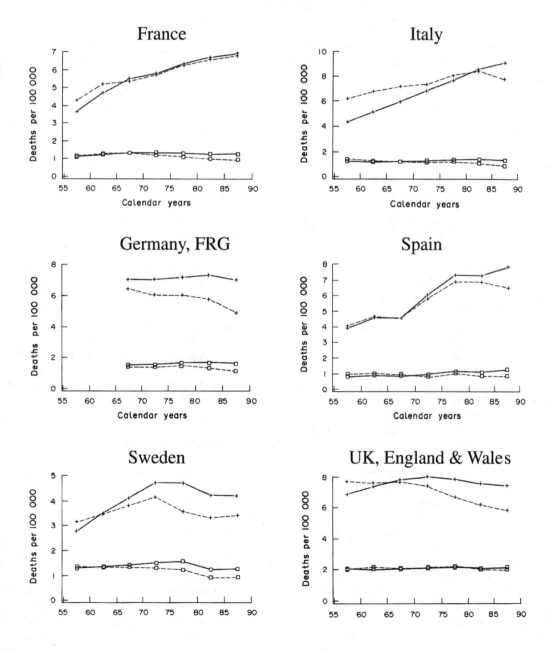

1987) was applied to mortality data, cohort values in men in most of western Europe increased up to the generations born around 1920–40, and declined thereafter (Figure 3a). Steady upward trends were however observed in Spain and Hungary. The pattern of cohort and period of death values were similar for women in several countries, although generally less consistent, possibly due to smaller absolute numbers (Figure 3b).

This pattern of cohort trends indicates that the generations with heaviest exposure to tobacco smoking, as well as occupational exposure to aromatic amines and other chemicals in most European countries, were those born in the first decades of the 20th century, with subsequent declines in most recent decades (La Vecchia et al., 1998).

Tobacco smoking

Cigarette smoking is undoubtedly the main recognized cause of bladder cancer not only in developed countries, but also in the few developing ones for which data are available (Bedwani et al., 1993, 1997). Smokers have a two- to four-fold increased risk for bladder cancer as compared to nonsmokers, and the risk increases with the number of cigarettes smoked and the duration of smoking. Furthermore, high-tar, black-tobacco cigarettes are associated with higher bladder cancer risk than low-tar, blond-tobacco types (Matanoski & Elliott, 1981; D'Avanzo et al., 1990) (Table 1).

More than two dozen case–control and several cohort studies have provided data on the smoking-bladder cancer relationship, and have consistently shown an elevated risk among smokers (Dolin, 1991). The largest study, based on 2992 cases and 5782 controls from 10 geographical areas of the United States (Hartge et al., 1987), found a relative risk (RR) of 2.9 for current and of 1.7 for former smokers. The RR declined to 1.4 after 30 or more years since stopping smoking. In another study of over 1800 cases from nine United States cities (Augustine et al., 1988), the RR was 2.5 for male heavy smokers, but the relation was less consistent for women.

Smokers of filtered low-tar cigarettes show a less strong association as compared to smokers of unfiltered high-tar cigarettes, with approximately a 30–40% lower risk. It is unclear, however, how much of this difference is due to the tar yield of cigarettes rather than to the type of tobacco, since

these two factors tend to be correlated. Black tobacco, in fact, has higher levels of aromatic amines, which are one of the major bladder carcinogenic components in tobacco smoking. For instance, in a case–control study from northern Italy (D'Avanzo et al., 1990), the RR was 3.8 for cigarette smokers of black tobacco, as compared to 2.7 for smokers of blond tobacco.

Smokers who have also been occupationally exposed to aromatic amines tend to have an additive component for the overall RR for bladder cancer, i.e. the RR for simultaneous exposure to both factors is closer to the sum than to the product of the individual risks (La Vecchia et al., 1990). This may also be related to the common constituents of genetic susceptibility, since slow acetylators are at increased risk for bladder cancer from both exposures (Bartsch et al., 1990; Vineis et al., 1990).

In terms of population-attributable risk, in Great Britain it was estimated that about 50% of bladder cancer cases could be attributed to cigarette smoking (85% of men and 27% of women, Moolgavkar & Stevens,1981). In the United States, the estimated proportion of bladder cancer associated with smoking was about half in men and about one-third in women (Hartge et al., 1987). In Italy, the proportion of bladder cancer attributable to tobacco smoking was of similar magnitude, on the basis of the number of smokers and relative risk estimates in case–control studies carried out in Turin and Milan (Vineis et al., 1983; D'Avanzo et al., 1990). In the latter study, the overall population-attributable risk was 50% (66% men, 17% women; D'Avanzo et al., 1995).

Occupational exposure to aromatic amines

A high risk of bladder carcinoma has been observed in dyestuff factory workers exposed to aromatic amines since the end of the 19th century. Involved in bladder carcinogenesis are 2-naphthylamine, benzidine and other aromatic amines, such as fuchsin, auramine and safranin (IARC, 1987).

It had been estimated that 5–10% of bladder carcinomas in Great Britain and North America were of occupational origin (Moolgavkar & Stevens, 1981). The proportion was probably greater in the past and in other heavily industrialized areas of the world, including for instance

Figure 3a. Age, period and cohort estimates for bladder cancer mortality among men in selected European countries, from La Vecchia *et al.*, 1998.

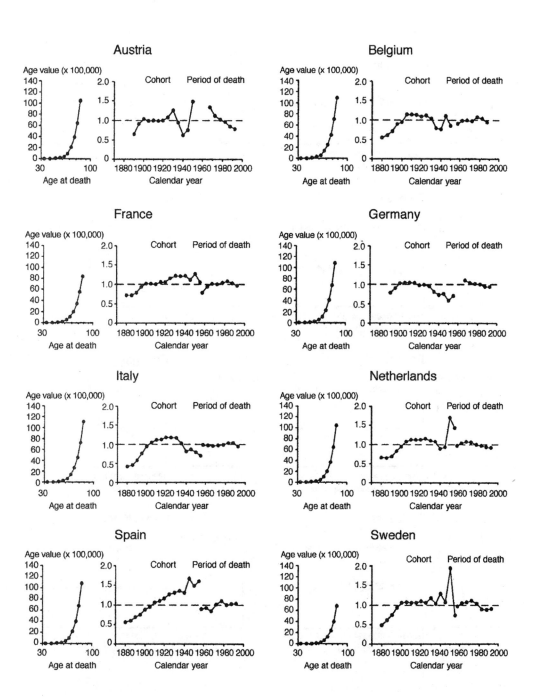

Figure 3a (contd).

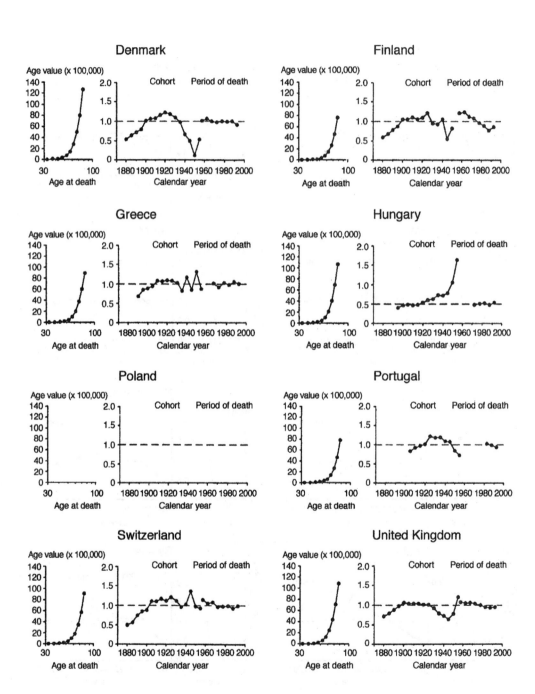

Figure 3b. Age, period and cohort estimates for bladder cancer mortality among women in selected European countries, from La Vecchia *et al.*, 1998.

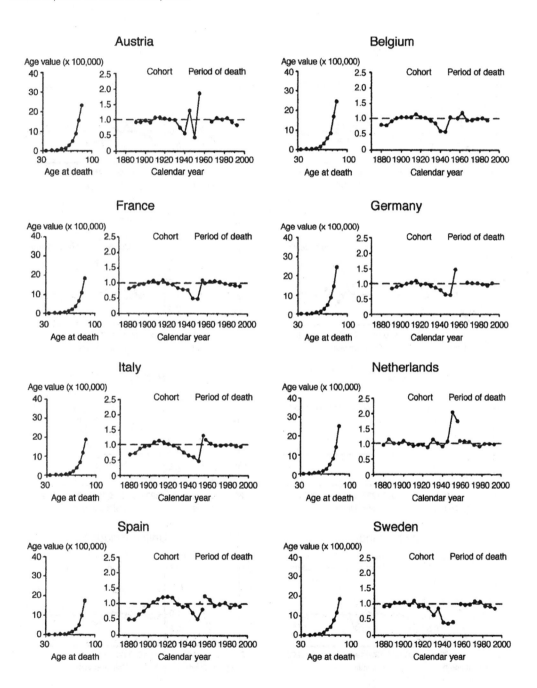

Figure 3b. (contd)

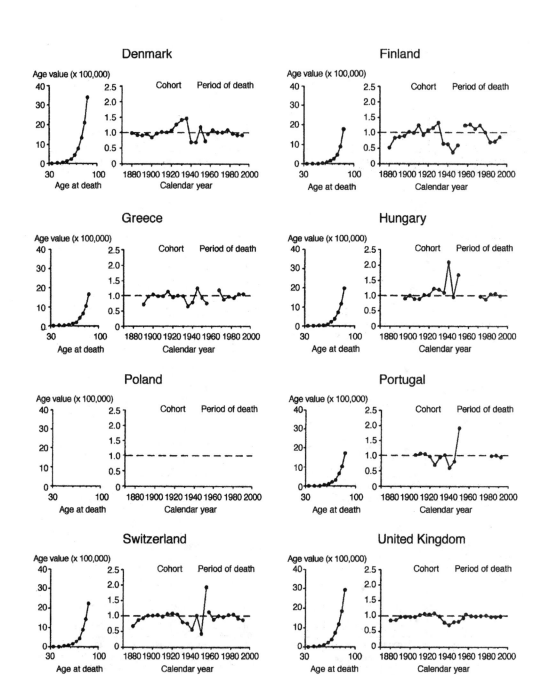

Table 1. Relative risk (RR) estimates (and 95% confidence intervals [CI]) of bladder cancer in relation to selected measures of exposure to tobacco smoking in a study of 337 cases and 392 controls from northern Italy[a]

	Bladder cancer	Controls	RR	(95% CI)
Never smokers	75	168	1[b]	
Ex-smokers	89	95	1.9	(1.2–3.1)
Current smokers				
< 20 cigarettes/day	73	60	2.9	(2.0–4.2)
≥ 20 cigarettes/day	100	69	3.9	(2.4–6.4)
Duration of smoking[c]				
< 30 years	56	84	1.8	(1.1–3.0)
≥ 30 years	187	119	3.5	(2.3–5.2)
Type of tobacco[c]				
Blond or mixed	205	187	2.7	(1.8–4.0)
Black	38	19	3.8	(2.0–7.4)

[a] From D'Avanzo *et al.* (1990)
[b] Reference category

central Europe (Levi *et al.*, 1993, 1994), and has likely been declining during the last few years (La Vecchia *et al.*, 1998).

Up to 1970, a group of dyestuff factory workers on the outskirts of Turin were exposed to naphthylamine, benzidine and other aromatic amines, and a study of hospital cases identified 23 bladder carcinomas (Rubino & Coscia, 1973). In this same cohort of workers, up to 1981, among 664 workers exposed to aromatic amines, 41 deaths from bladder carcinoma were registered (46 times the expected number). The data from this cohort provide therefore one of the few examples in human carcinogenesis in which the number of cases is so high as to allow the evaluation of duration of exposure, age at first exposure and time since last exposure in different models of carcinogenesis (Decarli *et al.*, 1985; Piolatto *et al.*, 1991).

The results obtained by applying two different models, multiplicative and additive (in other words assuming that the risk related to aromatic amines influences multiplicatively or additively the baseline risk), are shown in Table 2 with reference to categories arbitrarily chosen and showing, respectively, RR estimates and excess absolute risk.

On the basis of both models, the risk was higher in workers directly involved in the manufacture of aromatic amines than for those with irregular exposure. There was no marked effect of age at first exposure on the excess absolute risk of bladder carcinoma, but the RR was strongly and inversely associated with age at first exposure, even when duration and other variables were included in the model. Assuming that the process of carcinogenesis has several stages (the so-called 'multistage' carcinogenesis), this pattern of risk (i.e., an age independence on the excess absolute risk, and an inverse relationship of RR with age at first exposure) indicates an effect on one of the first stages of the carcinogenesis process (Armitage & Doll, 1961; Day & Brown, 1980).

The excess absolute risk increased considerably with duration of exposure, and continued to increase moderately even after exposure had stopped. The relative risk, however, diminished when exposure ceased, suggesting the existence also of an effect on one of the latter stages of the process. The results from the two models do not appear therefore to be contradictory when referred to the 'multistage' theory of carcinogenesis, even though they are not wholly consistent with a

Table 2. Relative and absolute excess bladder cancer risk estimates in workers exposed to aromatic amines according to different variables: data from a cohort of 664 workers of a dyestuff factory in northern Italy[a]

Variables	Multiplicative model Relative risk	Additive model Absolute excess risk
Age at first exposure		
< 25 years	1[b]	1[b]
25–34 years	0.42	1.05
≥ 35 years	0.17	1.77
Duration of exposure		
< 5 years	1[b]	1[b]
5–9 years	1.94	3.84
≥ 10 years	1.80	9.40
Job category		
Naphthylamine or benzidine manufacture	1[b]	1[b]
Naphthylamine or benzidine use	0.09	0.09
Intermittent contact with naphthylamine or benzidine	0.08	0.07
Fuchsin or safranin T manufacture	0.41	0.56
Time since last exposure		
During exposure	1[b]	1[b]
< 5 years	0.59	0.95
5–9 years	0.39	1.16
≥ 10 years	0.36	2.14

[a] From Decarli et al. (1985) and Piolatto et al. (1995), modified.
[b] Reference category

single stage effect, early or late, in the carcinogenesis process (Piolatto et al., 1991, 1995).

The results obtained by mathematical model fitting are of theoretical interest in that they provide information on the effects produced by carcinogens on a multistage process. In this model, it is assumed that only cells reaching the stage n have some likelihood of evolving to the $n + 1$ stage, and so on. The role of a carcinogen then would be to enhance such a likelihood. Carcinogens affecting early stages of the process (initiators) will influence the clinical appearance of the tumour after long periods (usually decades) since first exposure, due to the number of transitions required for the full process to be completed. Moreover, following the cessation of exposure, cancer incidence will continue to rise (Day & Brown, 1980; Hicks, 1980).

Different indications can be derived from a model that suggests a late-stage effect. This is considered to be a reversible phenomenon in the short–medium time frame (Hicks, 1980). In this case, absolute excess risk would be higher for older subjects, who are likely to have more cells in advanced transition stages. However, a late-stage effect is more readily preventable, since cessation of exposure will cause a substantial reduction in cancer incidence after a short interval.

The dyestuff worker study showed that aromatic amines probably act on more than one stage of the process of carcinogenesis, probably an early and a late one. According to a general role for preventing late-stage effects, removal of subjects known to have been exposed to bladder carcinogens from further exposure to aromatic amines and other bladder carcinogens, including tobacco, is a priority for prevention. However, since an early-stage effect was also suggested by the model of aromatic amines on bladder carcinogenesis, continuing surveillance of workers exposed to these chemicals in the past is of major importance. Thus, better understanding of the model of bladder carcinogenesis not only holds theoretical interest, but has also immediate implications for cancer prevention and public health.

Biomarkers of cancer susceptibility and exposure in risk assessment

Aromatic amines, like most other chemical carcinogens, require metabolic activation to reactive species that bind to DNA to exert their carcinogenic effect. Polymorphic distribution of the enzymes involved in the activation and/or deactivation of aromatic amines in humans has been regarded as an important determinant of individual susceptibility to their carcinogenic effects. Metabolic polymorphisms, genetically determined or arising from environmental factors, can mediate the formation of aromatic amine-DNA or haemoglobin adducts, that may be used to detect human exposure to these compounds. Biological markers of exposure in conjunction with markers of individual susceptibility may be predictive of bladder cancer risk.

The N-acetylation of aromatic amines and the O-acetylation of their N-hydroxy derivative are catalysed by acetyltransferases. Acetylation may result in detoxification, but, in some cases, acetylation causes activation to DNA-binding metabolites, as observed with the aryldiamine benzidine (Rothman et al., 1996; Zenser et al., 1996). N-acetyltransferase (NAT) activity in humans is coded by two distinct genes named NAT1 and NAT2 (Grant et al., 1989). The NAT2 enzyme has long been known to be polymorphic. In about 50% of Caucasians, termed slow acetylators, this enzyme activity is reduced. A number of point mutations in the NAT2 gene associated with the slow acetylator phenotype have been identified (Blum et al., 1991).

The relationship between acetylation phenotype and cancer susceptibility was first observed in a case–control study of bladder cancer, in which a large proportion of slow acetylators was detected among subjects occupationally exposed to aromatic amines, but not among smoke-related bladder cancer patients (Cartwright et al., 1982).

The high proportion of slow acetylators among occupationally exposed patients has been a matter of controversy (D'Errico et al., 1996). A significant excess of genotypic slow acetylators has also been reported in bladder cancer patients occupationally exposed to aromatic amines or who were cigarette smokers, thus confirming that the slow NAT2 genotype is a risk factor in bladder carcinogenesis (Risch et al., 1995; Okkels et al., 1997).

The NAT1 enzyme was considered to be monomorphic until some recent studies demonstrated the presence of a variant polyadenylation signal of the NAT1 gene (NAT1*10 allele) associated with higher enzyme activity (Bell et al., 1995). The activity of NAT1 is reportedly higher than that of NAT2 in the bladder and may increase the formation of DNA binding metabolites of aromatic amines within the target organ (Badawi et al., 1995). However, the NAT1 genotype has not been associated with increased risk of bladder cancer (Okkels et al., 1997).

The aromatic amine 4-aminobiphenyl (4-ABP), which is present in tobacco smoke, is thought to be relevant to bladder carcinogenesis. In line with the risks for bladder cancer observed in epidemiological studies, the levels of 4-ABP-haemoglobin adducts have been associated with smoking status and type of tobacco (Bryant et al., 1988) and with aromatic amine-DNA adducts in exfoliated urothelial cells (Talaska et al., 1991). The NAT2 phenotype is associated with levels of 4-ABP-haemoglobin adducts which were higher in subjects with the slow phenotype than in those with the rapid one (Bartsch et al., 1990; Vineis et al., 1990; Yu et al., 1994). The NAT2 phenotype did not affect DNA-benzidine adducts in exfoliated urothelial cells from exposed workers, suggesting a different activation pathway for aromatic mono- and diamines (Rothman et al., 1996).

The NAT1*10 genotype and phenotype correlated with higher levels of aromatic amine adducts in DNA from bladder mucosa. As expected, individuals with the slow NAT2 and the rapid NAT1 genotypes showed the highest adduct level (Badawi et al., 1995).

About 50% of Caucasians show an inherited deletion of two copies of the gene for the enzyme glutathione S-transferase M1, which is involved in the detoxification of a number of carcinogens. Several studies have suggested that individuals homozygous for the deleted genotype (*GSTM1* 0/0) are at higher risk of developing bladder cancer (Bell *et al.*, 1993; Brockmöller *et al.*, 1994). However, it was shown that the *GSTM1* deletion may not be a risk factor for bladder cancer development, but may be related to the bladder cancer patient survival (Okkels *et al.*, 1996).

Although 4-ABP or its metabolites have not been shown to be substrates for glutathione S-transferases, 4-ABP-haemoglobin adduct levels were higher in subjects carrying the *GSTM1* 0/0 genotype who were also slow acetylators (Yu *et al.*, 1995). It is thus evident that 4-ABP-DNA and haemoglobin adduct formation is significantly influenced by metabolic polymorphism, and might modify bladder cancer risk.

Hair dyes

Studies of occupational exposure to hair dyes up to 1992 were reviewed within the *IARC Monographs* programme (IARC, 1993). At least seven cohort and 11 case–control studies have included data on occupational exposure to hair dyes — among hairdressers, barbers and beauticians — and subsequent bladder cancer risk. The pooled RR estimate was 1.4 (183 observed versus 129 expected) for cohort studies, and some association was also observed in several case–control studies. These results are compatible with some moderate associa-tion between past professional exposure to hair dyes and subsequent bladder cancer risk, but errors and biases in observational epidemio-logical studies could be responsible, particularly since allowance for smoking was lacking or inad-equate in most studies. A major open question, moreover, is whether current exposure to modern hair dyes is still related to some excess risk, or whether the selective elimination of carcinogenic compounds over recent years has reduced any such risk to immeasurable levels. Only further surveil-lance and future studies will provide definite answers.

Five case–control studies included information on personal use of hair dyes and bladder cancer risk. None of these showed any excess bladder cancer risk among users of hair dyes (Table 3). Thus, the overall evidence from epidemiological studies allows the exclusion of any appreciable and measurable risk for bladder cancer from personal use of hair dyes (La Vecchia & Tavani, 1995).

Dietary factors

A role of diet and nutrition on bladder carcino-genesis is plausible, since most substances and metabolites, including carcinogens, are excreted through the urinary tract. Ecological studies have found positive correlations between fat and oil consumption and bladder cancer, but these are

Table 3. Summary results from selected case–control studies of bladder cancer providing information on personal use of hair dyes[a]

Reference, country	Sex	No. of cases	No. of exposed cases	Odds ratio
Howe *et al.* (1980), Canada	F	152	NR	0.7
	M	480	8	- (No exposed control)
Hartge *et al.* (1982), USA	F	733	443	0.9
	M	2249	172	1.1
Ohno *et al.* (1985), Japan	F	65	42	1.6
Claude *et al.* (1986), Germany	F	91	NR	No association
	M	340	NR	
Nomura *et al.* (1989), USA	F	66	41	1.5
	M	195	1.5	1.3

[a] From La Vecchia & Tavani (1996), modified

F, female; M, male; NR, not reported

only partly reflected in the international differences in bladder cancer rates, which are generally higher in Europe than in North America. At least 10 case–control and three cohort studies of bladder cancer including some information on dietary factors have been published over the last two decades, and these have recently been reviewed (La Vecchia & Negri, 1996).

Of seven studies which considered various types and measures of fruit and vegetable consumption, six found a reduced risk with increasing consumption, which was more consistent for vegetables, with RR estimates of between 0.5 and 0.7 for the highest versus the lowest consumption level. There is, therefore, suggestive evidence that a diet rich in fresh fruit and vegetables is a correlate — or an indicator — of reduced bladder cancer risk. No clear association emerged for other foods investigated, including meat and milk.

With reference to nutrients (Table 4), total fat intake was related to bladder cancer risk in three case–control studies, with RRs between 1.4 and 1.7 for the highest versus the lowest consumption level. However, no relation between fats and bladder cancer emerged in a cohort study on Japanese Americans in Hawaii (Nomura *et al.*, 1991). Similarly, no consistent association emerged between protein or carbohydrate consumption and bladder cancer risk.

Among micronutrients, vitamin A, and particularly carotenoids, showed a protective effect on bladder cancer risk in four case–control studies (Mettlin & Graham, 1979; La Vecchia *et al.*, 1989; Nomura *et al.*, 1991; Vena *et al.*, 1992), including one in which total calorie intake was measured, but they were not consistently related in two other studies. There were only scattered and inconclusive data on vitamin C and E (Risch *et al.*, 1988; Riboli *et al.*, 1991). One study suggested that calcium intake may be related to bladder cancer risk (Riboli *et al.*, 1991). Another, conducted in New York City, found an RR of 2.1 for the highest sodium consumption level (Vena *et al.*, 1992).

Table 4. Relationship between intake of various nutrients and bladder cancer risk. Main results from selected studies[a]

Reference, country	Nutrient	Relative risk estimate for level of intake[b]				
		1 (low)[c]	2	3	4	5 (high)
Steineck *et al.* (1990), Sweden	Fat	1	1.0	1.4	1.4	1.7
	Protein	1	0.9	1.0	1.2	1.4
	Carbohydrates	1	1.2	1.2	1.6	1.2
	Total energy	1	1.1	1.5	1.7	1.4
Riboli *et al.* (1991), Spain	Total fat	1	1.4	1.6	1.4	-
	Saturated fat	1	1.7	2.2	2.3	-
	Protein	1	1.1	1.2	1.5	-
	Carbohydrates	1	1.2	1.0	1.4	-
Vena *et al.* (1992), USA	Fat	1	1.3	1.2	1.4	-
	Protein	1	0.8	0.6	0.6	-
	Carbohydrates	1	1.0	1.0	1.0	-
	Total energy	1	1.3	1.6	1.8	-
Chyou *et al.* (1993), Hawaii	Fat	1	0.7	0.9	-	-
	Protein	1	0.7	0.9	-	-
	Carbohydrates	1	0.7	1.0	-	-
	Total energy	1	0.8	1.1	-	-

[a] From La Vecchia & Negri (1996), modified
[b] In some cases, summary relative risk is derived from published data.
[c] Reference category

Thus, available data on diet and bladder cancer remain inconclusive. This is at least partly attributable to the limited number of cohort studies, in which satisfactorily detailed and validated dietary questionnaires were used. Despite these limitations, available data suggest that a diet rich in fresh fruit and vegetables is a correlate of reduced bladder cancer risk. The role of specific nutrients remains open to debate.

Coffee drinking

Since the early 1970s, the possible association between coffee consumption and bladder cancer risk has been a topic of widespread interest. Cole (1971), in a case–control study from the Boston area reported an RR of 1.2 in men and 2.6 in women who drank coffee compared with non-drinkers. Since then, more than two dozen case–control studies have been published on the topic, the main results of which have been reviewed in detail, among others, in the IARC Monographs programme (1991).

Briefly, compared with non-consumers of coffee, the RR in most studies tended to be elevated in drinkers, but this increase was generally not dose- or duration-related.

This risk pattern was clear in the largest case–control study on bladder cancer based on 2982 cases and 5782 controls interviewed in a collaborative, population-based study in 10 geographical areas of the United States (Hartge *et al.* (1983). The RRs for ever versus never coffee drinkers, after simultaneous allowance for sex, age, race, geographical area and tobacco consumption, were 1.6 (95% confidence interval (CI), 1.2–2.2) for men, 1.2 (95% CI, 0.8–1.7) for women, and 1.4 (95% CI, 1.1–1.8) for both sexes combined. When various consumption levels were considered, the RR was 1.5 (95% CI, 1.1–1.9) for men who drank over 64 cups per week, but no consistent dose–risk relation was evident in either sex. Similarly, there was no association with duration of coffee drinking. No interaction or effect modification was observed with geographical area, race, occupation, artificial sweetener use or history of urinary tract infections. The authors noted that adjustment for smoking reduced the RR for ever versus never coffee drinking from 1.8 to 1.4, and that residual confounding by tobacco (or other correlates of coffee drinking) would only partly explain the apparent relation-

ship between bladder cancer and coffee drinking, which was still present when only subjects who claimed to be lifelong nonsmokers were considered.

On the basis of these findings, together with data from different parts of the world on the coffee–bladder cancer relation, it is possible to exclude confidently a strong association between coffee and bladder cancer, while at the same time it appears that coffee drinking may represent an indicator of risk. Whether this indicator is non-specific or includes some aspects of causality is still open to debate.

In biological terms, caffeine and the large number of other substances contained in coffee may have a wide spectrum of direct as well as indirect metabolic activities. It is therefore conceivable that even small amounts of coffee may induce changes in levels of carcinogens or anti-carcinogens in the bladder epithelium. On the other hand (although it is less likely), coffee drinking may systematically interfere with the likelihood of interview. These and other possible sources of error or bias may at first sight appear to be largely speculative. A considerable amount of epidemiological research, however, has systematically, and with remarkable consistency, shown an association between coffee and bladder cancer. Even apparently less plausible hypotheses should therefore be considered and, if possible, tested in future research (La Vecchia, 1993).

Saccharin and other artificial sweeteners

Large quantities of saccharin (i.e., a few percent of the diet) have been shown to cause bladder cancer in rodents, when administered after N-methyl-N-nitrosourea, and when given alone over more than one generation (US Congress Office of Technology Assessment, 1977; Doll & Peto, 1981; Silverman *et al.*, 1996).

A case–control study based on 408 cases (Howe *et al.*, 1977) showed a 60% increased risk for bladder cancer in men (but not women) who used artificial sweeteners. The issue attracted widespread interest at that time, but several subsequent epidemiological studies failed to provide any consistent evidence of association between saccharin or other artificial sweeteners consumed in various forms and human bladder cancer. The RRs were slightly above unity in some of these and slightly below unity in others, with no clear pattern.

The largest and most informative study included 3010 cases of bladder cancer and 5783 population controls from 10 areas of the USA (Hoover & Hartge Strasser, 1980): the overall RR associated with ever having used any form of artificial sweeteners was 1.02 (95% CI, 0.92–1.11). No association was observed in men (RR, 0.99) or women (RR, 1.07), nor according to type or form of artificial sweeteners, and there was no dose–risk relationship. This study also evaluated subgroups based on use of cigarettes and potential exposures to occupational carcinogens. Excesses of borderline significance were observed in nonsmoking women, smoking men, and heavily smoking women.

In contrast, a study from the Greater Boston area (Morrison & Buring, 1980) found an RR of 0.6 in smoking men and 1.5 in smoking women, although none of these estimates was significant. Similarly inconsistent results across strata of sex and smoking habits were observed in a study from Yorkshire, UK (Cartwright et al., 1981). The authors did not interpret these finding as suggestive of human carcinogenicity of saccharin. In another study, no association was observed in separate strata of histological type of bladder cancer (squamous-cell, adenocarcinoma, transitional-cell; Kantor et al., 1988).

In a study on postmortem material, no relation was found between the proportion of atypical nuclei in bladder epithelium and use of artificial sweeteners. Information on the latter was available for only 149 out of 282 patients. Proportions were unadjusted for tobacco smoke (Auerbach & Garfinkel, 1989).

A descriptive study from Denmark (Jensen & Kambi, 1982) provided no evidence of increased bladder cancer rates during the first 30–35 years of life associated with *in utero* saccharin exposure during the Second World War.

It is therefore now clear that saccharin — or other artificial sweeteners — in the doses commonly used, are not relevant human bladder carcinogens on an individual risk or public health level.

Urinary tract diseases

Infectious agents and other diseases of the urinary tract, which may cause chronic irritation and hence favour the action of specific carcinogens, have a major influence on bladder cancer risk in developing countries such as Egypt and Tanzania.

In these areas, there is a consistent relation between bladder carcinoma and bladder schistosomiasis, and a substantial proportion of bladder cancers are of squamous-cell type (Morrison & Cole, 1982; Kantor et al., 1984; Bedwani et al., 1993, 1997).

Urinary tract infections, moreover, may explain the relatively high bladder cancer rates in some southern Italian provinces where rates of other tobacco-related neoplasms are relatively low (Cislaghi et al., 1986). The proportion of cases in Italy attributable to infection is difficult to estimate, but is probably about 10% (La Vecchia et al., 1991; D'Avanzo et al., 1995). The strength of the association, however, remains open to discussion, because of difficulties in exposure assessment and definition among other factors.

In fact, the role of infectious agents other than schistosomiasis and of nonspecific cystitis or urinary calculi in bladder carcinogenesis is difficult to study epidemiologically, particularly because early symptoms of bladder cancer are similar to those of cystitis, and subjects with urinary tract conditions probably tend systematically to recall episodes of cystitis or other urinary tract conditions more accurately. Not surprisingly, therefore, published evidence is somewhat inconsistent, with RRs for urinary tract infections ranging from 1 (Kjaer et al., 1989) to 5 (Wynder et al., 1963) and for urinary tract stones from 1 (Kjaer et al., 1989) to 2.5 (Dunham et al., 1968).

With reference to urinary tract stones, the RR for bladder cancer was 2.2 in males in an early US study (Wynder et al., 1963), and around 1.5 in the large multicentric US study (Kantor et al., 1984). Three more recent case-control studies (González et al., 1991; La Vecchia et al., 1991; Sturgeon et al., 1994) found RRs between 1.2 and 1.4. Whether this reflects a causal association rather than recall bias is still unclear.

A Swedish record-linkage study, based on a cohort of 61,114 patients hospitalized for kidney or ureter stones and followed for up to 18 years (Chow et al., 1997), based on a total of 46 cases of renal pelvis or ureter cancer and 319 cases of bladder cancer, found a standardized incidence ratio of 2.5 for renal pelvis or ureter cancer and 1.4 for bladder cancer. The association was stronger in women. In a prospective cohort study of Japanese conducted in Hawaii, no relation was observed between serum uric acid and bladder cancer (Kolonel *et al.*, 1994).

Most findings, therefore, are consistent with a two- to three-fold elevated risk for urinary tract infections, although some of this apparent excess may be attributed to more accurate recall of urinary symptoms by bladder cancer cases. For urinary tract stones the association is moderate, and its causality remains open to discussion; this association may be stronger in women (La Vecchia *et al.*, 1991).

Published data also indicate that the role of urinary tract infections is probably related to one of the later stages of the process of carcinogenesis (Armitage & Doll, 1961).

Conclusions

There is ample scope for prevention and control of bladder cancer, including (*a*) avoidance of tobacco smoking; (*b*) close surveillance and avoidance of occupational exposures to aromatic amines and other related chemicals; (*c*) dietary changes, which have not yet, however, been satisfactorily defined; (*d*) stricter control of bladder and other urinary tract infections; and (*e*) identification of individuals who are susceptible to aromatic amine carcinogenesis.

Acknowledgement

This work was conducted within the framework of the CNR (Italian National Research Council) 'Clinical Applications of Oncological Research' (Contract No. 96.00759.PF39), and with the contribution of the Italian Association for Cancer Research, Milan. The Authors thank Mrs J. Baggott, M.P. Bonifacino and the G.A. Pfeiffer Memorial Library staff for editorial assistance.

References

Armitage, P. & Doll, R. (1961) Stochastic models for carcinogenesis. In: Neyman J., ed., *Proceedings of the 4th Berkeley Symposium on Mathematical Statistics and Probability*, Vol. 4, Berkeley, University of California, p. 19

Auerbach, O. & Garfinkel, L. (1989) Histologic changes in the urinary bladder in relation to cigarette smoking and use of artificial sweeteners. *Cancer*, **64**, 983–987

Augustine, A., Hebert, J.R., Kabat, G.C. & Wynder, E.L. (1988) Bladder cancer in relation to cigarette smoking. *Cancer Res.*, **48**, 4405–4408

Badawi, A.F., Hirvonen, A., Bell, D.A., Lang, N.P. & Kadlubar, F.F. (1995) Role of aromatic amine acetyltransferases, NAT1 and NAT2, in carcinogen-DNA adduct formation in the human urinary bladder. *Cancer Res.*, **55**, 5230–5237

Bartsch, H., Caporaso, N., Coda, M., Kadlubar, F., Malaveille, C., Skipper, P., Talaska, G., Tannenbaum, S.R. & Vineis, P. (1990) Carcinogen hemoglobin adducts, urinary mutagenicity, and metabolic phenotype in active and passive cigarette smokers. *J. Natl Cancer Inst.*, **82**, 1826–1831

Bedwani, R., El Khwsky, F., La Vecchia, C., Boffetta, P. & Levi, F. (1993) Descriptive epidemiology of bladder cancer in Egypt. *Int. J. Cancer*, **55**, 351–352

Bedwani, R., Renganathan, E., El Khwsky, F., Braga, C., Abu Seif, H.H., Abul Azm, T., Zaki, A., Franceschi, S., Boffetta, P. & La Vecchia, C. (1997) Schistosomiasis and the risk of bladder cancer in Alexandria, Egypt. *Br. J. Cancer*, **77**, 1186–1189

Bell, D.A., Taylor, J.A., Paulson, D.F., Robertson, C.N., Mohler, J.L. & Lucier, G.W. (1993) Genetic risk and carcinogen exposure: a common inherited defect of the carcinogen-metabolism gene glutathione S-transferase M1 (GSTM1) that increases susceptibility to bladder cancer. *J. Natl Cancer Inst.*, **85**, 1159–1164

Bell, D.A., Badawi, A.F., Lang, N.P., Ilett, K.F., Kadlubar, F.F. & Hirvonen, A. (1995) Polymorphism in the *N*-acetyltransferase 1 (NAT1) polyadenylation signal: association of NAT1*10 allele with higher *N*-acetylation activity in bladder and colon tissue. *Cancer Res.*, **55**, 5226–5229

Blum, M., Demierre, A., Grant, D.M., Heim, M. & Meyer, U.A. (1991) Molecular mechanism of slow acetylation of drugs and carcinogens in humans. *Proc. Natl Acad. Sci. USA*, **88**, 5237–5241

Brockmöller, J., Kerb, R., Drakoulis, N., Staffeldt, B. & Roots, I. (1994) Glutathione S-transferase M1 and its variants A and B as host factors of bladder cancer susceptibility: a case–control study. *Cancer Res.*, **54**, 4103–4111

Bryant, M.S., Vineis, P., Skipper, P.L. & Tannenbaum, S.R. (1988) Hemoglobin adducts of aromatic amines: associations with smoking status and type of tobacco. *Proc. Natl Acad. Sci. USA*, **85**, 9788–9791

Cartwright, R.A., Adib, R., Glashan, R. & Gray, B.K. (1981) The epidemiology of bladder cancer in West Yorkshire. A preliminary report on non-occupational aetiologies. *Carcinogenesis*, **2**, 343-347

Cartwright, R.A., Glashan, R.W., Rogers, H.J., Ahmad, R.A., Barham Hall, D., Higgins, E. & Kahn, M.A. (1982) Role of *N*-acetyltransferase phenotypes in bladder carcinogenesis: a pharmacogenetic epidemiological approach to bladder cancer. *Lancet*, ii, 842–845

Chow, W.-H., Lindblad, P., Gridley, G., Nyrén, O., McLaughlin, J.K., Linet, M.S., Pennello, G.A., Adami, H.-O. & Fraumeni, J.F., Jr (1997) Risk of urinary tract cancers following kidney or ureter stones. *J. Natl Cancer Inst.*, **89**, 1453–1457

Chyou, P.H., Nomura, A.M.Y. & Stemmermann, G.N. (1993) A prospective study of diet, smoking, and lower urinary tract cancer. *Ann. Epidemiol.*, **3**, 211–216

Cislaghi, C., Decarli, A., La Vecchia, C., Laverda, N., Mezzanotte, G. & Smans, M. (1986) *Dati, Indicatori e Mappe di Mortalità Tumorale, Italia 1975–77*, Bologna, Pitagora Editrice

Claude, J., Kunze, E., Frentzel-Beyme, R., Paczkowski, K., Schneider, J. & Schubert, H. (1986) Life-style and occupational risk factors in cancer of the lower urinary tract. *Am. J. Epidemiol.*, **124**, 578–589

Cole, P. (1971) Coffee-drinking and cancer of the lower urinary tract. *Lancet, i*, 1335–1337

D'Avanzo, B., Negri, E., La Vecchia, C., Gramenzi, A., Bianchi, C., Franceschi, S. & Boyle, P. (1990) Cigarette smoking and bladder cancer. *Eur. J. Cancer*, **26**, 714–718

D'Avanzo, B., La Vecchia, C., Negri, E., Decarli, A. & Benichou, J. (1995) Attributable risks for bladder cancer in northern Italy. *Ann. Epidemiol.*, **5**, 427–431

Day, N.E. & Brown, C.C. (1980) Multistage models and primary prevention of cancer. *J. Natl Cancer Inst.*, **64**, 977–989

Decarli, A. & La Vecchia, C. (1987) Age, period and cohort models: review of knowledge and implementation in GLIM. *Riv. Stat. Appl.*, **20**, 397–410

Decarli, A., Peto, J., Piolatto, G. & La Vecchia, C. (1985) Bladder cancer mortality of workers exposed to aromatic amines: analysis of models of carcinogenesis. *Br. J. Cancer*, **51**, 707–712

D'Errico, A., Taioli, E., Chen, X. & Vineis, P. (1996) Genetic metabolic polymorphisms and the risk of cancer: a review of the literature. *Biomarkers*, **1**, 149–173

Dolin, P.J. (1991) An epidemiological review of tobacco use and bladder cancer. *J. Smoking-Rel. Dis.*, **2**, 129–143

Doll, R. & Peto, R. (1981) The causes of cancer. Quantitative estimates of avoidable risks of cancer in the United States today. *J. Natl Cancer Inst.*, **66**, 1191–1308

Dunham, L.J., Rabson, A.S., Stewart, H.L., Frank, A.S. & Young, J.L. (1968) Rates, interview, and pathology study of cancer of the urinary bladder in New Orleans, Louisiana. *J. Natl Cancer Inst.*, **41**, 683–709

González, C.A., Errezola, M., Izarzugaza, I., López-Abente, G., Escolar, A., Nebot, M. & Riboli, E. (1991) Urinary infection, renal lithiasis and bladder cancer in Spain. *Eur. J. Cancer*, **27**, 498–500.

Grant, D.M., Lottspeich, F. & Meyer, U.A. (1989) Evidence for two closely related isozymes of arylamine N-acetyl-transferase in human liver. *FEBS Lett.*, **244**, 203–207

Hartge, P., Hoover, R., Altman, R., Austin, D.F., Cantor, K.P., Child, M.A., Key, C.R., Mason, T.J., Marrett, L.D., Myers, M.H., Narayana, A.S., Silverman, D.T., Sullivan, J.W., Swanson, G.M., Thomas, D.B. & West, D.W. (1982) Use of hair dyes and risk of bladder cancer. *Cancer Res.*, **42**, 4784–4787

Hartge, P., Hoover, R., West, D.W. & Lyon, J.L. (1983) Coffee drinking and risk of bladder cancer. *J. Natl Cancer Inst.*, **70**, 1021–1026

Hartge, P., Silverman, D., Hoover, R., Schairer, C., Altman, R., Austin, D., Cantor, K., Child, M., Key, C., Marrett, L.D., Mason, T.J., Meigs, J.W., Myers, M.H., Narayana, A., Sullivan, J.W., Swanson, G.M., Thomas, D. & West, D. (1987) Changing cigarette habits and bladder cancer risk: a case–control study. *J. Natl Cancer Inst.*, **78**, 1119–1125

Hicks, R.M. (1980) Multistage carcinogenesis in the urinary bladder. *Br. Med. Bull.*, **36**, 39–46

Hoover, R.N. & Hartge Strasser, P. (1980) Artificial sweeteners and human bladder cancer. Preliminary results. *Lancet, i*, 837–840

Howe, G.R., Burch, J.D., Miller, A.B., Morrison, B., Gordon, P., Weldon, L., Chambers, L.W., Fodor, G. & Winsor, G.M. (1977) Artificial sweeteners and human bladder cancer. *Lancet, ii*, 578–581

Howe, G.R., Burch, J.D., Miller, A.B., Cook, G.M., Esteve, J., Morrison, B., Gordon, P., Chambers, L.W., Fodor, G. & Winsor, G.M. (1980) Tobacco use, occupation, coffee, various nutrients, and bladder cancer. *J. Natl Cancer Inst.*, **64**, 701–713

IARC (1985) *IARC Monographs on the Evaluation of the Carcinogenic Risks of Chemicals to Humans*, Vol. 38, *Tobacco Smoking*, Lyon

IARC (1987) *IARC Monographs on the Evaluation of Carcinogenic Risks to Humans*, Suppl. 7, *Overall Evaluation of Carcinogenicity: An Updating of* IARC Monographs *Volumes 1 to 42*, Lyon

IARC (1991) *IARC Monographs on the Evaluation of Carcinogenic Risks to Humans*, Vol. 51, *Coffee, Tea, Mate and Methylxanthines*, Lyon

IARC (1993) *IARC Monographs on the Evaluation of Carcinogenic Risks to Humans*, Vol. 57, *Occupational Exposures of Hairdressers and Barbers and Personal Use of Hair Colourants; Some Hair Dyes, Cosmetic Colourants, Industrial Dyestuffs and Aromatic Amines*, Lyon

Jensen, O.M. & Kamby, C. (1982) Intra-uterine exposure to saccharin and risk of bladder cancer in man. *Int. J. Cancer*, **29**, 507–509

Kantor, A.F., Hartge, P., Hoover, R.N., Narayana, A.S., Sullivan, J.W. & Fraumeni, J.F., Jr (1984) Urinary tract infection and risk of bladder cancer. *Am. J. Epidemiol.*, 119, 510–515

Kantor, A.F., Hartge, P., Hoover, R.N. & Fraumeni, J.F., Jr (1988) Epidemiological characteristics of squamous cell carcinoma and adenocarcinoma of the bladder. *Cancer Res.*, 48, 3853–3855

Kjaer, S.K., Knudsen, J.B., Sorensen, B.L. & Jensen, O.M. (1989) The Copenhagen case–control study of bladder cancer. V. Review of the role of urinary-tract infection. *Acta Oncol.*, 28, 631–636

Kolonel, L.N., Yoshizawa, C., Nomura, A.M. & Stemmermann, G.N. (1994) Relationship of serum uric acid to cancer occurrence in a prospective male cohort. *Cancer Epidemiol. Biomarkers Prev.*, 3, 225–228

Kosary, C.L., Gloeckler Ries, L.A., Miller, B.A., Hankey, B.F., Harras, A. & Edwards, B.K., eds (1996) *SEER Cancer Statistics Review, 1973-1992. Tables and Graphs*, Bethesda, MD, US Department of Health and Human Services

La Vecchia, C. (1993) Coffee and cancer epidemiology. In: Garattini, S., ed., *Caffeine, Coffee, and Health*, New York, Raven Press, pp. 379–398

La Vecchia, C. & Decarli, A. (1996) Epidemiology of bladder cancer. In: Luciani, L., Debruyne, F.M.J. & Schalken, J.A., eds, *Basic Research in Urological Oncology*, Basel, Karger, pp. 86–96

La Vecchia, C. & Negri, E. (1996) Nutrition and bladder cancer. *Cancer Causes Control*, 7, 95–100

La Vecchia, C. & Tavani, A. (1995) Epidemiological evidence on hair dyes and the risk of cancer in humans. *Eur. J. Cancer Prev.*, 4, 31–43

La Vecchia, C., Negri, E., Decarli, A., D'Avanzo, B., Liberati, C. & Franceschi, S. (1989) Dietary factors in the risk of bladder cancer. *Nutr. Cancer*, 12, 93–101

La Vecchia, C., Negri, E., D'Avanzo, B. & Franceschi, S. (1990) Occupation and the risk of bladder cancer. *Int. J. Epidemiol.*, 19, 264–268

La Vecchia, C., Negri, E., D'Avanzo, B., Savoldelli, R. & Franceschi, S. (1991) Genital and urinary tract diseases and bladder cancer. *Cancer Res.*, 51, 629–631

La Vecchia, C., Lucchini, F., Negri, E., Boyle, P., Maisonneuve, P. & Levi, F. (1992) Trends of cancer mortality in Europe, 1955–1989: IV. Urinary tract, eye, brain and nerves, and thyroid. *Eur. J. Cancer*, 28A, 1210–1281

La Vecchia, C., Negri, E., Levi, F., Decarli, A. & Boyle, P. (1998) Cancer mortality in Europe: Effects of age, cohort of birth and period of death. *Eur. J. Cancer*, 34, 118–141

Levi, F., La Vecchia, C., Lucchini, F. & Boyle, P. (1993) Cancer incidence and mortality in Europe 1983-87. *Soz. Praventivmed.*, 34 (Suppl. 3), S155–S229

Levi, F., Lucchini, F. & La Vecchia, C. (1994) Worldwide patterns of cancer mortality, 1985–89. *Eur. J. Cancer Prev.*, 3, 109–143

Matanoski, G.M. & Elliott, E.A. (1981) Bladder cancer epidemiology. *Epidemiol. Rev.*, 3, 203–229

Mettlin, C. & Graham, S. (1979) Dietary risk factors in human bladder cancer. *Am. J. Epidemiol.*, 110, 255–263

Moolgavkar, S.H. & Stevens, R.G. (1981) Smoking and cancer of bladder and pancreas: risks and temporal trends. *J. Natl Cancer Inst.*, 67, 15–23

Morrison, A.S. & Burin, J.E. (1980) Artificial sweeteners and cancer of the lower urinary tract. *N. Engl. J. Med.*, 302, 537–541

Morrison, A.S. & Cole, P. (1982) Urinary tract. In: Schottenfeld, D., ed., *Cancer Epidemiology and Prevention*, Philadelphia, Saunders, pp. 925–937

Nomura, A., Kolonel, L.N. & Yoshizawa, C.N. (1989) Smoking, alcohol, occupation, and hair dye use in cancer of the lower urinary tract. *Am. J. Epidemiol.*, 130, 1159–1163

Nomura, A.M., Kolonel, L.N., Hankinn, J.H. & Yoshizawa, C.N. (1991) Dietary factors in cancer of the lower urinary tract. *Int. J. Cancer*, 48, 199–205

Ohno, Y., Aoki, K., Obata, K. & Morrison, A.S. (1985) Case–control study of urinary bladder cancer in metropolitan Nagoya. *Natl Cancer Inst. Monogr.*, 69, 229–234

Okkels, H., Sigsgaard, T., Wolf, H. & Autrup, H. (1996) Glutathione S-transferase μ as a risk factor in bladder tumours. *Pharmacogenetics*, 6, 251–256.

Okkels, H., Sigsgaard, T., Wolf, H. & Autrup, H. (1997) Arylamine N-acetyltransferase 1 (NAT1) and 2 (NAT2) polymorphisms in susceptibility to bladder cancer: the influence of smoking. *Cancer Epidemiol. Biomarkers Prev.*, 6, 225–231

Osmond, C. & Gardner, M.J. (1982) Age, period and cohort models applied to cancer mortality rates. *Stat. Med.*, 1, 245–259

Piolatto, G., Negri, E., La Vecchia, C., Pira, E., Decarli, A. & Peto, J. (1991) Bladder cancer mortality of workers exposed to aromatic amines: an updated analysis. *Br. J. Cancer*, 63, 457–459

Piolatto, G., Decarli, A. & La Vecchia, C. (1995) Bladder cancer of workers exposed to aromatic amines. In: *Encyclopedia of Environmental Control Technology*, Vol. 7, *High-Hazard Pollutants*, Houston, Gul, pp. 41–51

Riboli, E., Gonzales, C.A., Lopez-Abente, G., Errezola, M., Izarzugaza, I., Escolar, A., Nebot, M., Hemon, B. & Agudo, A. (1991) Diet and bladder cancer in Spain: a multi-centre case–control study. *Int. J. Cancer*, **49**, 214–219

Risch, H.A., Burch, J.D., Miller, A.B., Hill, G.B., Steele, R. & Howe, G.R. (1988) Dietary factors and the incidence of cancer of the urinary bladder. *Am. J. Epidemiol.*, **127**, 1179–1191

Risch, A., Wallace, D.M., Bathers, S. & Sim, E. (1995) Slow N-acetylation genotype is a susceptibility factor in occupational and smoking related bladder cancer. *Hum. Mol. Genet.*, **4**, 231–236

Ross, R.K., Jones, P.A. & Yu, M.C. (1996) Bladder cancer epidemiology and pathogenesis. *Semin. Oncol.*, **23**, 536–545

Rothman, N., Bhatnagar, V.K., Hayes, R.B., Zenser, T.V., Kashyap, S.K., Butler, M.A., Bell, D.A., Lakshmi, V., Jaeger, M., Kashyap, R., Hirvonen, A., Schulte, P.A., Dosemeci, M., Hsu, F., Parikh, D.J., Davis, B.B. & Talaska, G.T. (1996) The impact of interindividual variation in NAT2 activity on benzidine urinary metabolites and urothelial DNA adducts in exposed workers. *Proc. Natl Acad. Sci. USA*, **93**, 5084–5089

Rubino, G. & Coscia, G.C. (1973) Occupational neoplasms of the urinary tract (In Italian). *Il Cancro*, **23**, 151–159

Silverman, D.T., Morrison, A.S. & Devesa, S.S. (1996) Bladder cancer. In: Schottenfeld, D. & Fraumeni, J.F., Jr, eds, *Cancer Epidemiology and Prevention*, 2nd Ed., New York, Oxford University Press, pp. 1156–1179

Steineck, G., Hagman, U., Gerhardsson, M. & Norell, S.E. (1990) Vitamin A supplements, fried foods, fat and urothelial cancer. A case–reference study in Stockholm in 1985–1987. *Int. J. Cancer*, **45**, 1006–1011

Sturgeon, S.R., Hartge, P., Silverman, D.T., Kantor, A.F., Marston Linehan, W., Lynch, C. & Hoover, R.N. (1994) Associations between bladder cancer risk factors and tumor stage and grade at diagnosis. *Epidemiology*, **5**, 218–225

Talaska, G., Schamer, M., Skipper, P., Tannenbaum, S., Caporaso, N., Unruh, L., Kadlubar, F.F., Bartsch, H., Malaveille, C. & Vineis, P. (1991) Detection of carcino-gen-DNA adducts in exfoliated urothelial cells of cigarette smokers: association with smoking, hemoglobin adducts, and urinary mutagenicity. *Cancer Epidemiol. Biomarkers. Prev.*, **1**, 61–66

US Congress Office of Technology Assessment (1977) *Cancer Testing Technology and Saccharin*, Washington DC, US Government Printing Office

US Office on Smoking and Health (1982) *The Health Consequences of Smoking: Cancer. A Report of the Surgeon General of the Public Health Service*, Washington DC, US Government Printing Office

Vena, J.E., Graham, S., Freudenheim, J., Marshall, J., Zielezny, M., Swanson, M. & Sufrin, G. (1992) Diet in the epidemiology of bladder cancer in western New York. *Nutr. Cancer*, **18**, 255–264

Vineis, P., Frea, B., Uberti, E., Ghisetti, V. & Terracini, B. (1983) Bladder cancer and cigarette smoking in males: a case–control study. *Tumori*, **69**, 17–22

Vineis, P., Caporaso, N., Tannenbaum, S.R., Skipper, P.L., Glogowski, J., Bartsch, H., Coda, M., Talaska, G. & Kadlubar, F. (1990) Acetylation phenotype, carcinogen-hemoglobin adducts, and cigarette smoking. *Cancer Res.*, **50**, 3002–3004

Wynder, E.L., Onderdonk, J. & Mantel, N. (1963) An epidemiological investigation of cancer of the bladder. *Cancer*, **16**, 1388–1407

Yu, M.C., Skipper, P.L., Taghizadeh, K., Tannenbaum, S.R., Chan, K.K., Henderson, B.E. & Ross, R.K. (1994) Acetylator phenotype, aminobiphenyl-hemoglobin adduct levels, and bladder cancer risk in white, black, and Asian men in Los Angeles, California. *J. Natl Cancer Inst.*, **86**, 712–716

Yu, M.C., Ross, R.K., Chan, K.K., Henderson, B.E., Skipper, P.L., Tannenbaum, S.R. & Coetzee, G.A. (1995) Glutathione S-transferase M1 genotype affects aminobiphenyl-hemoglobin adduct levels in white, black and Asian smokers and nonsmokers. *Cancer Epidemiol. Biomarkers Prev.*, **4**, 861–864

Zenser, T.V., Lakshmi, V.M., Rustan, T.D., Doll, M.A., Deitz, A.C., Davis, B.B. & Hein, D.W. (1996) Human N-acetylation of benzidine: role of NAT1 and NAT2. *Cancer Res.*, **56**, 3941–3947

Corresponding author

Carlo La Vecchia
Istituto di Richerche Farmacologiche 'Mario Negri',
Istituto Di Statistica Medica E Biometria,
Universita degli Studi de Milano, Milan, Italy

Species Differences in Thyroid, Kidney and Urinary Bladder Carcinogenesis
C.C. Capen, E. Dybing, J.M. Rice and J.D. Wilbourn, eds
IARC Scientific Publications No. 147
International Agency for Research on Cancer, Lyon, 1999

Calculi, precipitates and microcrystalluria associated with irritation and cell proliferation as a mechanism of urinary bladder carcinogenesis in rats and mice

S. Fukushima and T. Murai

Introduction

A number of environmental agents which lack genotoxic activity act as promoters for urinary bladder carcinogenesis in rodents. Carcinogenesis due to chronic physical irritation has for many years attracted attention of researchers (Brand *et al.*, 1975) and a number of studies of this phenomenon in the urinary bladder have been performed.

In this chapter, the possible mechanisms linking formation of calculi, precipitates and microcrystalluria with urinary bladder cancer induction in rats and mice are discussed, concentrating particularly on new data for uracil and sodium ascorbate.

Urinary calculi and bladder cancer in rodents

The coexistence of carcinomas and calculi in the urinary bladders of rats and mice has been observed in carcinogenicity studies on a variety of chemical agents. In most strains of rats and mice, the spontaneous incidences of these lesions are low (Goodman *et al.*, 1979; Frith *et al.*, 1982; Maekawa *et al.*, 1983). However, two strains of rat, the Brown Norway and DA/Han, have high incidences of spontaneous bladder tumours that are often associated with the presence of calculi (Boorman, 1975; Deerberg *et al.*, 1985).

A number of older publications describe calculus formation in the urinary bladder following surgical treatment including implantation with cholesterol, paraffin wax or wood pellets, glass beads or chalk powder (Jull, 1951; Bonser *et al.*, 1953; Mobley *et al.*, 1966; Toyoshima & Leighton, 1975; Teelman & Niemann, 1979). In rodents, foreign bodies are thus associated with urinary bladder carcinogenesis (Clayson, 1974). However, in these studies, cytomorphological and proliferative reactions to the surgery itself led to difficulties in interpretation of the underlying mechanisms. From this point of view, models utilizing endogenous urinary calculus formation by non-genotoxic agents allow more precise investigation of cell proliferation due to physical irritation.

Herz *et al.* (1972) found uric acid urolithiasis in the dilated renal pelvic cavities, dilated ureters and enlarged urinary bladders of rats with surgical portacaval anastomosis (i.e., linking the portal vein to the vena cava). They suggested that this treatment resulted in alterations of renal tubule function, leading to a lowered pH with a consequent decrease in solubility of uric acid. Bladder carcinomas were observed in animals with portacaval shunts and chronic irritation by stones was suggested to be the most likely cause (Engelmann *et al.*, 1987). However, Mori and Yamaguchi (1989) suggested that tumour development after portacaval anastomosis in rats might be due to vitamin A deficiency rather than to bladder calculi or generation of urinary carcinogens, because this condition was correlated with increased urothelial ornithine decarboxylase activity. Schramek *et al.* (1993) reported sex-dependent urolithiasis in rats with portacaval shunts. Heidenreich and Engelmann (1993) suggested that hormonal alterations might contribute to sex-dependent stone formation in rats with portacaval anastomosis, because significantly decreased testosterone levels and increased oestradiol and glucagon levels in males and marked rises in testosterone and glucagon levels as well as a decrease in oestradiol levels in females were correlated with urolithiasis.

There are many chemicals which cause formation of endogenous urinary calculi or microcrystalluria when administered to rats and mice, as shown in Table 1 (Cohen & Ellwein, 1991). Ethylene glycol and its derivatives are converted to oxalic acid, which is then excreted through the kidney and forms urinary calcium oxalate calculi. Weil *et al.* (1965) reported the presence of calcium oxalate calculi in the urinary bladders of male rats treated with diethylene glycol but not in female rats, and that males but not females developed papillomas. They suggested that the calculi rather than the chemical administered were responsible for the tumorigenesis, because transplantation of the stones also induced urinary bladder tumours. Hueper and Payne (1963) similarly described calculi and tumour induction in the urinary bladders of mice fed polyoxyethylene-(8)-stearate. While

the authors claimed that the chemical or some impurity was the cause of tumour induction (because of the presence of a tumour in one female mouse lacking urinary bladder stones), bladder calculi are likely to be voided more easily by females than males because of the shorter urethra and the lack of curvature (Clayson *et al.*, 1995). Although conflicting views have been presented, it was concluded by Teelman and Nielmann (1979), who implanted multiple small glass beads surgically into the bladder lumina of male and female mice, that calculi were associated with tumour induction. Clayson (1979) reported that dietary xylitol and terephthalic acid induced formation of bladder stones and bladder tumours in rodents. Heck and Tyl (1985) reviewed work on terephthalic acid, dimethyl terephthalate and melamine which produce stone formation in the urinary bladder and associated tumours. These chemicals basically induce an epithelial hyperplastic response due to irritative stimulation by calculi (Frith *et al.*, 1984; Oyasu *et al.*, 1984; Heck & Tyl, 1985).

Uracil calculi and cancer induction in rats

Lalich (1966) first reported stone formation in the urinary bladder of rats after oral administration of uracil, a component of RNA. Subsequently, Shirai *et al.* (1986) demonstrated that oral administration of uracil induced mucosal papillomatosis, a severe, diffuse papillary hyperplasia of the urinary bladder, associated with yellowish-white and finely granular calculi (Figure 1), with a low incidence of urinary bladder carcinomas also being observed after a relatively short period of treatment. The calculi were found to consist of uracil itself.

In a two-year carcinogenicity test of uracil administered to Fischer 344 rats of both sexes, urinary bladder carcinomas, particularly transitional cell carcinomas, were observed at very high incidence in males, but at a low incidence in females (Fukushima *et al.*, 1992). All the carcinomas were papillary or polypoid, and non-invasive. No metastases to other organs were observed. In addition, all carcinomas were associated with the presence of a large number of urinary bladder calculi. In the renal pelvis, transitional cell carcinomas with formation of calculi were observed in 23% of males and 11% of females.

Dose-dependent increases in the incidence of urinary bladder tumours were observed in male

Table 1. Chemicals which form endogenous urinary calculi or microcrystalluria in mice and/or rats

Uracil
Thymine
Melamine
Uric acid
Homocysteine
Cysteine oxalates
Calcium oxalate
Calcium phosphate
Ethylene glycol and its
  derivatives
Biphenyl
4-Ethylsulfonylnaphthalene-1-sulfonamide
Oxamide
Acetazolamide
Terephthalic acid
Dimethyl terephthalate
Nitrilotriacetate
Polyoxyethylene-(8)-stearate
Glycine
Orotic acid

Adapted from Cohen & Ellwein (1991)

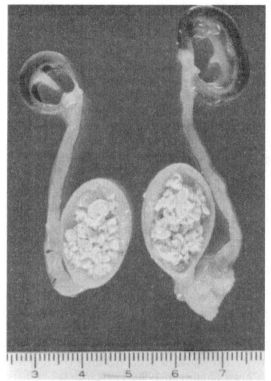

Figure. 1. Urinary bladder calculi in a rat treated with 3% uracil in the diet (provided by Dr T. Shirai)

Fischer 344 rats given 3, 1 or 0.3% uracil in the diet for 36 weeks followed by 4 weeks without the chemical, the total observation period being 40 weeks (Okumura *et al.*, 1991). A high incidence (11/15, 73%) of carcinomas was observed in the urinary bladder of 3% uracil-treated rats, but not in the 1% or 0.3% treatment groups, and no calculi were observed with these lower doses. Shirai *et al.* (1987) and Masui *et al.* (1989) previously detected low yields of urinary bladder carcinomas after treatment with 3% uracil for 20 weeks (1/10, 10%) and for 30 weeks (1/5, 20%). Wang *et al.* (1987) observed urinary bladder carcinomas at an incidence of 26% (6/23) after 20 weeks of uracil exposure followed by non-treatment for 20 weeks. These results imply that the induction of carcinomas in the urinary bladder requires both an adequate uracil concentration and time for tumour progression to occur.

The effects of sodium chloride (NaCl) on uracil administration provided clear mechanistic

evidence on the carcinogenicity of uracil in the rat urinary bladder (Fukushima *et al.*, 1992). Male Fischer 344 rats were given diets containing 3% uracil, 3% uracil plus 5% NaCl, 3% uracil plus 10% NaCl or only 10% NaCl for 36 weeks and then diet without chemicals for 4 weeks. Increased amounts of urine were observed in the NaCl-treated groups. The average food and water consumption were higher in groups given uracil plus NaCl, especially 10% NaCl, than in the group given uracil alone. The incidences of carcinomas and calculi of the urinary bladder were 75% and 81% for uracil alone, 6% and 6% for uracil plus 5% NaCl, and zero and zero for uracil plus 10% NaCl. Thus, the induction of carcinomas by uracil was cleary related to the presence of calculi in the urinary bladder.

Thymine (5-methyluracil) is also able to exert a similar effect in the rat urinary bladder (Okumura *et al.*, 1992). Male Fischer 344 rats were administered 3% or 1% thymine in the diet for 36 weeks followed by a 4-week period without the chemical. Exploratory laparotomy at week 36 revealed the formation of fine granuliform calculi in the urinary bladder in the 3% thymine group. Papillomas and carcinomas were induced in 9/20 (45%) rats compared with 1/20 (5%) rats of the 1% group, which had very limited calculi. The results indicate that the calculi induced by thymine are also directly related to urinary bladder carcinomas in rats.

Uracil calculi and cancer induction in mice

Sakata *et al.* (1988) reported calculus formation in the urinary bladder of mice following administration of uracil. Both male and female mice of two strains, Swiss and C3H, were given 3 or 1% uracil in their diet for 15 weeks. The higher dose (3%) induced epithelial proliferative changes of the urinary bladder with calculus formation by 10 weeks of administration and a more severe hyperplastic lesion (nodular and papillary hyperplasia) was observed in mice killed at week 15. Mice fed 1% uracil rarely had calculi or proliferative changes. The males tended to be more severely affected than the females, particularly those of the C3H strain. The pattern of proliferation was predominantly nodular type with downward growth.

The carcinogenicity of uracil in mice was confirmed in a long-term study (Fukushima *et al.*, 1992). Male and female B6C3F$_1$ mice were given a diet containing 0 (control) or 3% (weeks 1 to 6) and then 2.5% (weeks 7 to 96) uracil. The total observation period was 96 weeks. Gross observation of the urinary bladders revealed thickening of the wall in the uracil-treated groups, but no polypoid or papillary lesions were seen on the luminal surface of the urinary bladder. Transitional cell carcinomas were histologically observed with a high incidence in females, but at a low incidence in males. No papillomas were found in either sex of any group. In addition, no renal pelvic tumours were observed in the uracil-treated mice. The incidences of calculi in the urinary bladder of uracil-treated groups could not be determined exactly at the time of autopsy, and no calculi were found in the urinary bladder in any fixed preparation, because they disappeared during three weeks' fixation with formalin.

Melamine calculi and cancer induction in rats

Melamine (2,4,6-triamino-s-triazine) is used in the manufacture of melamine-formaldehyde amino resins, found in household goods such as buttons and electrical equipment. Short-term mutagenicity and related tests have found it to be non-genotoxic. In a two-year carcinogenicity study, Melnick et al. (1984) observed transitional cell carcinomas in the urinary bladder at an incidence of 16% (8/49) in male Fischer 344 rats given 0.45% melamine in the diet, but not in females (0%, 0/46). Seven of eight rats with carcinomas had urinary bladder calculi and the overall incidence of calculi (93%) was much higher in the melamine-dosed group than in controls (4%).

Okumura et al. (1992) also examined the carcinogenicity of melamine in male Fischer 344 rats administered doses of 0.3, 1 or 3% in the diet for 36 weeks followed by 4 weeks without the chemical. Urinary bladder carcinomas were induced in 79% (15/19) of the 3% group, 5% (1/20) of the 1% group, and 0% (0/20) of the 0.3% melamine-treated rats. A significant correlation between calculus formation estimated by exploratory laparotomy at experimental week 36 and tumour incidence at week 40 was observed.

As was the case with uracil, an inhibitory effect of NaCl on carcinogenicity of melamine for the urinary bladder in rats was clearly shown by Ogasawara et al. (1995). In Fischer 344 male rats given 3% melamine alone in the diet, the incidence of urinary bladder carcinomas was 90%, whereas no such lesions were evident in animals given 3% melamine plus 10% NaCl. The water intake, used as an index of urinary output, was increased by NaCl treatment and calculus formation resulting from melamine administration was suppressed. The main constituents of the calculi were determined to be melamine itself and uric acid (total content 61–81%) in equal molar ratios. The results from all experiments indicate that carcinoma induction in the rat urinary bladder by melamine is directly due to irritative stimulation by calculi, as with uracil.

Urinary calculi and cell proliferation

The initiating mechanism of calculi induced by non-genotoxic agents in the bladder remains uncertain, but some hypotheses have been suggested. In a review by Clayson et al. (1995), three possibilities for initiating factors were proposed: (1) the excess mitosis in a normally quiescent tissue may lead to mutation, (2) inflammation through the accretion of phagocytes in the tissue may lead to excessive oxidative DNA damage (Cohen & Ellwein, 1990, 1991), or (3) a urinary constituent derived from the metabolism of natural constituents of the food supply may act as an initiator.

Shirai et al. (1986, 1989) found that dietary administration of uracil at a concentration of 3% quickly induced bladder mucosal papillomatosis secondary to the formation of urinary calculi in all treated rats (Figure 2). Surprisingly, although urinary calculi and bladder papillomatosis, which showed papillary projections of epithelial proliferation, were severe and extensive, they disappeared when the treatment with uracil stopped; the bladder mucosa returned to normal. Thus, uracil calculi induce a reversible hyperplasia of the urinary bladder epithelium. 5-Bromo-2'-deoxyuridine (BrdU) or proliferating cell nuclear antigen (PCNA) labelling indices in the epithelium were high during uracil treatment but quickly returned to normal after removal of the chemical insult (Shirai et al., 1989, 1995; Otori et al., 1997). Interestingly, cyclin D1-positive cells were observed immunohistochemically in hyperplastic epithelium of the urinary bladder in rats during uracil administration, but not when the treatment

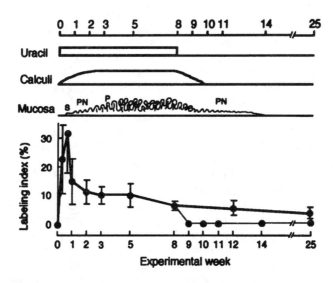

Figure 2. Time sequence in the development and disappearance of calculi and epithelial proliferative lesions. S, simple hyperplasia; PN, papillary or nodular hyperplasia; P, papilloma. (Contributed by Dr T. Shirai)

was stopped (Otori *et al.*, 1997). In addition, PCNA-positive cells were present mainly at the top to middle of the papillary projections in papillomatosis. On the other hand, areas positive for anti-Le^y(BM-1/JIMRO), an important marker of apoptosis, were mainly located at the bottom to middle of the papillary projections. It is speculated that areas of PCNA-positive cells are in direct contact with the calculi, while BM-1 positive cells are secondarily induced. The results confirm that irritation by the calculi simultaneously increases both cell proliferation and apoptosis in papillomatosis. When the uracil treatment is continued, the level of apoptosis is weaker than that of proliferation, resulting in papillary hyperplasia. On the other hand, when urinary calculi disappeared one week after the uracil treatment was stopped, PCNA-positive cells had almost disappeared and apoptosis was still markedly increased. In disappearing papillomatosis, the surface epithelium was found to be clearly stained with BM-1 and nick-end labelling, markers of apoptosis. Although clear erosion and ulcers are not observed in the urinary bladders of animals given uracil, the hyperplastic response is likely to be regenerative in nature. However, the degree of proliferation due to uracil-induced

calculi appears to be more marked than is generally observed in regenerative processes induced by ulcers (Shirai *et al.*, 1978). Therefore, further studies are required to elucidate the mechanism of the cell proliferation due to calculi. Uracil itself is not cytotoxic for the urinary bladder.

To evaluate the mechanism of the appearance of uracil-induced papillomatosis, Fukushima *et al.* (unpublished data) examined changes in the activity and localization of ornithine decarboxylase (ODC), a key enzyme in polyamine biosynthesis, and epithelial proliferation accompanying the sequential bladder epithelial changes following administration and withdrawal of uracil. ODC activity during uracil administration was maintained at a high level compared to normal epithelium, but this activity sharply decreased after cessation of uracil treatment. Accumulation of ODC protein could be observed in the proliferating bladder epithelium by immunohistochemical examination and Western blotting analysis, and even after cessation of treatment, protein binding to anti-ODC antibody remained mildly elevated. Sequential changes of PCNA-positive cells in the epithelium during the development and disappearance of papillomatosis correlated with ODC activity. ODC mRNA was also strongly expressed in the proliferating epithelium of rats treated with uracil and weakly in normal epithelium, in accordance with the findings for ODC protein. These data demonstrate that cell proliferation in the development of papillomatosis is closely associated with increased polyamine production, and moreover suggest that ODC activity is up-regulated in a post-translational step.

Sakata *et al.* (1988) examined DNA synthesis in the urinary bladder epithelium of male and female Swiss and C3H mice treated with 3 or 1% uracil in the diet using [*methyl*-³H]thymidine. The labelling indices were significantly increased in both strains and sexes treated with 3% uracil as compared to controls, and in males compared to females at week 10, but not week 15. Clayson and Pringle (1966) reported that the rate of mitosis in the urothelium of the mouse bladder with paraffin wax or cholesterol pellets was 20–30-fold higher than that of normal bladder. The increase in the rate of cellular proliferation is probably the result of the damaging effect of the implanted bladder concretions (Clayson *et al.*, 1995).

Gene alterations in urinary bladder carcinomas induced by uracil treatment alone or in two-stage carcinogenesis models

Exposure to a genotoxic carcinogen may cause cell cycle arrest at the G1 check-point involving negative cell cycle regulators such as p53, p21$^{waf1/cip1}$ and pRB. Under conditions of continuous exposure to a genotoxic carcinogen, cells with abnormalities in such negative regulators might be expected to enter S phase and thus possess a growth advantage over the cells retained in the G1 phase. In experimental rat urinary bladder carcinomas induced by continuous exposure to the genotoxic carcinogen N-nitroso-n-butyl(4-hydroxybutyl)amine (BBN), *p53* mutations are frequent (Masui *et al.*, 1994, 1996). Chronic stimulation of proliferation increases the fixing of DNA damage in epithelial cells as mutations (Cohen & Ellwein, 1990). This implies that the frequency of spontaneous initiated and putative preneoplastic foci increases with enhanced cell proliferation due to longer or more intense calculus stimulation. However, tumours associated with uracil alone may lack such mutations (Fukushima *et al.*, unpublished data), and indeed, infrequent

alteration of the *p53* gene in tumours produced in a two-stage rat urinary bladder carcinogenesis model has been reported by Asamoto *et al.* (1994). These authors also indicated that cells with a *p53* mutation may not have any particular advantage under the influence of a promoter as confirmed by our recent results (Lee *et al.*, 1997). Thus *p53* mutation is not a critical event. Furthermore, *H-ras* mutations are not observed in uracil-induced urinary bladder carcinomas of rats. The search for alternative control pathways must therefore continue.

Promotion of urinary bladder carcinogenesis by sodium and potassium salts

A list of sodium and potassium salts which show promoting effects on urinary bladder carcinogenesis is given in Table 2 (see also Cohen, this volume). The mechanism by which sodium or potassium salts might affect proliferation of urinary bladder epithelial cells remains to be defined.

As summarized in Table 3, there is an apparent relationship between promoting potential and fluctuation in urinary parameters, particularly pH and sodium or potassium concentration. Parent acids of sodium salts, *per se*, do not show

Table 2. Sodium salts which have promoting activity in the second stage of urinary bladder carcinogenesis

Compound	References
Sodium saccharin	Hicks *et al.*, 1975; Cohen *et al.*, 1979
Sodium L-ascorbate	Fukushima *et al.*, 1983a
Sodium o-phenylphenate	Fukushima *et al.*, 1983b
Sodium erythorbate	Fukushima *et al.*, 1984
Sodium bicarbonate	Fukushima *et al.*, 1986a
Sodium citrate	Fukushima *et al.*, 1986b
Sodium phenobarbital	Diwan *et al.*, 1989
Sodium barbital	Diwan *et al.*, 1989
Sodium chloride	Shibata *et al.*, 1992
Sodium succinate	Otoshi *et al.*, 1993
Trisodium phosphate	Shibata *et al.*, 1992
Potassium carbonate	Fukushima *et al.*, 1987
Tripotassium phosphate	Shibata *et al.*, 1992

Table 3. Summary of relation between changes in urinary parameters and promoting potential

Test chemicals	Promoting potential	Fluctuation in urinary parameters			Increase of crystals
		pH	Electrolyte	Total ascorbic acid	
Ascorbic acid + $NaHCO_3$	+++	↑	Na ↑	↑	++
Ascorbic acid	–	↓	↔	↑	±
$NaHCO_3$	+	↑	Na ↑, Ca ↑, P ↓	↔	+ ~ ++
Na ascorbate	++~ +++	↑	Na ↑, Mg ↓	↑	+ +
Na ascorbate + NH_4Cl	±	↔	Na ↑, Cl ↑	↑	+ ~ ++
NH_4Cl	–	↓	Na ↓, Cl ↑	↔	±
K_2CO_3	±	↑	K ↑, Cl ↓	↔	ND
Ascorbic acid + K_2CO_3	+++	↑	K ↑, Cl ↓	↑	ND
$CaCO_3$	-	↑	Ca ↑, Mg ↓	↔	ND
Ascorbic acid + $CaCO_3$	-	↔	Ca ↑, Mg ↓	↑	ND
$MgCO_3$	-	↔	Ca ↑, Mg ↑, P ↓	↔	ND
Ascorbic acid + $MgCO_3$	–	↔	Ca ↑, Mg ↑, P ↓	↑	ND

For further details, see Fukushima *et al.* (1986a) and Fukushima *et al.* (1987)

ND, not detected, but calculus formation was not observed.

promoting activity or increase the urinary pH and sodium ion concentration (Fukushima *et al.*, 1986b). However, a combination of L-ascorbic acid plus sodium bicarbonate or potassium carbonate did reveal co-promoting activity associated with urinary changes (Fukushima *et al.*, 1987). Other cations, such as calcium and magnesium, in the urine did not show any promoting activity (Fukushima *et al.*, 1987). Cohen *et al.* (1991a) also reported that calcium carbonate alone did not exert a promoting effect. Sodium hippurate was negative under increase of urinary sodium ion concentration without elevation of urinary pH in the tumour promotion bioassays, although the mechanism remains to be clarified.

The hypothesis has been suggested that physical irritation by precipitates or microcrystalluria

formed in the urinary bladder of rats given sodium saccharin is related to proliferation of urinary bladder epithelium (Cohen *et al.*, 1991b). Analysis of urine from rats given non-genotoxic sodium or potassium salts has revealed increases in the urinary pH as well as in the concentrations of sodium or potassium ions. These factors could be relevant to the promoting mechanism. However, Cohen *et al.* (1995) have reported the presence of precipitates in urine of rats given not only sodium saccharin but also sodium L-ascorbate, sodium erythorbate, sodium bicarbonate, sodium chloride and sodium citrate, but not sodium *o*-phenylphenate (S.M. Cohen, personal communication).

Cohen and Lawson (1995) paid particular attention to amorphous precipitates, which are formed under relatively high pH in the urine of rats administered sodium salts, as a significant factor in proliferation of urinary bladder epithelium. This is of considerable importance in the context of the human hazard potential of the artificial sweetener, sodium saccharin. In addition, other salts acting as promoters also induce cell proliferation in the bladder epithelium (Shibata et al., 1989, 1992; Cohen et al.,1995).

Influence of physical stimulation of the urinary bladder epithelium as a factor responsible for sex, strain and species differences

Kurata et al. (1986) suggested that interaction between high urinary sodium concentration and the existence of urinary crystals might be an important factor related to promoting activity, since biphenyl induced the formation of characteristic stones and a high sodium concentration in the urine without altering urinary pH. Shirai et al. (1987) and Masui et al. (1989) similarly found strong promoting activity of urinary calculi in BBN- and N-methyl-N-nitrosourea-initiated urinary bladder carcinogenesis in rats.

A fundamental hypothesis proposed by Cohen et al. (1991b) was that a combination of a high pH brought about by ingestion of sodium saccharin plus a high concentration of urinary proteins results in precipitation and formation of microcrystals, including silicate, which may act as microabrasives that injure urinary bladder epithelium, leading to compensatory regenerative hyperplasia. Okamura et al. (1992) showed that silicate urolithiasis induced by tetraethylorthosilicate induces microscopic changes in urinary bladder epithelium similar to those observed in rats given sodium saccharin. They pointed to α_{2u}-globulin, a characteristic urinary protein in male rats as the key substance. This hypothesis fitted the finding that sodium saccharin exerts promoting activity in male rats but not in female rats or in mice. Mice have low levels of urinary protein and do not produce α_{2u}-globulin (Hard, 1995), while female rats have very much lower levels of this protein than males (Vandoren et al., 1983). Cohen et al. (1995) suggested that a similar mechanism might be responsible for the promoting effects of sodium salts including sodium L-ascorbate, glutamate and bicarbonate, after demonstrating that these can also cause precipitate formation. The above hypothesis is strengthened by evidence gained with NCI-Black-Reiter (NBR) rats, which lack the ability to synthesize α_{2u}-globulin and are less prone to the urothelial hyperplasia induced by sodium saccharin than intact or castrated male Fischer 344 rats (Garland et al., 1994). This hypothesis might explain the lack of carcinogenic activity of saccharin in humans, which do not produce α_{2u}-globulin. Recently, Uwagawa et al. (1997) demonstrated that sodium L-ascorbate had no promoting effect on urinary bladder carcinogenesis in NBR male rats, which do exhibit a proliferative response to uracil equivalent to that seen with Fischer 344 rats (Uwagawa et al., 1994).

Thus, this hypothesis is very attractive to explain sex and species differences observed in the case of sodium saccharin and possibly other sodium salts, and is especially important with regard to human risk assessment, but there are some difficulties (Clayson et al., 1995; Hard, 1995). Recently Murai et al. (unpublished data) found promoting activity of sodium L-ascorbate in bladder carcinogenesis of female rats which lack urinary α_{2u}-globulin. This result indicates the need for further investigation of promotion mechanisms.

Clayson et al. (1995) questioned whether the rate of cellular proliferation induced by sodium saccharin is sufficient to induce genetic changes leading to cancer. Arnold and Clayson (1985) speculated another mechanism for the carcinogenicity of sodium saccharin. They claimed that permeability of cell membranes to sodium saccharin might differ between the neonatal stage and early maturity and its penetration into epithelial cells might induce genomic changes through unequal inhibition of enzymes concerned with DNA synthesis. In addition to the effects of sodium saccharin administered during the neonatal stage on cellular proliferation, endogenous mitogens such as epidermal growth factors whose synthesis is regulated by sex hormones might affect two-generation bioassays of sodium saccharin.

Strain, sex or species differences in promoting activity of sodium salts

The promoting activity of sodium salts described above has been observed in males of a limited number of rat strains. However, strain differences in promotion of urinary bladder carcinogenesis by sodium saccharin or sodium L-ascorbate have been observed (Ito *et al.*, 1983; Mori *et al.*, 1987, 1991; Uwagawa *et al.*, 1994; Murai *et al.*, 1997a; Uwagawa *et al.*, 1997). Tamano *et al.* (1993) reported that B6C3F$_1$ mice are resistant to agents that promote bladder tumorigenesis in rats, including sodium L-ascorbate, in spite of significant increases in urinary pH value and sodium ion concentration after four weeks' initiation with BBN. The initiation period seems to be important in relation to promoting activity in other species because after six weeks' administration of BBN to the Mongolian gerbil, 2-*tert*-butyl-4-hydroxyanisole (BHA), which is known to be a promoter of rat urinary bladder tumours, did not show any promoting activity. However, after 20 weeks' administration of BBN, promoting activity of sodium L-ascorbate was found in this species (Mori *et al.*, unpublished observations). Hamsters and monkeys also fail to show a promoting response to sodium saccharin and female rats do not respond to sodium saccharin to the same extent as male rats (IARC, 1980; Ellwein & Cohen, 1990), although sodium L-ascorbate does have promoting activity in female rats.

Anatomical relationships of bladders in humans versus rats

DeSesso (1995) suggested that the disparity of tumour incidence between humans and rats might be related to anatomical aspects of the bladder rather than to any species difference in tissue susceptibility. Thus, objects within the lumen of the bladder, which are greatly influenced by gravity, will come to rest on the most inferior surface of the bladder and the difference in facility of excretion of such objects could be attributed to the difference in anatomical location of the bladder. In man, the internal urethral orifice is located at the bottom of the bladder in the ordinary standing or sitting position. On the other hand, in rats the bladder is normally parallel to the ground, with the orifice to one side. Thus objects in the bladder are liable to be excreted by humans, while in rats they may persist for longer periods. The ventral dome of the bladder of rats might therefore be expected to be more affected by calculi, precipitates or microcrystalluria. Cohen *et al.* (1990) reported that hyperplasia was observed in the wall of the ventral dome of the bladder of rats

given sodium saccharin. DeSesso (1995) also speculated that the epithelium of the urinary bladder might become damaged if crystals or microcrystals are trapped in the crypts that are formed as the asymmetric unit membrane invaginates into the supranuclear region of the superficial cells.

Dietary and genetic influences on promoting activity of sodium salts

Since dietary and genetic factors have been reported to have considerable influence on chemical-induced carcinogenesis, Mori *et al.* (1987) investigated the modifying effects of diet and strain on promoting activity of sodium L-ascorbate in two-stage urinary bladder carcinogenesis assays in male F344/DuCrj (F344) and LEW/Crj (LEW) rats after BBN initiation. Two kinds of commercial basal diet (Oriental MF (M) and Clea CA-1 (C)) were used. The relative promoting effects of sodium L-ascorbate on bladder carcinogenesis were: F344 strain–M diet > LEW strain–C diet > F344 strain–C diet = LEW strain–M diet. In both strains and with both diets, increases in urinary pH and in the concentrations of sodium ions and total ascorbic acid showed no obvious correlation with the strength of promotion. Garland *et al.* (1989) observed a similar dietary influence on promotion by sodium saccharin. Moreover, Garland *et al.* (1989) and Okamura *et al.* (1991) showed that the low urinary pH associated with consumption of the AIN-76A diet eliminated the promoting activity of sodium saccharin.

Possible role of precipitate or crystal formation in promotion of urinary bladder carcinogenesis in rats

As described above (Mori *et al.*, 1987), susceptibility to sodium L-ascorbate promotion differs among strains of rats, with Fischer 344 and LEW animals being sensitive. In contrast, ODS/Shi-od/od (ODS, Osteogenic Disorder Shionogi, genotype: od/od) rats, which lack the ability to synthesize L-ascorbic acid, are not sensitive (Mori *et al.*, 1991), although they are sensitive to BBN (Mori *et al.*, 1990). However, heterozygotes (+/od) and normal (+/+) ODS rats, which can synthesize L-ascorbic acid, are also resistant to sodium L-ascorbate promotion, when compared with Fischer 344 and LEW rats (Mori *et al.*, 1991). Recently, Mori *et al.* (1997)

further showed that ODS rats are resistant to the modifying effects of sodium bicarbonate and/or L-ascorbic acid on two-stage urinary bladder carcinogenesis. Thus other genetic factors may play an important role in promotion by sodium L-ascorbate of two-stage urinary bladder carcinogenesis and genes other than that at the *od* locus in ODS rats might be involved. ODS rats were developed from a sister strain of the WS/Shi (WS) strain, established by full-sibling mating of Wistar rats introduced in 1952 to Aburahi Lab., Shionogi & Co., Ltd., from the Faculty of Agriculture of Tokyo University, Japan. Therefore, some loci of biochemical markers in ODS rats are shared by the WS strain (Makino *et al.*, 1990). Three experiments were performed to examine strain differences in sensitivity of rats to the promoting effects of sodium L-ascorbate on the development of urinary bladder tumours (Murai *et al.*, 1997a). In the first experiment, WS, ODS and LEW rats were given 0.05% BBN in their drinking water and subsequently fed basal M diet with or without a 5% sodium L-ascorbate supplement. In LEW rats, the sodium L-ascorbate treatment increased the induction of neoplastic lesions in the urinary bladder, whereas WS and ODS-od/od animals did not show this response. Equivalent increases in urinary pH and sodium concentration were observed in all three strains. In the second experiment, WS and Fischer 344 rats were maintained on two kinds of commercial basal diet (M and C), during the administration of sodium L-ascorbate. In Fischer rats, feeding M diet during the promotion period yielded significantly more neoplastic lesions than the C diet, but in WS rats no influence of diet was apparent. Urinary parameters did not differ between the two strains. In the third experiment, strain differences in biosynthesis of α_{2u}-globulin were assessed in ODS, WS and Fischer 344 rats. Immunohistochemical analysis of renal tubules and Western blotting analysis of urine revealed the presence of α_{2u}-globulin without any significant variation between the three strains. Moreover, Murai *et al.* (1997b) observed that female Fischer 344 rats, which have low biosynthesis of α_{2u}-globulin, are sensitive to the promoting activity of sodium L-ascorbate to the same extent as male Fischer 344 rats. These data suggest that differences in susceptibility to promotion are indeed due to genetic factors, as Mori *et al.* (1991) proposed,

rather than to dietary factors or the ability to synthesize α_{2u}-globulin. However, further studies are needed to confirm this hypothesis, because other urinary precipitates such as calcium phosphate may exert such effects (Clayson *et al.*, 1995).

Previous reports have suggested that different levels of protein in the urine between male and female rats are related to the proliferative stimulus of sodium saccharin on the rat urinary bladder epithelium, and that the sex-dependence of nephropathy is mostly attributable to the presence of α_{2u}-globulin, which occurs exclusively in urine of males (Hard, 1995). In the experiment described above, LEW and ODS rats both exhibited mild nephropathy, whereas lesion development was more marked in the WS strain. Moreover, the total protein level in the urine of ODS rats did not differ from those of Fischer 344 or LEW rats, while slightly higher values in WS rats were gained with test sticks, which indicate urinary protein levels. Thus, urinary α_{2u}-globulin and protein levels in general may not always be critical for the urinary bladder tumour-promoting activity of sodium L-ascorbate. Moreover, Fukushima *et al.* (1983a) reported no correlation between the number of crystals in urinary sediments and the occurrence of neoplastic lesions in experimental rats after BBN initiation. Indeed, from results of our studies, as summarized in Table 3, no clear relationship between increased crystal formation and promoting activity was noted, while simultaneous increases in sodium or potassium ion concentration and pH were positively correlated with promoting activity as long as they occurred together. In contrast, treatments causing an increase in either the urinary pH or the sodium ion concentration alone did not lead to clear promoting activity (Fukushima *et al.*, 1983b).

Imaida *et al.* (1983) indicated that the membrane potential of the epithelium in the early stage of urinary bladder carcinogenesis is significantly increased by sodium saccharin. Since the apical membrane potential of the cell depends largely on the permeability to sodium ions, this presumably reflects the activity of the sodium ion channel, which is essential for sodium ion transport across the urinary bladder epithelium. Moreover, amiloride (an inhibitor of Na^+/H^+ exchange) can inhibit both the promoting effects and the increase of BrdU labelling index, which is an indicator of cell proliferation, induced by sodium L-ascorbate, whereas ouabain (an inhibitor of Na+/K+ ATPase) does not influence the promoting effects (Murai *et al.*, 1996, 1997c). We therefore speculate that increases of sodium or potassium in urine may stimulate Na+/H+ exchange activity and bring about a rise in intracellular sodium or potassium concentration and pH, resulting in increased DNA synthesis. However, there is conflicting evidence regarding the membrane potential (Gatzy *et al.*, 1989; Asamoto *et al.*, 1992) and further experiments are needed to clarify this point.

Genetic factors relating to the promoting mechanisms of microcrystals or precipitates

While microcrystal or precipitate formation could explain the response to sodium saccharin in different species, this hypothesis cannot be universally applied to other compounds. The mechanism underlying promotion by sodium saccharin might also differ from the case with other sodium salts, because in a two-generation study it was itself found to induce bladder tumours (Arnold *et al.*, 1980). Two-generation investigations of other sodium salts have not been reported.

Several reports of race, population and family variation in human urinary bladder cancer have pointed to an important role of genetic factors in urinary bladder carcinogenesis (Fraumeni & Thomas, 1967; Herring *et al.*, 1979; Lynch *et al.*, 1979; Kiemeney & Schoenberg, 1996; Schoenberg *et al.*, 1996).

Mori *et al.* (1992) showed that susceptibility to the promoting effects of sodium L-ascorbate is inherited as a dominant autosomal trait, by examining hybrids between sensitive (Fischer 344 and LEW) and resistant (WS) parents. We are now paying special attention to the information encoded by the inherited genes. These might be related to Na+/H+ exchange, as Rotin *et al.* (1989) suggested from observation of in vivo growth retardation in an Na+/H+ exchange-deficient mutant-derived human bladder carcinoma cell line. Genetic factors contributing to the sensitivity to sodium salts of organic acids might be essential for promotion to occur.

Conclusions

Information concerning factors modifying the development of bladder carcinomas has been accumulated through experimental animal studies. However, the mechanisms of promotion by urinary calculi, precipitates and microcrystalluria have still to be elucidated in detail and, as discussed in this paper, there is much conflicting evidence.

Cell proliferation due to uracil treatment is thought to be regenerative hyperplasia due to cell necrosis. However, the degree of proliferation observed with uracil-induced calculi appears to be more marked than that generally apparent in regenerative processes. Indeed, an unknown mitogenic mechanism seems also to act, since gene analysis of tumours induced by uracil alone revealed an absence of *p53* or *H-ras* gene mutation. This result seems to be in conflict with the usually accepted view (Cohen & Ellwein, 1990) that all such chronic stimulation increases the fixing of DNA damage in epithelial cells as mutations.

Clayson *et al.* (1995) pointed out that the cell proliferation induced by sodium saccharin would not be expected to be a major component of cancer induction in the urinary bladder. Indeed, the degree of promoting activity appears to differ between chemicals associated with pronounced urolithiasis and others such as sodium salts, in that the former can induce carcinomas without initiation but the latter usually do not, except for sodium saccharin.

For more reliable evaluation of human risk, the species, sex and strain differences as well as differences in physiology and anatomy must be taken into consideration. As described above, the susceptibility to sodium salts remains to be elucidated for many strains or species. Differences are regulated by DNA and analysis of genes governing responses to non-genotoxic carcinogens in experimental animals clearly warrant further study in order to facilitate extrapolation of animal data to humans.

References

Arnold, D.L. & Clayson, D.B. (1985) Saccharin–a bitter sweet case. In: Clayson, D.B., Krewski, D. & Munro, I., eds, *Toxicological Risk Assessment*, Volume 2, *General Criteria and Case Studies*, Boca Baton, FL, CRC Press, pp. 227–243

Arnold, D.L., Moodie, C.A., Grice, H.C., Charbonneau, S.M., Stavric, B., Collins, B.T., McGuire, P.F., Zawidzka, Z.Z. & Munro, I.C. (1980) Long-term toxicity of ortho-toluenesulfonamide and sodium saccharin in the rat. *Toxicol. Appl. Pharmacol.*, **52**, 113–152

Asamoto, M., Irnaida, K., Hasegawa, R., Hotta, K. & Fukishima, S. (1992) Change of membrane potential in rat urinary bladder epithelium treated with sodium L-ascorbate. *Cancer Lett.*, **63**, 1–5

Asamoto, M., Mann, A.M. & Cohen, S.M. (1994) p53 Mutation is infrequent and might not give a growth advantage in rat bladder carcinogenesis in vivo. *Carcinogenesis*, **15**, 455–458

Bonser, G.M., Clayson, D.N. & Jull, J.W. (1953) The induction of tumours of the bladder epithelium in rats by the implantation of paraffin wax pellets. *Br. J. Cancer*, **7**, 456–459

Boorman, G.A. (1975) High incidence of spontaneous urinary bladder and ureter tumours in the Brown Norway rat. *J. Natl Cancer Inst.*, **52**, 1005–1008

Brand, K.G., Buoen, L.C., Johnson, K.H. & Brand, I. (1975) Etiological factors, stages, and the role of the foreign body in foreign body tumorigenesis. *Cancer Res.*, **35**, 279–286

Clayson, D.B. (1974) Bladder carcinogenesis in rats and mice: possibility of artifacts. *J. Natl Cancer Inst.*, **52**, 1685–1689

Clayson, D.B. (1979) Bladder carcinogenesis in rats and mice: possibility of artifacts. *Natl Cancer Inst. Monogr.*, **52**, 519–524

Clayson, D.B. & Pringle, J.A.S. (1966) The influence of a foreign body on the induction of tumours of the bladder epithelium of the mouse. *Br. J. Cancer*, **20**, 564–568

Clayson, D.B., Fishbein, L. & Cohen, S.M. (1995) Effects of stones and other physical factors on the induction of rodent bladder cancer. *Food Chem. Toxicol.*, **33**, 771–784

Cohen, S.M. & Ellwein, L.B. (1990) Cell proliferation in carcinogenesis. *Science*, **249**, 1007–1011

Cohen, S.M. & Ellwein, L.B. (1991) Genetic errors, cell proliferation, and carcinogenesis. *Cancer Res.*, **51**, 6493–6505

Cohen, S.M. & Lawson, T.A. (1995) Rodent bladder tumors do not always predict for humans. *Cancer Lett.*, **93**, 9–16

Cohen, S.M., Arai, M., Jacobs, J.B. & Friedell, G.H. (1979) Promoting effect of saccharin and DL-tryptophan in urinary bladder carcinogenesis. *Cancer Res.*, **39**, 1207–1217

Cohen, S.M., Fisher, M.J., Sakata, T., Cano, M., Schoenig, G.P., Chappel, C. I. & Garland, E.M. (1990) Comparative

analysis of the proliferative response of the rat urinary bladder to sodium saccharin by light and scanning electron microscopy and autoradiography. *Scanning Microscopy*, **4**, 135–142

Cohen, S.M., Ellwein, L.B., Okamura, T., Masui, T., Johansson, S.L., Smith, R.A., Wehner, J.M., Khachab, M., Chappel, C.I., Shoenig, G.P., Emerson, J.L. & Garland, E.M. (1991a) Comparative bladder tumor promoting activity of sodium saccharin, sodium ascorbate, related acids, and calcium salts in rats. *Cancer Res.*, **51**, 1766–1777

Cohen, S.M., Cano, M., Earl, R.A., Carson, S.D. & Garland, E.M. (1991b) A proposed role for silicates and protein in the proliferative effects of saccharin on the male rat urothelium. *Carcinogenesis*, **12**, 1551–1555

Cohen, S.M., Cano, M., Garland, E.M., John, M.St. & Arnold, L.L. (1995) Urinary and urothelial effects of sodium salts in male rats. *Carcinogenesis*, **16**, 343–348

Deerberg, F., Rehm, S., & Jostmeyer, H.H. (1985) Spontaneous urinary bladder tumors in DA/Han rats: a feasible model of human bladder cancer. *J. Natl Cancer Inst.*, **75**, 1113–1121

DeSesso, J.M. (1995) Anatomical relationships of urinary bladders compared: their potential role in the development of bladder tumours in humans and rats. *Food Chem. Toxicol.*, **33**, 705–714

Diwan, B.A., Hagiwara, A., Ward, J.M. & Rice, J.M. (1989) Effects of sodium salts of phenobarbital and barbital on development of bladder tumors in male F344/NCr rats pretreated with either N-[4-(5-nitro-2-furyl)-2-thia-zolyl]formamide or N-nitrosobutyl-4-hydroxybuty-lamine. *Toxicol. Appl. Pharmacol.*, **98**, 269–277

Ellwein, L.B. & Cohen, S.M. (1990) The health risks of saccharin revisited. *Crit. Rev. Toxicol.*, **20**, 311–326

Engelmann, U., Schramek, P., Baum, H.P., Wertmann, B., Grun, M., & Jacobi, G.H. (1987) Bladder carcinogenesis in portacaval shunt rats. *Urol. Int.*, **42**, 165–169

Fraumeni, J.F. & Thomas, L.B. (1967) Malignant bladder tumors in a man and his three sons. *JAMA.*, **201**, 507–509

Frith, C.H., Farmer, J.H., Greeman, D.L. & Shaw, D.W. (1982) Biological and morphological characteristics of urinary bladder neoplasms induced in BALB/c female mice with 2-acetylaminofluorene. In: Staffa, J.A. & Mehlman, M.A., eds, *Innovations in Cancer Risk Assessment (EDO1 Study)*, Pathotox, Park Forest, IL, pp. 103–120

Frith, C.H., West, R.W., Stanley, J.W. & Jackson, C.D. (1984) Urothelial lesions in mice given 4-ethylsulfonyl-naphthalene-1-sulfonamide, acetazolamide and oxamide. *J. Environ. Pathol. Toxicol. Oncol.*, **5**, 25–38

Fukushima, S., Imaida, K., Sakata, T., Okamura, T., Shibata, M.-A. & Ito, N. (1983a) Promoting effects of sodium L-ascorbate on two-stage urinary bladder carcinogenesis in rats. *Cancer Res.*, **43**, 4454–4457

Fukushima, S., Kurata, Y., Shibata, M., Ikawa, E. & Ito, N. (1983b) Promoting effect of sodium *o*-phenylphenate and *o*-phenyphenol on two-stage urinary bladder carcinogenesis in rats. *Gann.*, **74**, 625–632

Fukushima, S., Kurata, Y., Shibata, M., Ikawa, E. & Ito, N. (1984) Promotion by ascorbic acid, sodium erythorbate and ethoxyquin of neoplastic lesions in rats initiated with N-butyl-N-(4-hydroxybutyl) nitrosamine. *Cancer Lett.*, **23**, 29–37

Fukushima, S., Shibata, M.-A., Shirai, T., Tamano, S. & Ito, N. (1986a) Roles of urinary sodium ion concentration and pH in promotion by ascorbic acid of urinary bladder carcinogenesis in rats. *Cancer Res.*, **46**, 1623–1626

Fukushima, S., Thamavit, W., Kurata, Y. & Ito, N. (1986b) Sodium citrate: a promoter of bladder carcinogenesis. *Gann.*, **77**, 1–4

Fukushima, S., Shibata, M.-A., Shirai, T., Kurata, Y., Tamano, S. & Imaida, K. (1987) Promotion by L-ascorbic acid of urinary bladder carcinogenesis in rats under conditions of increased urinary K ion concentration and pH. *Cancer Res.*, **47**, 4821–4824

Fukushima, S., Tanaka, H., Asakawa, E., Kagawa, M., Yamamoto, A. & Shirai, T. (1992) Carcinogenicity of uracil, a nongenotoxic chemical, in rats and mice and its rationale. *Cancer Res.*, **52**, 1675–1680

Garland, E.M., Sakata, T., Fisher, M.J., Masui, T. & Cohen, S.M. (1989) Influences of diet and strain on the proliferative effect on the rat urinary bladder induced by sodium saccharin. *Cancer Res.*, **49**, 3789–3794

Garland, E.M., St. John, M., Asamoto, M., Eklund, S.H., Mattson, B.J., Johnson, L.S., Cano, M. & Cohen, S.M. (1994) A comparison of the effects of sodium saccharin in NBR rats and in intact and castrated male F344 rats. *Cancer Lett.*, **78**, 99–107

Gatzy, J.T., Ayers, T.A., Bond, J.M. & Harper, C. (1989) Effects of Na saccharin feeding and urine on barrier properties of excised rat urinary bladder. *Toxicol. Appl. Pharmacol.*, **100**, 424–439

Goodman, D.G., Ward, J.M., Squire R.A., Chu, K.C. & Linhart, M.S. (1979) Neoplastic and nonneoplastic lesions in aging F344 rats. *Toxicol. Appl. Pharm.*, **48**, 237–248

Hard, G.C. (1995) Species comparison of the content and composition of urinary proteins. *Food Chem. Toxicol.*, **33**, 731–746

Heck, H.D. & Tyl, R.W. (1985) The induction of bladder stones by terephthalic acid, dimethyl terephthalate, and melamine (2,4,6-triamino-*s*-triazine) and its relevance to risk assessment. *Regul. Toxicol. Pharmacol.*, **5**, 294–313

Heidenreich, A. & Engelmann, U. (1993) Sex-dependent urolithiasis in the portacaval shunt rat. 2. Hormones and stone formation. *Urol. Int.*, **51**, 198–203

Herring, D.W., Cartwright, R.A. & Williams, D.D.R. (1979) Genetic associations of transitional cell carcinoma. *Br. J. Urol.*, **51**, 73–77

Herz, R., Sauter, V. & Bircher, J. (1972) Fortuitous discovery of urate nephrolithiasis in rats subjected to portacaval anastomosis. *Experientia*, **28**, 27–28

Hicks, R.M., Wakefield, J.St.J. & Chowaniec, J. (1975) Evaluation of a new model to detect bladder carcinogens and co-carcinogens; results obtained with saccharin, cyclamate and cyclophosphamide. *Chem. Biol. Interactions*, **11**, 225–233

Hueper, W.C. & Payne, W.W. (1963) Polyoxyethylene-(8)-stearate: carcinogenic studies. *Arch. Environ. Health*, **6**, 484–502

IARC (1980) *IARC Monographs on the Evaluation of the Carcinogenic Risk of Chemicals to Humans*, Volume **22**, *Some Non-Nutritive Sweeting Agents*, Lyon, France, pp. 111–170

Imaida, K., Oshima, M., Fukushima, S., Ito, N. & Hotta, K. (1983) Membrane potentials of urinary bladder epithelium in F344 rats treated with N-butyl-N-(4-hydroxybutyl)nitrosamine or sodium saccharin. *Carcinogenesis*, **4**, 659–661

Ito, N., Fukushima, S., Shirai, T. & Nakanishi, K. (1983) Effects of promoters on N-butyl-N-(4-hydroxybutyl)nitrosamine-induced urinary bladder carcinogenesis in the rat. *Environ. Health Perspect.*, **50**, 61–69

Jull, J.W. (1951) The induction of tumours of the bladder epithelium in mice by the direct application of a carcinogen. *Br. J. Cancer*, **5**, 328–330

Kiemeney, L. & Schoenberg, M. (1996) Familial transitional cell carcinoma. *J. Urol.*, **156**, 867–872

Kurata, Y., Asamoto, M., Hagiwara, A., Masui, T. & Fukushima, S. (1986) Promoting effects of various agents in rat urinary bladder carcinogenesis initiated by N-butyl-N-(4-hydroxybutyl)nitrosamine. *Cancer Lett.*, **32**, 125–135

Lalich, J.J. (1966) Experimentally induced uracil urolithiasis in rats. *J. Urol.*, **95**, 83–86

Lee, C.C.R.,Yamamoto, S., Wanibuchi, H., Wada, S., Sugimura, K., Kishimoto, T. & Fukushima, S. (1997) Cyclin D1 overexpression in rat two-stage bladder carcinogenesis and its relationship with oncogenes, tumor suppressor genes and cell proliferation. *Cancer Res.*, **57**, 4765–4776

Lynch, H.T., Walzak, M.P., Fried, R., Domina, A.H. & Lynch J.F. (1979) Familial factors in bladder carcinoma. *J. Urol.*, **122**, 458–461

Maekawa, A., Kurokawa, Y., Takahashi, M., Kokubo, T., Ogiu, T., Onodera, H., Tanigawa, H., Ohno, Y., Furakawa, F. & Hayashi, Y. (1983) Spontaneous tumors in F344/DuCrj rats. *Gann*, **74**, 365–372

Makino, S., Yamashita, H., Harada, M., Konishi, T. & Hayashi, Y. (1990) Genetic monitoring of the ODS rat. In: Fujita, T., Fukase, M. & Konishi, T., eds, *Vitamin C and the Scurvy-Prone ODS Rat*, Amsterdam, Elsevier, pp. 29–34

Masui, T., Mann, A.M., Garland, E.M. & Cohen, S.M. (1989) Strong promoting activity by uracil on urinary bladder carcinogenesis and a possible inhibitory effect on thyroid tumorigenesis in rats initiated with N-methyl-N-nitrosourea. *Carcinogenesis*, **10**, 1471–1474

Masui, T., Don, I., Takada, N., Ogawa, K., Shirai, T. & Fukushima, S. (1994) p53 Mutations in early neoplastic lesions of the urinary bladder in rats treated with N-butyl-N-(4-hydroxybutyl)nitrosamine. *Carcinogenesis*, **15**, 2379–2381

Masui, T., Dong, Y., Yamamoto, S., Takada, N., Nakanishi, H., Inada, K., Fukushima, S. & Tatematsu, M. (1996) p53 Mutations in transitional cell carcinomas of the urinary bladder in rats treated with N-butyl-N-(4-hydroxybutyl)-nitrosamine. *Cancer Lett.*, **105**, 105–112

Melnick, R.L., Boorman, G.A., Haseman, J.K., Montali, R.J. & Huff, J. (1984) Urolithiasis and bladder carcinogenicity of melamine in rodents. *Toxicol. Appl. Pharm.*, **72**, 292–303

Mobley, T.L., Coyle, J.K., al-Hussaini, M. & McDonald, D.F. (1966) The role of chronic mechanical irritation in experimental urothelial tumorigenesis. *Invest. Urol.*, **3**, 325–333

Mori, K. & Yamaguchi, Y. (1989) Pre-neoplastic changes in rat urothelium following portacaval anastomosis. *J. Surg. Oncol.*, **42**, 80–91

Mori, S., Kurata, Y., Takeuchi, Y., Toyama, M., Makino, S. & Fukushima, S. (1987) Influences of strain and diet on the promoting effects of sodium L-ascorbate in two-stage urinary bladder carcinogenesis in rats. *Cancer Res.*, **47**, 3492–3495

Mori, S., Murai, T., Takeuchi, Y., Toyama, M., Makino, S., Konishi, T., Hayashi, Y., Kurata, Y. & Fukushima, S. (1990) Dose response of N-butyl-N-(4-hydroxybutyl)-nitrosamine on urinary bladder carcinogenesis in mutant ODS rats lacking L-ascorbic acid synthesizing ability. *Cancer Lett.*, **49**, 139–145

Mori, S., Murai, T., Takeuchi, Y., Hosono, M., Ohhara, T., Makino, S., Hayashi, Y., Shibata, M.-A., Kurata, Y.,

Hagiwara, A. & Fukushima, S. (1991) No promotion of urinary bladder carcinogenesis by sodium L-ascorbate in male ODS/Shi-od/od rats lacking L-ascorbic acid-synthesizing ability. *Carcinogenesis*, **12**, 1869–1873

Mori, S., Makino, S., Murai, T., Hosono, M., Takeuchi, Y., Ohhara, T., Takeda, R., Hayashi, Y. & Fukushima, S. (1992) Inherited susceptibility to sodium L-ascorbate urinary bladder tumor promotion in male rats (Abstract). In: *First Conference of International Federation of Societies of Toxicologic Pathologists*, p. 62

Mori, S., Murai, T., Hosono, M., Machino, S., Makino, S., Chou, C. & Fukushima, S. (1997) Lack of promotion of urinary bladder carcinogenesis by sodium bicarbonate and/or L-ascorbic acid in male ODS/SHi-od/od rats synthesizing alpha 2 mu-globulin but not L-ascorbic acid. *Food Chem. Toxicol.*, **35**, 783–787

Murai, T., Mori, S., Takeda, R., Wanibuchi, H. & Fukushima, S. (1996) (Abstract) Inhibition due to amiloride on sodium L-ascorbate promotion in urinary bladder carcinogenesis by N-butyl-N-(4-hydroxybutyl)-nitrosamine in F344 rats. In: *Proceedings of the Japanese Cancer Association*, 55th Annual Meeting, p. 246

Murai, T., Mori, S., Hosono, M., Takashima A., Machino, S., Oohara, T., Yamashita, H., Makino, S., Matsuda, T., Wanibuchi, H. & Fukushima, S. (1997a) Strain differences in sensitivity to the promoting effect of sodium L-ascorbate in a two-stage rat urinary bladder carcinogenesis model. *Jpn. J. Cancer Res.*, **88**, 245–253

Murai, T., Mori, S. & Fukushima, S (1997b) (Abstract) The relationship between α_{2u}-globulin and sodium L-ascorbate promotion of bladder carcinogenesis in male and female F344 rats. In: *Proceedings of the Japanese Cancer Association*, 56th Annual Meeting, p. 87

Murai, T., Mori, S. & Fukushima, S (1997c) Influence of amiloride and ouabain on the promoting effects of sodium L-ascorbate (author's translation) (Abstract). In: *Proceedings of the Japanese Society of Pathology*, 86th Meeting, p. 235

Ogasawara, H., Imaida, K., Ishiwata, H., Toyoda, K., Kawanishi, T., Uneyama, C., Hayashi, S., Takahashi, M. & Hayashi Y. (1995) Urinary bladder carcinogenesis induced by melamine in F344 male rats: correlation between carcinogenicity and urolith formation. *Carcinogenesis*, **16**, 2773–2777

Okamura, T., Garland, E.M., Masui, T., Sakata, T., St. John, M. & Cohen, S.M. (1991) Lack of bladder tumor promoting activity in rats fed sodium saccharin in AIN-76A diet. *Cancer Res.*, **51**, 1778–1782

Okamura, T., Garland, E.M., Johnson, L.S., Cano, M., Johansson, S.L. & Cohen, S.M. (1992) Acute urinary tract toxicity of tetraethylorthosilicate in rats. *Fundam. Appl. Toxicol.*, **18**, 425–441

Okumura, M., Shirai, T., Tamano, S., Ito, M., Yamada, S. & Fukushima, S. (1991) Uracil-induced calculi and carcinogenesis in the urinary bladder of rats treated simultaneously with N-butyl-N-(4-hydroxybutyl)nitrosamine. *Carcinogenesis*, **12**, 35–41

Okumura, M., Hasegawa, R., Shirai, T., Ito, M., Yamada, S. & Fukushima, S. (1992) Relationship between calculus formation and carcinogenesis in the urinary bladder of rats administered the non-genotoxic agents thymine or melamine. *Carcinogenesis*, **13**, 1043–1045

Otori, K., Yano, Y., Takada, N., Lee, C.C., Hayashi, S., Otani, S. & Fukushima, S. (1997) Reversibility and apoptosis in rat urinary bladder papillomatosis induced by uracil. *Carcinogenesis*, **18**, 1485–1489

Otoshi, T., Iwata, H., Yamamoto, S., Murai, T., Yamaguchi, S., Matsui-Yuasa, I., Otani, S. & Fukushima, S. (1993) Severity of promotion by sodium salts of succinic acid in rat urinary bladder carcinogenesis correlates with sodium ion concentration under conditions of equal urinary pH. *Carcinogenesis*, **14**, 2277–2281

Oyasu, R., Iwasaki, T. & Ozono, S. (1984) Diffuse papillomatosis of rat urinary bladder occurring in association with vesical calculi. *J. Urol.*, **132**, 1012–1015

Rotin, D., Steele-Norwood, D., Grinstein, S. & Tannock, I. (1989) Requirement of the Na^+/H^+ exchanger for tumor growth. *Cancer Res.*, **49**, 205–211

Sakata, T., Masui, T., St. John, M. & Cohen, S. (1988) Uracil-induced calculi and proliferative lesions of the mouse urinary bladder. *Carcinogenesis*, **9**, 1271–1276

Schramek, P., Heidenreich, A. & Engelmann, U.H. (1993) Sex-dependent urolithiasis in the portacaval shunt rat. Part I. *Urol. Int.*, **50**, 77–81

Schoenberg, M., Kiemeney, L., Walsh, P.C., Griffin, C.A. & Sidransky, D. (1996) Germline translocation t(5;20)(p15;q11) and familial transitional cell carcinoma. *J. Urol.*, **155**, 1035–1036

Shibata, M.A., Yamada, M., Asakawa, E., Hagiwara, A. & Fukushima, S. (1989) Responses of rat urine and urothelium to bladder tumor promoters: possible roles of prostaglandin E2 and ascorbic acid synthesis in bladder carcinogenesis. *Carcinogenesis*, **10**, 1651–1656

Shibata, M.A., Tamano, S., Shirai, T., Kawabe, M. & Fukushima, S. (1992) Inorganic alkalizers and acidifiers under conditions of high urinary Na^+ or K^+ on cell proliferation and two-stage carcinogenesis in the rat bladder. *Jpn. J. Cancer Res.*, **83**, 821–829

Shirai, T., Cohen, S.M., Fukushima, S., Hananouchi, M. & Ito, N. (1978) Reversible papillary hyperplasia of the rat urinary bladder. *Am. J. Pathol.*, **91**, 33–48

Shirai, T., Ikawa, E., Fukushima, S., Masui, T. & Ito, N. (1986) Uracil-induced urolithiasis and the development of reversible papillomatosis in the urinary bladder of F344 rats. *Cancer Res.*, **46**, 2062–2067

Shirai, T., Tagawa, Y., Fukushima, S., Imaida, K. & Ito, N. (1987) Strong promoting activity of reversible uracil-induced urolithiasis on urinary bladder carcinogenesis in rats initiated with N-butyl-N-(4-hydroxybutyl)-nitrosamine. *Cancer Res.*, **47**, 6726–6730

Shirai, T., Fukushima, S., Tagawa, Y., Okumura, M. & Ito, N. (1989) Cell proliferation induced by uracil — calculi and subsequent development of reversible papillomatosis in the rat urinary bladder. *Cancer Res.*, **49**, 378–383

Shirai, T., Shibata, M., Takahashi, S., Tagawa,Y., Imaida, K. & Hirose, M. (1995) Differences in cell proliferation and apoptosis between reversible and irreversible mucosal lesions associated with uracil-induced urolithiasis in N-butyl-N-(4-hydroxybutyl)-nitrosamine-pretreated rats. *Carcinogenesis*, **16**, 501–505

Tamano, S., Asakawa, E., Boomyaphiphat, P., Masui, T. & Fukushima, S. (1993) Lack of promotion of N-butyl-N-(4-hydroxybutyl)nitrosamine-initiated urinary bladder carcinogenesis in mice by rat cancer promoters. *Teratog. Carcinog. Mutag.*, **13**, 89–96

Teelmann, K. & Niemann, W. (1979) The short term fate of dischargeable glass beads implanted surgically in the mouse urinary bladder. *Arch. Toxicol.*, **42**, 51–61

Toyoshima, K. & Leighton, J. (1975) Bladder calculi and urothelial hyperplasia with papillomatosis in the rat following insertion of chalk powder in the bladder cavity with subsequent trauma of the bladder wall. *Cancer Res.*, **35**, 3786–3791

Uwagawa, S., Saito, K., Okuno, Y., Kawasaki, H., Yoshitake, A., Yamada, H. & Fukushima, S. (1994) Lack of induction of epithelial cell proliferation by sodium saccharin and sodium L-ascorbate in the urinary bladder of NCI-Black-Reiter (NBR) male rats. *Toxicol. Appl. Pharmacol.*, **127**, 182–186

Uwagawa, S., Saito, K., Seki, T., Kawasaki, H., Takaba, K., Wanibuchi, H. & Fukushima, S. (1997) Lack of promotion effects of sodium L-ascorbate on urinary bladder carcinogenesis in NCI-Black-Reiter (NBR) male rats initiated with N-butyl-N-(4-hydroxybutyl)nitrosamine. *J. Toxicol. Pathol.*, **10**, 103–107

Vandoren, G., Mertens, B., Heyns, W., Van Baelen, H., Rombauts, W. & Verhoeven, G. (1983) Different forms of alpha 2u-globulin in male and female rat urine. *Eur. J. Biochem.*, **134**, 175–181

Wang, C.Y., Kamiryo, Y., Hayashida, S. & Croft, W.A. (1987) Production of urinary tract tumors by co-administration of uracil and N-[4-(5-nitro-2-furyl)-2-thiazolyl]formamide in F344 rats. *Cancer Lett.*, **34**, 249–255

Weil, C.S., Carpenter, C.P. & Smyth, H.F., Jr (1965) Urinary bladder response to diethylene glycol. Calculi and tumors following repeated feeding and implants. *Arch. Environ. Health*, **11**, 569–581

Corresponding authors

S. Fukushima & T. Murai
Department of Pathology,
Osaka City University Medical School
1-4-54 Asahi-machi, Abeno-ku,
Osaka 545-8585, Japan

Species Differences in Thyroid, Kidney and Urinary Bladder Carcinogenesis
C.C. Capen, E. Dybing, J.M. Rice and J.D. Wilbourn, eds
IARC Scientific Publications No. 147
International Agency for Research on Cancer, Lyon, 1999

Calcium phosphate-containing urinary precipitate in rat urinary bladder carcinogenesis

S.M. Cohen

Introduction

In 1970, Bryan *et al.* (1970) reported that sodium saccharin incorporated in cholesterol pellets which were then surgically implanted into the mouse urinary bladder produced an increased incidence of cancer. Thus began a saga, that has already lasted nearly three decades, of attempts to ascertain the potential cancer hazard to humans of this commonly used sweetener (Arnold *et al.*, 1983; Ellwein & Cohen, 1990). The form of saccharin used in animal experiments to produce bladder cancer has been the sodium salt, administered as high doses in the diet. The sodium and calcium salts are consumed by humans.

Tumours formed after ingestion of high doses of sodium saccharin are produced only in rats (Frederick *et al.*, 1989; Ellwein & Cohen, 1990). The tumours produced in mice by implantation of sodium saccharin-containing cholesterol pellets appear to be formed after the rapid leaching of the chemical from the pellet; the coarse pellet, no longer containing saccharin, acts as an abrasive, leading to significant urothelial necrosis, regeneration and ultimately bladder cancer (DeSesso, 1989). Oral administration of high doses of sodium saccharin to mice does not produce a proliferative effect in the urothelium (Fukushima *et al.*, 1983a; Frederick *et al.*, 1989; Arnold *et al.*, 1995).

Administration of sodium saccharin in a standard two-year bioassay in rats, beginning at six to eight weeks of age, has not produced bladder cancer (Arnold *et al.*, 1983; Ellwein & Cohen, 1990). However, increased incidence of bladder cancer has been observed when lifetime administration to rats is begun before conception (two-generation bioassay) (Schoenig *et al.*, 1985; Ellwein & Cohen, 1990), at the time of birth (Schoenig *et al.*, 1985) or before five weeks of age (Arnold *et al.*, 1980). The male rat is significantly more susceptible to the urothelial effects of sodium saccharin than the

female, with female rats showing no effect in most studies (Arnold *et al.*, 1980; Ellwein & Cohen, 1990). The dose–response curve for sodium saccharin carcinogenicity in a two-generation bioassay is extremely steep, with a no-effect level at 1% of the diet (Schoenig *et al.*, 1985).

In contrast to its lack of carcinogenicity even at high doses in a standard two-year bioassay, sodium saccharin administered to mature rats at high doses after a brief treatment with a known bladder carcinogen produces high incidences of bladder tumours. Agents which have been used to pre-treat rats before sodium saccharin administration include intravesical *N*-methyl-*N*-nitrosourea (MNU) (Hicks *et al.*, 1973), *N*-[4-(5-nitro-2-furyl)-2-thiazolyl]formamide (FANFT) (Cohen *et al.*, 1979), *N*-butyl-*N*-(4-hydroxybutyl)nitrosamine (BBN) in the drinking-water (Nakanishi *et al.*, 1980a), cyclophosphamide (CP) by intraperitoneal injection (Cohen *et al.*, 1982) and freeze ulceration (Cohen *et al.*, 1982). Similarly to two-stage carcinogenesis in mouse skin and rat liver, treatment with sodium saccharin may be started after administration of the bladder carcinogen or it may be delayed; the longest interval between the two treatments has been 18 weeks (Hasegawa *et al.*, 1985). As in the two-generation bioassay, the dose–response curve is steep, with a no-effect level of 1% (Nakanishi *et al.*, 1980b). Tests of sodium saccharin in mice using the two-stage model of carcinogenesis and 2-acetylaminofluorene (2-AAF) as the initial carcinogen treatment gave negative results (Frederick *et al.*, 1989). The dietary levels used in mouse experiments were similar to those used in rat studies, resulting in higher doses on a mg/kg bw basis.

Strains of rats have different susceptibilities to the urothelial effects of sodium saccharin and other sodium salts, with Wistar rats being less susceptible than Fischer 344 or Sprague–Dawley rats

(Fukushima *et al.*, 1983a; Mori *et al.*, 1987; Murai *et al.*, 1997), NBR rats being only slightly susceptible (Garland *et al.*, 1994a; Uwagawa *et al.*, 1994) and ACI rats having particularly high sensitivity (Mori *et al.*, 1987). However, it is likely that the ACI strain is not optimal for evaluation of chemicals as bladder carcinogens since there is considerable hyperplasia in the ACI rat bladder even in control animals. It is unclear whether this spontaneous proliferation is due to parasitic contamination, urinary calculus formation or some other unidentified mechanism.

Although other forms of saccharin have not been investigated as extensively as sodium saccharin, it is clear that the acid form of the chemical (acid saccharin) is without effect on the rat urothelium (Hasegawa & Cohen, 1986; West *et al.*, 1986; Cohen *et al.*, 1991a).

Carcinogenicity of other sodium salts

Following the report by Fukushima *et al.* (1983b) demonstrating that sodium ascorbate also increased bladder tumour incidence in male rats when administered after BBN, the issue of saccharin carcinogenicity was extended to a broader class of chemicals, the sodium salts of organic acids. As in the case of sodium saccharin, the male rat is more susceptible to the effects of sodium ascorbate than the female, the mouse is without urothelial effects (Tamano *et al.*, 1993), the doses required are similar to those for sodium saccharin (Cohen *et al.*, 1995a) and the parent acid, ascorbic acid, is without effect on the urothelium (Fukushima *et al.*, 1983b; Shioya *et al.*, 1994). In the standard two-year bioassay, sodium ascorbate does not produce an increased incidence of bladder cancer; however, as with sodium saccharin, administration of high doses of sodium ascorbate to male rats following a two-generation protocol produces an increased incidence of bladder tumours (Cohen *et al.*, unpublished observations).

Subsequently, several sodium salts of other organic acids (Table 1) have been identified as having an effect on the bladder urothelium of male rats, either increasing urothelial proliferation following administration at high doses or increasing the incidence of bladder tumours when administered after pretreatment with a bladder carcinogen such as FANFT or BBN (Fukushima *et al.*, 1984, 1986; DeGroot *et al.*, 1988; Ellwein & Cohen, 1990; Cohen *et al.*, 1991a; Shibata *et al.*, 1991; Otoshi

Table 1. Sodium salts producing proliferative effects in the rat bladder when administered at high doses in the diet

Saccharin	Citrate	Erythorbate
Ascorbate	Succinate	Phosphate
Glutamate	Bicarbonate	
Aspartate	Chloride	

et al., 1993; Lina *et al.*, 1994; Kitamura *et al.*, 1996). Monosodium glutamate has been studied at high doses in the diet, producing an increased incidence of urothelial proliferation (DeGroot *et al.*, 1988), but not bladder cancer in a two-year bioassay (Owen *et al.*, 1978). Sodium and potassium bicarbonates and carbonates produced increased urothelial proliferation in short-term bioassays (Fukushima *et al.*, 1991; Cohen *et al.*, 1995b), with increased incidences of bladder tumours if administered for more than two and a half years rather than the standard two years (Lina *et al.*, 1994). Glutamic acid, in contrast to the corresponding acids of other sodium salts, has shown some evidence of causing increased proliferation of the urothelium (DeGroot *et al.*, 1988).

Hypotheses concerning mechanisms of action

Any hypothesis that is offered to explain the effects of administering saccharin and other sodium salts on the bladder must be consistent with the findings in a number of animal models (see Table 2).

During the past three decades, several mechanisms have been suggested for the carcinogenicity of sodium salts in rats (Table 3), beginning with the classical approach of possible interaction of

Table 2. Key observations regarding the carcinogenicity of sodium salts

Do not react with DNA

Increase bladder cancer in rats, but not in mice or monkeys

Positive in two-generation bioassay but not standard two-year bioassay

Male rats are more susceptible than female rats

High doses are required

Sodium salt positive, parent acid negative

Table 3. Suggested mechanisms by which sodium salts produce bladder urothelial proliferative effects in rats
Reaction with DNA
Formation of urinary calculi
Carcinogenic contaminant
Alteration of urinary physiology

saccharin or a possible metabolite with DNA (Arnold & Boyes, 1989). Sodium saccharin, like the other sodium salts, is a salt of a moderately strong acid with a pK_a of approximately 2.0 (Williamson *et al.*, 1987). Thus, under physiological conditions, essentially all of the administered chemical is ionized and present as a strong anion, not a cation as required for reactivity with DNA. No DNA binding was detected following administration of high doses of sodium saccharin to rats (Lutz & Schlatter, 1977), as expected given the chemistry of the molecule. Furthermore, in rats, as in humans, there is no evidence that the saccharin molecule is metabolized (Sweatman *et al.*, 1981).

In general, assays involving point mutations, such as the Ames assay, have given negative results, even with extremely high doses of sodium saccharin (Arnold & Boyes, 1989). Assays involving evaluation of chromosomal aberrations have shown some positive results, but only at extremely high concentrations. At these concentrations, it is possible that cytotoxicity is involved or, more likely, an osmotic effect (Ashby & Ishidate, 1986), as positive results are also produced with equimolar concentrations of sodium chloride or potassium chloride. A direct evaluation of genotoxicity by sodium saccharin administration in the target tissue, the rat urothelium, has been made using a combination in-vivo–in-vitro assay for unscheduled DNA synthesis (Zukowski *et al.*, 1994). This assay is positive for aromatic amines, which are known bladder carcinogens in humans and in rats, but negative for non-genotoxic compounds such as sodium saccharin.

In summary, the strongly nucleophilic nature of the saccharin anion and the anions of other sodium salts producing similar urothelial effects in rats, the lack of reactivity with DNA of the anion or any potential metabolite and the lack of DNA

binding or DNA damage in the target tissue provide considerable evidence against a genotoxic mechanism for the carcinogenicity of sodium salts such as sodium saccharin or sodium ascorbate.

A second possibility that has been suggested is that the carcinogenicity of sodium saccharin and related salts is due to contamination by a highly carcinogenic contaminant (Ball *et al.*, 1978; Arnold *et al.*, 1980). For sodium saccharin, this has been extensively investigated: a two-generation bioassay evaluation of *ortho*-toluene sulfonamide, the major contaminant of sodium saccharin preparations synthesized by the Remsen–Fahlberg procedure, gave negative results (Arnold *et al.*, 1980). The likelihood of this or other contaminants being responsible for the carcinogenic effects of saccharin or other sodium salts is minimal, not only on the basis of these direct bioassays, but also because the types of contaminant are different when saccharin is synthesized by the Maumee procedure (which does not generate *ortho*-toluene sulfonamide) (Cohen *et al.*, 1979), and the contaminants in sodium ascorbate and other sodium salts are totally unlike those in sodium saccharin.

A third possibility is that the bladder cancer is produced as a result of the formation of urinary tract calculi. Formation of calculi is a well established mechanism by which certain chemicals produce bladder cancer in rodents, especially in rats (Clayson *et al.*, 1995). Administration of extremely high doses of ascorbic acid to humans has been suggested to produce urinary tract calculi composed of calcium oxalate in a relatively small number of individuals, although the evidence is controversial (Wandzilak *et al.*, 1994). Administration of acid saccharin to rats at very high doses has occasionally produced urinary tract calculi composed of saccharin (Cohen *et al.*, unpublished observations). However, the administration to rodents of sodium ascorbate, sodium saccharin or other sodium salts has not been associated with the development of urinary tract calculi. In the bioassays in which sodium saccharin produced bladder cancer in rats, the incidences of calculi in the test groups were similar to those in controls (Arnold *et al.*, 1980; Schoenig *et al.*, 1985; Ellwein & Cohen, 1990).

A major issue regarding the carcinogenicity of sodium salts is whether the anion itself is involved in the carcinogenic process in the target tissue, the urothelium, or whether the administration of high doses of these sodium salts greatly alters urinary physiology and composition leading to a secondary process by which bladder cancer is produced (Hasegawa & Cohen, 1986; Williamson *et al.*, 1987; Fisher *et al.*, 1989). As is discussed further below, the evidence strongly suggests that after feeding high doses of the salts, tumours are produced indirectly by alteration of the urinary composition rather than by the anion itself. Evidence for this includes the observation that even administration of enormous doses of sodium ascorbate to rats leads to only a slight increase in urinary ascorbate concentrations (total ascorbate, including dehydroascorbate) (Fukushima *et al.*, 1983b; Shioya *et al.*, 1994), in contrast to the situation in humans. Rats are able to synthesize ascorbic acid, unlike humans for whom it is a dietary essential. The metabolism and excretion of ascorbate in rats also differ quantitatively from those in humans.

In addition, the proliferative and tumorigenic effects of these salts have little correlation with the urinary concentration of the anion (Renwick, 1993). For example, administration of acid saccharin or sodium saccharin (or ascorbic acid and sodium ascorbate) produces similar levels of the anion in the urine and yet the sodium salt produces a proliferative effect, whereas the acid does not (Fukushima *et al.*, 1983b; Hasegawa & Cohen 1986; Shioya *et al.*, 1994).

In summary, the evidence suggests that sodium salts produce bladder cancer by an indirect mechanism by altering the composition of the urine as a physiological response to administration of high levels of a sodium salt. The chemicals do not produce cancer by direct reactivity with DNA or by direct interaction of the chemical or a metabolite with the urothelium.

Urinary precipitate, cytotoxicity and consequent regeneration

Although administration of high concentrations of sodium salts does not appear to cause genotoxic effects in the bladder epithelium, it does produce an increase in proliferation (Fukushima & Cohen, 1980; Cohen *et al.*, 1990). No statistically significant increase is observed at 1% of the diet for sodium saccharin or sodium ascorbate, the no-effect level for carcinogenicity (Cohen *et al.*, 1995a,c). The extent of proliferation is relatively slight, with an increase in number of cells (hyperplasia) approximately 5–10 times greater than controls. This is evident by light microscopy as simple hyperplasia (Figure 1) which is predominantly present in the dome of the bladder initially, but then becomes more diffuse. Occasionally, nodular and papillary hyperplasia is also present. The rate of cell proliferation is also increased 2–10 times, as detected by labelling index following a one-hour pulse of tritiated thymidine or bromodeoxyuridine. The hyperplastic effect is detectable approximately four weeks after administration of these compounds, but the labelling index is already increased one week after administration has begun (Fukushima & Cohen, 1980).

Increased proliferation was present during the neonatal period in a two-generation type of bioassay, as well as later in life (Cohen *et al.*,

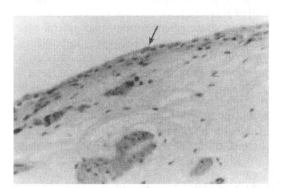
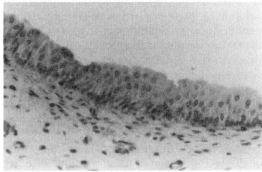

Figure 1. (Left) Normal bladder urothelium (arrow) of a control-fed male rat. x 400.
(Right) Simple hyperplasia of the bladder urothelium in a male rat fed 7.5% sodium saccharin in the diet for 10 weeks beginning at 5 weeks of age. x 400.

1995a,c). It is also present if administration begins at 6–8 weeks of age, as in a standard two-year bioassay. This is in apparent contradiction to the need for neonatal exposure for tumour production, since tumours are not produced if administration of the sodium salt begins at 6–8 weeks of age and continues for two years. However, this is a quantitative rather than a qualitative issue (Ellwein & Cohen, 1988). Based on the number of cell divisions that occur, a detectable statistically significant increase in bladder tumour incidence in a standard two-year bioassay with 50 animals per group would not be expected. Instead, the increase in tumour incidence is estimated to be only about 1%.

The requirement that treatment begins during the neonatal period for tumorigenicity to be observed is likely to be due to the difference in proliferation of the normal bladder during this time period compared to the adult bladder epithelium (Cohen et al., 1988). In the adult (4–6 weeks of age) rodent bladder epithelium, as in primates, the labelling index is generally less than 0.1% following a one-hour pulse of the label. In contrast, the bladder epithelium during gestation is a rapidly proliferating tissue with a labelling index of approximately 10%. Nearly every bladder epithelial cell is dividing every day in the prenatal bladder. This rapidly decreases immediately after birth. By seven days of age, the labelling index has decreased to approximately 1–1.5%, and it further decreases to less than 0.1% by approximately four weeks of age. Simple calculations suggest that approximately one-third of the total cell divisions in the normal urothelium of the bladder have occurred by four weeks of age (Ellwein & Cohen, 1988). Thus, administration of high doses of sodium saccharin or sodium ascorbate during this period leads to an increase in the proliferative rate of an already rapidly proliferating urothelium. In addition, since this occurs early in the life span of the animal, there is maximal time for continued expansion during the remainder of the animal's lifetime.

The effect of further increasing the already rapid proliferation during the neonatal period can be replicated by causing a burst of proliferation by simply ulcerating the bladder (Cohen et al., 1982; Murasaki & Cohen, 1983; Hasegawa et al., 1985). If no further treatment is given, the bladder

epithelium returns to normal within 4–6 weeks of ulceration and, after two years, no tumours are produced. However, if sodium saccharin is administered after ulceration, bladder tumours are produced. The number of cell replications occurring following ulceration has been estimated, and it is similar to that achieved by administration of the sodium salt during the neonatal period. Ulceration produced by application of a frozen rod or by administration of cyclophosphamide gives similar quantitative effects on cell replication and tumorigenesis (Cohen et al., 1982).

Extensive cell kinetic analyses and modelling procedures have indicated that increased cell replication can readily explain the quantitative aspects of tumorigenesis with sodium salts, including the requirement for neonatal period treatment in contrast to a standard two-year bioassay (Ellwein & Cohen, 1988).

Increased cell replication can be produced either by direct mitogenesis, which usually involves effects on hormones and/or growth factors, or by toxic effects with consequent regeneration (Cohen & Ellwein, 1990, 1991; Cohen, 1995a). Light microscopic observations of the bladders of animals fed high doses of sodium salts revealed little evidence of toxicity. However, examination by scanning electron microscopy showed necrosis of the superficial cell layer (Figure 2), beginning in the dome of the bladder and then spreading more diffusely (Cohen et al., 1990). However, complete erosion of the bladder epithelium does not occur nor is there ulceration, so there is no accompanying inflammatory response. Nevertheless, to replace the cells which are destroyed and exfoliated, there is regenerative hyperplasia, which, as indicated above, is quite mild, reflecting the mild nature of the toxicity. The extent of hyperplasia and the increase in labelling index are greater in male rats than in female rats (Garland et al., 1994b). The toxicity and regeneration occur only at high doses, with a no-effect level for sodium saccharin and sodium ascorbate of 1% of the diet (Cohen et al., 1990, 1995a,c).

Although calculi are not formed following administration of high doses of sodium salts, recent evidence suggests that a urinary amorphous-appearing precipitate (Figure 3) develops (Arnold et al., 1980; West & Jackson, 1981; Cohen et al., 1991b, 1995b). This is a high-dose

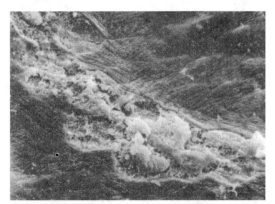

Figure 2. Necrosis of the superficial cell layer of the urothelium of a male rat fed 7.5% sodium saccharin in the diet for 10 weeks beginning at 5 weeks of age. x 460.

phenomenon only, with a no-effect level of 1% of the diet in rats fed sodium saccharin or sodium ascorbate. No precipitate forms when the corresponding acids are fed. The prerequisite changes in the urine for precipitate formation include overall high ionic density of the urine (high osmolality), high protein concentration, pH ≥ 6.5 and adequate levels of calcium and phosphate for precipitation of calcium phosphate. Although urinary osmolality and protein concentration in rats fed high levels of sodium salts are decreased compared to controls, they are still significantly higher than those in humans.

The major component of this precipitate is calcium phosphate, as determined by X-ray reflective spectroscopy and micro-analytical chemical analyses. The phosphate appears to be present as the mono- and di-basic forms. Little if any magnesium is present in the precipitate. Magnesium ammonium phosphate crystals are normal constituents of urine. The small amount of magnesium that appears in the precipitate is probably due to contamination by these crystals. In addition, some form of silicon-containing material is also present in the precipitate, along with a relatively small amount of protein, including α_{2u}-globulin (Cohen *et al.*, 1991b). Relatively large amounts of mucopolysaccharides are present in the precipitate, and the most common mucopolysaccharide appears to be heparan sulfate.

The precipitate in rats administered sodium saccharin contains small amounts of saccharin, as detected by chemical analysis and by infrared spectroscopy. However, there is little ascorbate present in the precipitate in rats fed high doses of sodium ascorbate. This difference between the two sodium salts may be related to the extremely high concentrations of saccharin in the urine following administration of any salt form of saccharin (200 mM after administration of 5% sodium saccharin), in contrast to the relatively low levels of ascorbate (3–4 mM) following administration of 7% sodium ascorbate in the diet (Fukushima *et al.*, 1983b; Hasegawa & Cohen, 1986; Shioya *et al.*, 1994).

In vitro, calcium phosphate is an essential ingredient of tissue culture medium for epithelial and other cells, and is usually present at a concentration of approximately 1 mM or less (Cohen *et al.*, 1995d). At these concentrations, the calcium phosphate is entirely soluble. If the concentration is increased to levels at which precipitation occurs (approximately 5 mM), there is cytotoxicity to bladder epithelial cells. Thus, it is likely that the calcium phosphate-containing precipitate in the urine of rats fed high concentrations of the sodium salts is cytotoxic to the urothelium, leading to erosion of the superficial cell layer of the bladder epithelium and consequent regenerative hyperplasia. The overall mechanism for the bladder carcinogenicity of sodium salts is summarized in Figure 4.

Influence of urinary protein

The presence of high concentrations of protein in the urine appears to be a prerequisite for the formation of the urinary precipitate and for the urothelial proliferation effects in rats fed high doses of sodium salts. The exact mechanism by which protein contributes to this process is not clear, but may be related to its functioning as a nucleus for initiating formation of the precipitate rather than actually participating in the growth of the precipitate once it has begun. Protein is present in the precipitate, but generally accounts for less than 5% of the total weight of the precipitate (Cohen *et al.*, 1991b).

Rats have extraordinarily high levels of protein in the urine, at mg/mL levels rather than the usual μg/mL levels occurring in humans (Olson *et al.*, 1990; Hard, 1995). In female rats, the high levels of urinary protein largely consist of albumin. The male rat has even higher concentrations of urinary

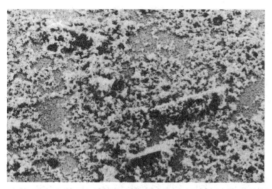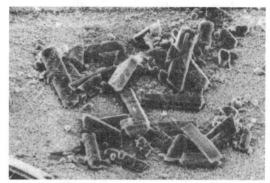

Figure. 3. (Left) A few MgNH$_4$PO$_4$ crystals with calcium phosphate-containing precipitate from the urine of a male rat fed 7.5% sodium saccharin in the diet for 4 weeks beginning at 5 weeks of age. x 300.
(Right) MgNH$_4$PO$_4$ crystals in control urine with their typical shape. x 460

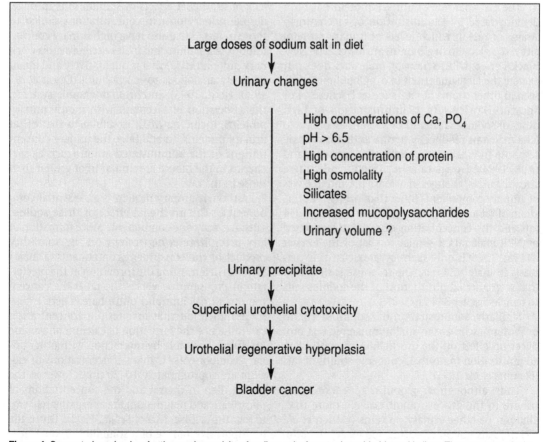

Large doses of sodium salt in diet

↓

Urinary changes

High concentrations of Ca, PO$_4$
pH > 6.5
High concentration of protein
High osmolality
Silicates
Increased mucopolysaccharides
Urinary volume ?

↓

Urinary precipitate

↓

Superficial urothelial cytotoxicity

↓

Urothelial regenerative hyperplasia

↓

Bladder cancer

Figure 4. Suggested mechanism for the carcinogenicity of sodium salts for rat urinary bladder epithelium. The parameters in the urine must all be at critical levels for the cytotoxic precipitate to form.

protein because of the presence of α_{2u}-globulin, from the age of approximately six weeks (Hard, 1995).

The anions of the carcinogenic sodium salts have been shown to associate closely with urinary proteins by co-elution in chromatographic systems (Cohen et al., 1991b, 1995b). However, the anions do not appear to be covalently bound, and the association does not appear to be of the same type as occurs with chemicals known to produce kidney tumours in male rats due to binding to α_{2u}-globulin (Lehman-McKeeman, unpublished observations). The anions associate with albumin, but also to a quantitatively greater extent with α_{2u}-globulin. It is possible that this close association of these anions with the protein contributes to the formation of the precipitate.

The essential role of urinary protein has been demonstrated by administration of saccharin to strains of rats in which levels of urinary protein, either α_{2u}-globulin or albumin, are lower. The NCI-Black-Reiter (NBR) strain of male rats does not excrete the large quantities of α_{2u}-globulin that are seen in other strains of rats, such as Fischer 344 or Sprague–Dawley rats. Administration of high doses of sodium saccharin or sodium ascorbate to NBR male rats produces a significantly lower toxic response than is seen in Fischer 344 rats (Garland et al., 1994a; Uwagawa et al., 1994). Under these circumstances, changes in urinary pH and in levels of urinary components other than proteins in this strain of rat are comparable to those in Fischer 344 rats and the concentration of saccharin excreted by NBR male rats is similar to that of the Fischer 344 rat. There is only slight cytotoxicity or hyperplasia in male NBR rats. The response is similar to that seen after administration of the sodium salts to female Fischer 344 rats.

Similarly, administration of sodium saccharin or sodium ascorbate to analbuminaemic rats produces no effect on the urothelium in contrast to administration to normal, congenic strains of rats (Homma et al., 1991).

Thus, although α_{2u}-globulin appears to contribute to the process quantitatively more than albumin or other urinary proteins (Cohen et al., 1991b), it is not an effect unique to α_{2u}-globulin, and urothelial toxicity and proliferation can occur, albeit only slightly, in the absence of α_{2u}-globulin, as seen in female rats or in male NBR rats.

The involvement of high levels of urinary protein, such as albumin, in addition to α_{2u}-globulin, helps to explain why the proliferative effect of sodium saccharin and sodium ascorbate can be seen in the neonatal male rat before excretion of high concentrations of α_{2u}-globulin begins, usually at approximately six weeks of age. Essentially, during the first six weeks of life, the male and female rats are similar in their response to these sodium salts (Cohen et al., 1995a,c). Once α_{2u}-globulin production and excretion begins in male rats, the response becomes significantly greater in males than in females. The effect in female rats is dependent on the high concentrations of albumin rather than the even higher protein concentrations due to α_{2u}-globulin in the adult male.

A difficulty arises, however, in explaining the lack of urothelial effects of sodium salts in mice, despite urinary protein concentrations similar to those in rats. Mice also have high urinary concentrations of albumin, and males excrete a mouse urinary protein (MUP) that is qualitatively and quantitatively analogous to α_{2u}-globulin (Olson et al., 1990; Hard, 1995). In chromatographic systems, the association of saccharin with mouse urinary proteins, including MUP, is similar to that of rat urinary proteins. In addition, the urinary concentrations of the administered anion (such as saccharin) in the mouse are similar to or greater than those in the rat.

Although urinary protein is an essential component of the urothelial effect of these sodium salts, it is only one component. Since formation of any precipitate is dependent on the solubility product of the constituent components, a major factor in determining the formation of the precipitate in mouse urine versus the rat is the concentrations of calcium and phosphate. There is also some indication that magnesium concentration can influence the formation of calcium phosphate precipitate, possibly by interaction with other urinary components. Urinary concentrations of calcium are approximately 10–20 times lower in the mouse than in the rat and the concentrations of phosphate and magnesium are approximately two to four times lower (Arnold et al., 1995). Given the multiplicative nature of a solubility product, it is clear that these significant differences in concentrations of calcium and phosphate quantitatively contribute to the lack of precipitate formation and urothelial proliferative effect in the mouse, in contrast to the rat.

Effect of urinary pH

For all of the salts, listed in Table 1, for which the corresponding acid has been tested, the latter form is without effect on the urothelium of the male rat, the most sensitive sex–species tested (West *et al.*, 1986; Ellwein & Cohen, 1990; Cohen *et al.*, 1991a; Shioya *et al.*, 1994). With most diets used in rodent bioassays, the urinary pH in the controls ranges from 6.5 to 7.5. Administration of sodium saccharin has little effect on the urinary pH, whereas administration of some of the other sodium salts, such as sodium ascorbate and sodium citrate, leads to a higher urinary pH than the controls (Cohen *et al.*, 1995b). Administration of the saccharin acid leads to a significant decrease in the urinary pH, usually to levels less than 6.0.

It is essential in determining the effect of urinary pH that freshly voided specimens be analysed and that the effect be determined during the night or early in the morning, within 2–3 h after the lights have been turned on in the animal room (Fisher *et al.*, 1989; Cohen, 1995b). Rodents are nocturnal animals, eating and drinking at night and sleeping during the day. During the hours of consumption and shortly thereafter, there is a rise in the urinary pH, which then rapidly decreases once the rats stop eating, becoming quite acidic (pH 5.0–6.0) during the lighted hours.

Formation of the calcium phosphate-containing precipitate in rat urine does not generally occur if the urinary pH is below 6.5. Thus, when the parent acid is administered, producing a urinary pH of 6.0 or less, the precipitate cannot form and, consequently, there is no cytotoxicity, regenerative hyperplasia or tumour formation. This can be demonstrated further by administration of high concentrations of the sodium salt with comparatively high levels of ammonium chloride (Garland *et al.*, 1989; Cohen *et al.*, 1991a; Shioya *et al.*, 1994; Cohen *et al.*, 1995a,b). The resulting marked acidification of the urine completely inhibits the formation of the calcium phosphate-containing precipitate, as well as completely inhibiting the cytotoxic, proliferative and tumorigenic effects of the sodium salt. Similarly, administration of the sodium salt in AIN-76A semi-synthetic diet generally results in a urinary pH of less than 6.0

(Fisher *et al.*, 1989; Garland *et al.*, 1989; Okamura *et al.*, 1991). It appears that the casein, the source of protein in this commonly used semi-synthetic diet, produces a markedly acidic urine, even in controls (pH < 6.0). If albumin is substituted for casein in the diet, the urinary pH attains the levels usually seen in control animals on other diets, such as Purina, Prolab, Oriental M or Clea, and a proliferative response is seen with the sodium salts. It is not the effect of the sodium salts on urinary pH in comparison to controls that is important but rather the specific level of pH that occurs in the urine of the animals administered the sodium salt. Thus, in some experiments, sodium saccharin administration has produced urinary pH slightly lower, rather than slightly higher, than in the controls but the pH is still above 6.5, and a urothelial proliferative response still occurs.

Sodium hippurate is chemically and toxicokinetically similar to the other sodium salts listed in Table 1. However, when it was administered to male rats at high levels in the diet either alone or after exposure to BBN, there was no proliferative response in the bladder (Fukushima *et al.*, 1983c; Schoenig *et al.*, 1985). The doses of sodium hippurate used were comparable to those producing toxic effects with the other sodium salts listed in Table 1, but administration of sodium hippurate at these doses gave a urinary pH less than 6.3. Thus, given the necessity for a urinary pH of at least 6.5, no precipitate can form, and consequently no cytotoxicity, regenerative hyperplasia or tumour formation occurs. Some investigators have claimed that a rise in urinary pH by itself can lead to urothelial proliferation in the rat and ultimately the development of tumours. However, this appears not to be the case, since administration of high concentrations of calcium carbonate in the diet produces a urinary pH of approximately 8.0, and yet there is no proliferative or tumorigenic effect in male rats (Cohen *et al.*, 1991a). Similarly, a rodent diet commonly used in Europe, Altromin 1321, routinely produces a urinary pH of 8.0 or higher, but has no effect on the urothelium of the control-fed rats (Cohen *et al.*, 1994).

Effect of urinary volume and other factors

A consequence of administration of high levels of sodium salts in the diet is an increase in water excretion accompanied by an increase in water ingestion (Fisher *et al.*, 1989; Cohen *et al.*, 1995b). This leads to an overall dilution of urinary components, with decreases in osmolality and creatinine levels. Occasionally, however, such as following administration of sodium saccharin, urinary calcium, phosphate and magnesium concentrations remain similar to those in the controls or even increase slightly despite the dilutional effect caused by increased water excretion (Schoenig & Anderson, 1985). A consequence of the increase in urinary excretion, which is usually in the range of two- to three-fold, is that the bladder becomes distended. It remains unclear whether this contributes to the carcinogenicity of these sodium salts or whether it is a coincidental event (Anderson, 1988). Clearly, urinary volume and urinary bladder distension alone are inadequate to explain the effects, since administration of diuretics, such as furosemide (US National Toxicology Program, 1989), produces even greater urinary volumes and distension than do the sodium salts, and yet there is no increase in urothelial proliferation or tumorigenicity.

It has also been suggested that increased sodium by itself leads to the proliferative effects seen with the sodium salts (Otoshi *et al.*, 1993; Shioya *et al.*, 1994). However, this fails to explain the differences between male and female rats, which excrete similar concentrations of sodium in the urine following administration of identical sodium salt levels in the diet (Schoenig & Anderson, 1985) and also fails to explain the differences between rats and mice, again since the urinary sodium concentrations are similar. Nevertheless, it does appear that an increase in sodium ingestion and excretion enhances the proliferative and tumorigenic effects of the sodium salts by unknown mechanisms.

Although the sodium salts have been studied most extensively, a few potassium salts have also been investigated, including potassium saccharin (Hasegawa & Cohen, 1986) and potassium bicarbonate (Fukushima *et al.*, 1991; Lina *et al.*, 1994). In general, the effect on the urothelium is less with the potassium salts than with the sodium salts, despite similar effects on urinary pH, volume and other components of the urine. Administration of high levels of calcium salts tends to produce only a slight proliferative effect on the urothelium (Hasegawa & Cohen, 1986; Cohen *et al.*, 1991a).

This is probably related to the urinary pH usually being 6.5 or lower when these calcium salts are administered. However, if they are co-administered with an agent that increases the urinary pH, there is a corresponding increase in proliferation and tumorigenicity.

As is apparent from the above discussion of the effects of urinary protein, pH, volume, osmolality, calcium, phosphate and possibly sodium, administration of these sodium salts at high levels in the diet produces a pleiotropic effect on the urine and it is the combination of effects that leads ultimately to the production of the calcium phosphate-containing precipitate and the bladder urothelial effects. It is essential that all of these components be present at critical levels for the effect to occur. It appears that mucopolysaccharides also contribute to the effect, as they are the major organic component of the precipitate. Preliminary investigations have shown that there is little mucopolysaccharide in normal rat urine, whereas the amount in the urine of rats ingesting high levels of sodium saccharin is considerable.

Other constituents of the diet that might influence the effect of the sodium salts on the urine include the level of silicates (Cohen *et al.*, 1991b). Administration of high levels of silicates is known to produce highly cytotoxic crystals in the urine of rats and domesticated animals (Emerick *et al.*, 1963). The contribution of these silicates present in the urinary precipitate to the urinary tract effects of sodium salts is unknown.

ortho-Phenylphenol and its sodium salt

Another apparent exception to the generalities above for sodium salts is *ortho*-phenylphenol (OPP). The parent acid, OPP, is a relatively weak acid with a pK_a of approximately 9. In contrast to acid saccharin, ascorbic acid or glutamic acid, it produces a significant proliferative response in the urothelium of male rats and ultimately produces bladder cancer (Hiraga & Fujii, 1984). This appears to be specific to the male rat, although there is a slight proliferative effect in female rats (Wahle *et al.*, 1997). The carcinogenic effect is seen only at high doses ($\geq$ 8000 ppm of the diet) and there is no effect on the urothelium in mice. Similar doses of the sodium salt of OPP produce a greater effect on the urothelium than does the acid (Fujii *et al.*, 1987). Although this combination of effects bears some resemblance to those of the other sodium salts mentioned above, the carcinogenicity of the acid OPP itself contrasts with lack of urothelial effects seen with the corresponding acids of the other sodium salts described above.

Administration of OPP or its sodium salt at high levels in the diet produces cytotoxicity and regenerative hyperplasia of the rat urothelium but, in contrast to the salts listed in Table 1, no urinary solids (calculi, microcrystalluria or calcium phosphate-containing precipitate) are produced (Cohen et al., 1997). The toxicity is similar quantitatively to that observed with the sodium salts discussed above, but must be due to the chemical itself or, more likely, its metabolites.

There have been suggestions that, although OPP is not genotoxic, its semiquinone or quinone metabolites might be genotoxic and form DNA adducts. However, in vivo, formation of DNA adducts following OPP administration has been observed only in examination of the whole rat bladder by ^{32}P-postlabelling techniques (Ushiyama et al., 1992) and in the DNA of mouse skin following direct application of extraordinarily high levels of OPP to the skin (Pathak & Roy, 1992). We have investigated the rat urothelium, the target tissue of OPP, following administration of doses as high as 12 500 ppm, and found no evidence of OPP–DNA adducts by ^{32}P-postlabelling techniques (Cohen et al., 1997).

Extrapolation to humans

In extrapolating findings in rodents to humans, an evaluation is required of both the effect of dose and the effect of species extrapolation (Cohen & Ellwein, 1990, 1991, 1992; Cohen, 1995a). As described above, the toxicity of sodium salts is a high-dose phenomenon; formation of the urinary precipitate, cytotoxicity, increased proliferation and tumorigenicity are all dependent on dietary levels of sodium saccharin or sodium ascorbate greater than 1%. This is not too surprising given the fact that all of the sodium salts listed in Table 1 except saccharin are natural compounds which are normal components of the diet and/or are formed during intermediary metabolism. Some are essential ingredients of the human diet, such as ascorbate, phosphate and chloride. Based on mechanistic considerations, the effect of the sodium salts appears to be a rat-specific phenomenon, with the effect being greater in males than in

females. The lack of an effect in mice is due to the significantly lower urinary concentrations of calcium, phosphate and possibly magnesium. With respect to primates, both non-human and human, the major differences in the urine compared to rats are in urinary protein concentrations and osmolality (Takayama et al., 1998). Urinary protein concentration is 100–1000 times higher in rodents than in healthy humans, although it can reach much higher concentrations in patients with the nephrotic syndrome, levels approaching those seen in rats. No protein qualitatively or quantitatively similar to α_{2u}-globulin or MUP occurs in primates (Olson et al., 1990; Hard, 1995). At the urinary protein concentrations seen in primate urine, including humans, there is no co-chromatographic association of these anions with the urinary proteins (Takayama et al., 1998). In the urine of monkeys administered sodium saccharin at a dose of 25 mg/kg bw, we found no evidence of formation of the urinary precipitate (Takayama et al., 1998). Preliminary investigations in humans have also failed to show the formation of this precipitate following administration of sodium saccharin.

In addition to differences in urinary protein concentration, the overall density of the urine in rodents is significantly higher than that in humans (Cohen, 1995b). The usual urinary osmolality in rodents is between 1400 and 2000 mosmol/kg and can reach higher levels. In contrast, humans generally have urinary osmolality of 50–500 mosmol/kg and, theoretically, it has been estimated that it cannot be higher than approximately 1200 mosmol/kg in humans.

Thus, on a purely mechanistic basis, it is expected that primates would not be responsive to the cytotoxic, proliferative or tumorigenic effects of the sodium salts, even at extremely high doses.

A recently completed study involving administration to monkeys of sodium saccharin in the diet at levels of 25 mg/kg bw for 18–23 years showed no cytotoxic or proliferative effect on the urothelium in males or females (Takayama et al., 1998). Similarly, an epidemiological evaluation of the proliferative response in humans ingesting artificial sweeteners failed to show an effect on bladder epithelial proliferation (Auerbach & Garfinkel, 1989).

In addition, there have been many epidemiological evaluations of sodium saccharin in humans and these have failed to demonstrate any significant increased incidence of bladder cancer (Elcock & Morgan, 1993). Thus, based on the epidemiology of tumorigenic or proliferative effects, extensive investigations in other species and an understanding of the mechanisms involved, the urothelial carcinogenicity of sodium salts is a rat-specific high-dose phenomenon. Therefore, there appears to be no carcinogenic hazard associated with human consumption of these sodium salts, despite frequent and commonly high levels of ingestion, especially of those that are naturally occurring.

References

Anderson, R.L. (1988) A hypothesis of the mechanism of urinary bladder tumorigenesis in rats ingesting sodium saccharin. *Food Chem. Toxicol.*, 26, 637–644

Arnold, D.L. & Boyes, B.G. (1989) The toxicological effects of saccharin in short-term genotoxicity assays. *Mutat. Res.*, 221, 69–132

Arnold, D.L., Moodie, C.A., Grice, H.C., Charbonneau, S.M., Stavric, B., Collins, B.T., McGuire, P.F., Zawidzka, Z.Z. & Munro, I.C. (1980) Long-term toxicity of ortho-toluenesulfonamide and sodium saccharin in the rat. *Toxicol. Appl. Pharmacol.*, 52, 113–152

Arnold, D.L., Krewski, D. & Munro, I.C. (1983) Saccharin: a toxicological and historical perspective. *Toxicology*, 27, 179–256

Arnold, L.L., Anderson, T., Cano, M., St. John, M., Mattson, B., Wehner, J. & Cohen, S.M. (1995) A comparison of urinary chemistry changes in male and female rats and mice treated with sodium saccharin (Abstract). *Toxicologist*, 15, 201

Ashby, J. & Ishidate, M., Jr (1986) Clastogenicity *in vitro* of the Na, K, Ca, and Mg salts of saccharin; and of magnesium chloride; consideration of significance. *Mutat. Res.*, 163, 63–73

Auerbach, O. & Garfinkel, L. (1989) Histologic changes in the urinary bladder in relation to cigarette smoking and use of artificial sweeteners. *Cancer*, 64, 983–987

Ball, L.M., Williams, R.T & Renwick, A.G. (1978) The fate of saccharin impurities. The excretion and metabolism of [14C]toluene-4-sulphonamide and 4-sulphamoyl[14C]-benzoic acid in the rat. *Xenobiotica*, 8, 183–190

Bryan, G.T., Erturk, E. & Yoshida, O. (1970) Production of urinary bladder carcinomas in mice by sodium saccharin. *Science*, 168, 1238–1240

Clayson, D.B., Fishbein, L. & Cohen, S.M. (1995) Effects of stones and other physical factors on the induction of rodent bladder cancer. *Food Chem. Toxicol.*, 33, 771–784

Cohen, S.M. (1995a) Role of cell proliferation in regenerative and neoplastic disease. *Toxicol. Lett.*, 82/83, 15–21

Cohen, S.M. (1995b) The role of urinary physiology and chemistry in bladder carcinogenesis. *Food Chem. Toxicol.*, 33, 715–730

Cohen, S.M. & Ellwein, L.B. (1990) Cell proliferation in carcinogenesis. *Science*, 249, 1007–1011

Cohen, S.M. & Ellwein, L.B. (1991) Genetic errors, cell proliferation, and carcinogenesis. *Cancer Res.*, 51, 6493–6505

Cohen, S.M. & Ellwein, L.B. (1992) Risk assessment based on high-dose animal exposure experiments. *Chem. Res. Toxicol.*, 5, 742–748

Cohen, S.M., Arai, M., Jacobs, J.B. & Friedell, G.H. (1979) Promoting effect of saccharin and DL-tryptophan in urinary bladder carcinogenesis. *Cancer Res.*, 39, 1207–1217

Cohen, S.M., Murasaki, G., Fukushima, S. & Greenfield, R.E. (1982) Effect of regenerative hyperplasia on the urinary bladder: carcinogenicity of sodium saccharin and N-[4-(5-nitro-2-furyl)-2-thiazolyl]formamide. *Cancer Res.*, 42, 65–71

Cohen, S.M., Cano, M., Sakata, T. & Johansson, S.L. (1988) Ultrastructural characteristics of the fetal and neonatal rat urinary bladder. *Scanning Microscopy*, 2, 2091–2104

Cohen, S.M., Fisher, M.J., Sakata, T., Cano, M., Schoenig, G.P., Chappel, C.I. & Garland, E.M. (1990) Comparative analysis of the proliferative response of the rat urinary bladder to sodium saccharin by light and scanning electron microscopy and autoradiography. *Scanning Microscopy*, 4, 135–142

Cohen, S.M., Ellwein, L.B., Okamura, T., Masui, T., Johansson, S.L., Smith, R.A., Wehner, J.M., Khachab, M., Chappel, C.I., Schoenig, G.P., Emerson, J.L. & Garland, E.M. (1991a) Comparative bladder tumor promoting activity of sodium saccharin, sodium ascorbate, related acids and calcium salts in rats. *Cancer Res.*, 51, 1766–1777

Cohen, S.M., Cano, M., Earl, R.A., Carson, S.D. & Garland, E.M. (1991b) A proposed role for silicates and protein in the proliferative effects of saccharin on the male rat urothelium. *Carcinogenesis*, 12, 1551–1555

Cohen, S.M., Cano, M., Johnson, L.S., St. John, M.K., Asamoto, M., Garland, E.M., Thyssen, J.H., Sangha, G.K. & van Goethem, D.L. (1994) Mitogenic effects of propoxur on male rat bladder urothelium. *Carcinogenesis*, 15, 2593–2597

Cohen, S.M., Garland, E.M., Cano, M., St. John, M.K., Khachab, M. & Arnold, L.L. (1995a) Effects of sodium ascorbate, sodium saccharin and ammonium chloride on the male rat urinary bladder. *Carcinogenesis*, **16**, 2743–2750

Cohen, S.M., Cano, M., Garland, E.M., St. John, M. & Arnold, L.L. (1995b) Urinary and urothelial effects of sodium salts in male rats. *Carcinogenesis*, **16**, 343–348

Cohen, S.M., Cano, M., St. John, M.K., Garland, E.M., Khachab, M. & Ellwein, L.B. (1995c) Effect of sodium saccharin on the neonatal rat bladder. *Scanning Microscopy*, **9**, 137–148

Cohen, S.M., Mann, A., Lear, C.L., Mattson, B. & Arnold, L.L. (1995d) Toxicity of calcium phosphate precipitate and urinary amorphous precipitate toward rat bladder epithelial cells (Abstract). *Proc. Am. Assoc. Cancer Res.*, **36**, 178

Cohen, S.M., Arnold, L.L., St. John, M.K., Cano, M., Smith, R.A., Sangha, G. & Christenson, R. (1997) Urothelial proliferation induced by high dose of o-phenylphenol (OPP) in male rats (Abstract). *Proc. Am. Assoc. Cancer Res.*, **38**, 465

DeSesso, I.M. (1989) Confounding factors in direct bladder exposure studies. *Comments Toxicol.*, **3**, 317–334

DeGroot, A.P., Feron, V.J. & Immel, H.R. (1988) Induction of hyperplasia in the bladder epithelium of rats by a dietary excess of acid or base: implications for toxicity/carcinogenicity testing. *Food Chem. Toxicol.*, **26**, 425–434

Elcock, M. & Morgan, R.W. (1993) Update on artificial sweeteners and bladder cancer. *Reg. Toxicol. Pharmacol.*, **17**, 35–43

Ellwein, L.B. & Cohen, S.M. (1988) A cellular dynamics model of experimental bladder cancer: analysis of the effect of sodium saccharin in the rat. *Risk Anal.*, **8**, 215–221

Ellwein, L.B. & Cohen, S.M. (1990) The health risks of saccharin revisited. *Crit. Rev. Toxicol.*, **20**, 311–326

Emerick, R.J., Kugel, E.E. & Wallace, V. (1963) Urinary excretion of silica and the production of siliceous urinary calculi in rats. *Am. J. Vet. Res.*, **24**, 610–613

Fisher, M.J., Sakata, T., Tibbels, T.S., Smith, R.A., Patil, K., Khachab, M., Johansson, S.L. & Cohen, S.M. (1989) Effect of sodium saccharin and calcium saccharin on urinary parameters in rats fed Prolab 3200 or AIN-76 diet. *Food Chem. Toxicol.*, **27**, 1–9

Frederick, C.B., Dooley, K.L., Kodell, R.L., Sheldon, W.G. & Kadlubar, F.F. (1989) The effect of lifetime sodium saccharin dosing on mice initiated with the carcinogen 2-acetylaminofluorene. *Fundam. Appl. Toxicol.*, **12**, 346–357

Fujii, T., Nakamura, K. & Hiraga, K. (1987) Effects of pH on the carcinogenicity of o-phenylphenol and sodium o-phenylphenate in the rat urinary bladder. *Food Chem. Toxicol.*, **25**, 359–362

Fukushima, S. & Cohen, S.M. (1980) Saccharin-induced hyperplasia of the rat urinary bladder. *Cancer Res.*, **40**, 734–736

Fukushima, S., Arai, M., Nakanowatari, J., Hibino, T., Okuda, M. & Ito, N. (1983a) Differences in susceptibility to sodium saccharin among various strains of rats and other animal species. *Gann (Jpn. J. Cancer Res.)*, **74**, 8–20

Fukushima S., Imaida, K., Sakata, T., Okamura, T., Shibata, M. & Ito, N. (1983b) Promoting effects of sodium L-ascorbate on two-stage urinary bladder carcinogenesis in rats. *Cancer Res.*, **43**, 4454–4457

Fukushima, S., Hagiwara, A., Ogiso, T., Shibata, M. & Ito, N. (1983c) Promoting effects of various chemicals in rat urinary bladder carcinogenesis initiated by N-nitroso-n-butyl-(4-hydroxybutyl)amine. *Food Chem Toxicol.*, **21**, 59–68

Fukushima, S., Kurata, Y., Shibata, M.-A., Ikawa, E. & Ito, N. (1984) Promotion by ascorbic acid, sodium erythorbate and ethoxyquin of neoplastic lesions in rats initiated with N-butyl-N-(4-hydroxybutyl)nitrosamine. *Cancer Lett.*, **23**, 29–37

Fukushima, S., Thamavit, S., Kurata, W. & Ito, N. (1986) Sodium citrate: a promoter of bladder carcinogenesis. *Jpn. J. Cancer Res.*, **77**, 1–4

Fukushima, S., Kurata, Y., Hasegawa, R., Asamoto, M., Shibata, M.A. & Tamano, S. (1991) L-Ascorbic acid amplification of bladder carcinogenesis promotion by K_2CO_3. *Cancer Res.*, **51**, 2548–2551

Garland, E.M., Sakata, T., Fisher, M.J., Masui, T. & Cohen, S.M. (1989) Influences of diet and strain on the proliferative effect on the rat urinary bladder induced by sodium saccharin. *Cancer Res.*, **49**, 3789–3794

Garland, E.M., St. John, M., Asamoto, M., Eklund, S.H., Mattson, B.J., Johnson, L.S., Cano, M. & Cohen, S.M. (1994a) A comparison of the effects of sodium saccharin in NBR rats and in intact and castrated male F344 rats. *Cancer Lett.*, **78**, 99–107

Garland, M.D., Mattson, B.J., Cano, M., St. John, M. & Cohen, S.M. (1994b) A comparison of the urinary and bladder changes produced by sodium saccharin treatment in male and female F344 rats (Abstract). *Toxicologist*, **14**, 129

Hard, G.C. (1995) Species comparison of the content and composition of urinary proteins. *Food Chem. Toxicol.*, **33**, 731–746

Hasegawa, R. & Cohen, S.M. (1986) The effect of different salts of saccharin on the rat urinary bladder. *Cancer Lett.*, 30, 261–268

Hasegawa, R., Greenfield, R.E., Murasaki, G., Suzuki, T. & Cohen, S.M. (1985) Initiation of urinary bladder carcinogenesis in rats by freeze ulceration with sodium saccharin promotion. *Cancer Res.*, 45, 1469–1473

Hicks, R.M., Wakefield, J.S. & Chowaniec, J. (1973) Co-carcinogenic action of saccharin in the chemical induction of bladder cancer. *Nature*, 243, 347–349

Hiraga, K. & Fujii, T. (1984) Induction of tumors of the urinary bladder in F344 rats by dietary administration of o-phenylphenol. *Food Chem. Toxicol.*, 22, 865–870

Homma, Y., Kondo, Y., Kakizoe, T., Aso, Y. & Nagase, S. (1991) Lack of bladder carcinogenicity of dietary sodium saccharin in analbuminaemic rats, which are highly susceptible to N-nitroso-n-butyl-(4-hydroxybutyl)amine. *Food Chem. Toxicol.*, 29, 373–376

Kitamura, M., Konishi, N., Kitahori, Y., Fukushima, Y., Yoshioka, N. & Hiasa, Y. (1996) Promoting effect of monosodium aspartate, but not glycine, on renal pelvis and urinary bladder carcinogenesis in rat induced by N-butyl-N-(4-hydroxybutyl)nitrosamine. *Toxicol. Pathol.*, 24, 573–579

Lina, B.A.R., Hollanders, V.M.H. & Kuijpers, M.H.M. (1994) The role of alkalizing and neutral potassium salts in urinary bladder carcinogenesis in rats. *Carcinogenesis*, 15, 523–527

Lutz, W.K. & Schlatter, C. (1977) Saccharin does not bind to DNA of liver or bladder in the rat. *Chem.-Biol. Interact.*, 19, 253–257

Mori, S., Kurata, Y., Takeuchi, Y., Toyama, M., Makino, S. & Fukushima, S. (1987) Influences of strain and diet on the promoting effects of sodium L-ascorbate in two stage urinary bladder carcinogenesis in rats. *Cancer Res.*, 47, 3492–3495

Murai, T., Mori, S., Honsono, M., Takashima, A., Machino, S., Oohara, T., Yamashita, H., Makino, S., Matsuka, T., Wanibuchi, H. & Fukushima, S. (1997) Strain differences in sensitivity to the promoting effect of sodium-L-ascorbate in a two-stage rat urinary bladder carcinogenesis model. *Jpn. J. Cancer Res.*, 88, 245–253

Murasaki, G. & Cohen, S.M. (1983) Effect of sodium saccharin on urinary bladder epithelial regenerative hyperplasia following freeze ulceration. *Cancer Res.*, 43, 182–187

Nakanishi, K., Hirose, M., Ogiso, T., Hasegawa, R., Arai, M. & Ito, N. (1980a) Effects of sodium saccharin and caffeine on the urinary bladder of rats treated with N-butyl-N-(4-hydroxybutyl)nitrosamine. *Gann (Jpn. J. Cancer Res.)*, 71, 490–500

Nakanishi, K., Hagiwara, A., Shibata, M., Imaida, K., Tatematsu, M. & Ito, N. (1980b) Dose response of saccharin in induction of urinary bladder hyperplasias in Fischer 344 rats pretreated with N-butyl-N-(4-hydroxybutyl)nitrosamine. *J. Natl Cancer Inst.*, 65, 1005–1010

Okamura, T., Garland, E.M., Masui, T., Sakata, T., St. John, M. & Cohen, S.M. (1991) Lack of bladder tumor promoting activity in rats fed sodium saccharin in AIN-76A diet. *Cancer Res.*, 51, 1778–1782

Olson, M.J., Johnson, J.T. & Reidy, C.A. (1990) A comparison of male rat and human urinary proteins; implications for human resistance to hyaline droplet nephropathy. *Toxicol. Appl. Pharmacol.*, 102, 524–536

Otoshi, T., Iwata, H., Yamamoto, S., Murai, T., Yamaguchi, S., Matsui-Yuasa, I., Otani, S. & Fukushima, S. (1993) Severity of promotion by sodium salts of succinic acid in rat urinary bladder carcinogenesis correlates with sodium ion concentration under conditions of equal urinary pH. *Carcinogenesis*, 14, 2277–2281

Owen, G., Cherry, C.P., Prentice, D.E. & Worden, A.N. (1978) The feeding of diets containing up to 4% monosodium glutamate to rats for 2 years. *Toxicol. Lett.*, 1, 221–226

Pathak, D.N. & Roy, D. (1992) Examination of microsomal cytochrome P450 catalyzed *in vitro* activation of o-phenylphenol DNA binding metabolite(s) by ^{32}P-postlabeling technique. *Carcinogenesis*, 13, 1593–1597

Renwick, A.G. (1993) A data-derived safety (uncertainty) factor for the intense sweetener, saccharin. *Food Add. Contam.*, 10, 337–350

Schoenig, G.P. & Anderson, R.L. (1985) The effects of high dietary levels of sodium saccharin on mineral and water balance and related parameters in rats. *Food Chem. Toxicol.*, 23, 465–474

Schoenig, G.P., Goldenthal, E.I., Geil, R.G., Frith, C.H., Richter, W.R. & Carlborg, F.W. (1985) Evaluation of the dose response and *in utero* exposure to saccharin in the rat. *Food Chem. Toxicol.*, 23, 475–490

Shibata, M.A., Kagawa, M., Kawabe, M., Hagiwara, A. & Fukushima, S. (1991) Comparative promoting activities of phosphate salts on rat two-stage bladder carcinogenesis under conditions of equivalent urinary Na+ or K+ levels. *Teratog. Carcinog. Mutag.*, 11, 305–316

Shioya, S., Nagami-Oguihara, R., Oguihara, S., Kimura, T., Imaida, K. & Fukushima, S. (1994) Roles of bladder distension, urinary pH and urinary sodium ion concentration in cell proliferation of urinary bladder epithelium in rats ingesting sodium salts. *Food Chem. Toxicol.*, 32, 165–171

Sweatman, T.W., Renwick, A.G. & Burgess, C.D. (1981) The pharmacokinetics of saccharin in man. *Xenobiotica*, **11**, 531–540

Takayama, S., Sieber, S.M., Adamson, R.H., Thorgeirsson, U.P., Dalgard, D.W., Arnold, L.L., Cano, M., Eklund, S. & Cohen, S.M. (1998) Lack of effect of sodium saccharin on monkey urine and urinary bladder in a long-term study. *J. Natl Cancer Inst.*, **90**, 19–25

Tamano, S., Asakawa, E., Boomyaphiphat, P., Masui, T. & Fukushima, S. (1993) Lack of promotion of *N*-butyl-*N*-(4-hydroxybutyl)nitrosamine-initiated urinary bladder carcinogenesis in mice by rat cancer promoters. *Teratog. Carcinog. Mutag.*, **13**, 89–96

Ushiyama, K., Nagai, F., Nakagawa, A. & Kano, I. (1992) DNA adduct formation by o-phenylphenol metabolite *in vivo* and *in vitro*. *Carcinogenesis*, **13**, 1469–1473

US National Toxicology Program (1989) *NTP Technical Report on the Toxicology and Carcinogenesis Studies of Furosemide (CAS No. 5431-9)* (NTP Technical Report Series, No. 356), U.S. Department of Health and Human Services, Public Health Service, National Institutes of Health, Research Triangle Park, NC

Uwagawa, S., Saito, K., Okuno, Y., Kawasaki, H., Yoshitake, A., Yamada, H. & Fukushima, S. (1994) Lack of induction of epithelial cell proliferation by sodium saccharin and sodium L-ascorbate in the urinary bladder of NCI-black-Reiter (NBR) male rats. *Toxicol. Appl. Pharmacol.*, **127**, 182–186

Wahle, B.S., Christenson, W.R., Lake, S.G., Elcock, L.E., Moore, K.D., Sangha, G.K. & Thyssen, J.H. (1997) Technical grade ortho-phenylphenol: a combined chronic toxicity/oncogenicity testing study in the rat. *The Toxicologist, Fundam. Appl. Toxicol.*, **36** (Suppl. 1), Abstract 1733, p. 341

Wandzilak, T.R., D'Andre, S.D., Davis, P.A. & Williams, H.E. (1994) Effect of high dose vitamin C on urinary oxalate levels. *J. Urol.*, **151**, 834–837

West, R. W. & Jackson, D.C. (1981) Saccharin effects on the urinary physiology and urothelium of the rat when administered in diet or drinking water. *Toxicol. Lett.*, **7**, 409–416

West, R.W., Sheldon, W.G., Gaylor, D.W., Haskin, M.G., Delongchamp, R.R. & Kadlubar, F.F. (1986) The effects of saccharin on the development of neoplastic lesions initiated with *N*-methyl-*N*-nitrosourea in the rat urothelium. *Fundam. Appl. Toxicol.*, **7**, 585–600

Williamson, D.S., Nagel, D.L., Markin, R.S. & Cohen, S.M. (1987) Effect of pH and ions on the electronic structure of saccharin. *Food Chem. Toxicol.*, **25**, 211–218

Zukowski, K., Debiec-Rychter, M., Van Goethem, D.L., Sangha, G.K., Thyssen, J.H. & Wang, C.Y. (1994) A UDS system for differentiating genotoxic and nongenotoxic bladder carcinogenesis in the rat. *Proc. Am. Assoc. Cancer Res.*, **35**, 684

Corresponding author

S.M. Cohen

University of Nebraska Medical Center, Department of Pathology and Microbiology, 600 South 42nd Street, Omaha, Nebraska 68198-3135, USA

Species Differences in Thyroid, Kidney and Urinary Bladder Carcinogenesis
C.C. Capen, E. Dybing, J.M. Rice and J.D. Wilbourn, eds
IARC Scientific Publications No. 147
International Agency for Research on Cancer, Lyon, 1999

Appendix 1

Agents that induce epithelial neoplasms of the urinary bladder, renal cortex and thyroid follicular lining in experimental animals and humans:

Summary of data from IARC Monographs Volumes 1-69

J. D. Wilbourn, C. Partensky and J. M. Rice

Introduction

The *IARC Monographs on the Evaluation of Carcinogenic Risks to Humans* are critical summaries of the published scientific evidence for cancer in humans as a result of exposures to selected environmental agents and for carcinogenicity of those agents to animals in bioassays. Other data relevant to carcinogenic hazard identification are also critically reviewed and summarized. Agents are chosen for evaluation on the basis of two criteria: there must be evidence or suspicion of carcinogenicity in humans or in experimental animals, and there must be human exposure. A total of 836 chemicals and mixtures, biological and physical agents, and lifestyle and occupational exposures have been evaluated in volumes 1 to 69 of the *Monographs*. Each *Monograph* concludes with an evaluation, which is the consensus or majority opinion of invited scientific experts as to the strength of the total evidence for carcinogenicity to humans. Criteria for strength of the evidence for carcinogenicity in humans and in animals (*sufficient, limited, inadequate,* or *evidence suggesting lack of carcinogenicity*), and definitions of the groups (1, 2A, 2B, 3, and 4) that comprise the overall evaluations, are summarized in Tables 1 and 2, respectively. These criteria and definitions are published in the Preamble to the *Monographs* which is printed at the beginning of each volume in the series. The Preamble is revised from time to time, and in 1992 provision was made for inclusion of evidence relating to mechanisms of carcinogenicity in reaching final, overall

evaluations of carcinogenic risk to humans (IARC, 1992).

It must be stressed that the IARC criteria for *sufficient* evidence of carcinogenicity to animals place great emphasis on reproducibility. Evidence for carcinogenicity of any agent that is positive in only a single bioassay, no matter how well conducted, is rarely considered more than *limited* by IARC working groups. Those agents for which evidence of carcinogenicity is *sufficient* in humans or in animals or both, or for which there is *limited* evidence in humans and *sufficient* evidence in animals, and which are associated causally with epithelial tumours of urinary bladder, renal cortex, or thyroid follicular epithelium are listed in Tables 3, 4, and 5, respectively.

These tables were prepared by first utilizing an electronic data base to identify agents associated with tumours at one or more of the selected organ sites, and then cross-checking with the *Monographs* entries for each agent. Where human data are inadequate, only agents that met the criterion of *sufficient* evidence for carcinogenicity in animals were included in the tables. In effect, that restricts the agents included in Tables 3-5 to those in Groups 1, 2A, and 2B of the IARC classification system (Table 2). The resulting tables indicate how often tumours of a given organ site have contributed to IARC evaluations; whether there is or is not concordance between cancer sites in humans and animals for a given agent; and whether more than one organ site played a role in the evaluation of evidence of carcinogenicity. A number of agents

Table 1. Criteria for carcinogenic hazard evaluation in the IARC Monographs on the Evaluation of Carcinogenic Risks to Humans

Degrees of evidence for carcinogenicity in humans

Sufficient:
A positive relation has been observed between the exposure and human cancer in studies in which chance, bias and confounding can be ruled out with reasonable confidence.

Limited:
A positive relation has been observed for which a causal interpretation is credible, but chance, bias or confounding could not be ruled out with reasonable confidence.

Inadequate:
Available studies are of insufficient quality, consistency or statistical power to permit a conclusion regarding the presence or absence of a causal association; or no data on cancer in humans are available.

Evidence suggesting lack of carcinogenicity:
Several adequate studies covering the full range of human exposures exist that are mutually consistent in not showing a positive association between the agent and any cancer studied, at any level of exposure (inevitably limited to the cancer sites, conditions and levels of exposure and length of observation covered by the available studies).

Degrees of evidence for carcinogenicity in experimental animals

Sufficient:
A causal relationship has been established between the agent and an increased incidence of malignant neoplasms or of an appropriate combination of benign and malignant neoplasms in (a) two or more species of animals or (b) in two or more independent studies in one species carried out at different times or in different laboratories or under different protocols. Exceptionally, a single study in one species may provide sufficient evidence when malignant neoplasms occur to an unusual degree with regard to incidence, site, type of tumour or age at onset.

Limited:
Data suggest a carcinogenic effect but are limited for making a definitive evaluation because (a) evidence is restricted to a single experiment; (b) there are unresolved questions regarding the adequacy of the design, conduct, or interpretation of the study; or (c) the agent increases the incidence only of benign neoplasms or of lesions of uncertain neoplastic potential, or of certain neoplasms which may occur spontaneously in high incidences in certain strains.

Inadequate:
The studies cannot be interpreted as showing either presence or absence of a carcinogenic effect because of major qualitative or quantitative limitations; or no data in experimental animals are available.

Evidence suggesting lack of carcinogenicity:
Adequate studies involving at least two species are available which show that, within the limits of the tests used, the agent or mixture is not carcinogenic. Such a conclusion is inevitably limited to the species, tumour sites and levels of exposure studied.

Table 2. Overall evaluations[a] of carcinogenicity in the IARC Monographs on the Evaluation of Carcinogenic Risk to Humans	
Group 1 Carcinogenic to humans	*Sufficient evidence* of cancer in humans
Group 2A Probably carcinogenic to humans	*Limited evidence* of cancer in humans; *Sufficient evidence* of carcinogenicity in experimental animals
Group 2B Possibly carcinogenic to humans	*Inadequate evidence* of cancer in humans; *Sufficient evidence* of carcinogenicity in experimental animals
Group 3 Not classifiable as to carcinogenicity to humans	*Inadequate evidence* of cancer in humans; Less than *sufficient evidence* of carcinogenicity in experimental animals

Exceptionally, agents for which evidence of carcinogenicity is *inadequate* in humans but *sufficient* in experimental animals may be placed in this category when there is strong evidence that the mechanism of carcinogenicity in experimental animals does not operate in humans.

Group 4 Probably not carcinogenic to humans	Evidence in both humans and experimental animals *suggesting lack of carcinogenicity*

[a] Overall evaluations of 2A, 2B, and 3 may be adjusted upward or downward on the basis of other relevant data including mechanisms of carcinogenicity. The definitions provided for Groups 1, 2A, 2B, 3 and 4 are the ones most generally used, but additional combinations of human, animal, and mechanistic evidence may also serve to place an agent in Groups 1, 2A, 2B, or 3; for details, see the Preamble to the *IARC Monographs*.

were carcinogenic at a chosen organ site in only one sex of a given species; this information is not captured in the tables. For ease of comparison among the tables, the same set of footnotes is used in all three, although some are not applicable throughout.

A number of chemicals that did not meet the criteria for listing in Tables 3-5 are nonetheless of considerable interest in the context of this volume. These are discussed individually in the text.

Epithelial Neoplasms of the Urinary Bladder

Thirty-eight agents that are carcinogenic to the urinary bladder by systemic exposure in humans, animals, or both are summarized in Table 3. These

comprise 5% of all agents evaluated in *IARC Monographs* Volumes 1-69. Substances that are carcinogenic to the urinary bladder of rats or mice only when incorporated into pellets of inert material and implanted into the lumen of the bladder, such as some of the polynuclear aromatic hydrocarbons and their heterocyclic analogues, are not included in Table 3. For fifteen of these 38 agents, there is *limited* or *sufficient* evidence of carcinogenicity in humans at one or more organ sites including the urinary bladder. Six of the 38 agents are complex mixtures, and for 5 of these evidence for carcinogenicity to the urinary bladder is only from epidemiological studies of exposed humans: diesel engine exhaust, coal tars and coal tar pitches, untreated or mildly treated mineral

Table 3. Some agents (chemicals, mixtures and parasites) producing urinary bladder neoplasms (IARC Monographs. Volumes 1–69)

Agent	Vol., page	Suppl. 7, page	Evidence of carcinogenicity H	A	Group	Human	Mouse	Rat	Hamster	Dog	Other
ortho-Aminoazotoluene	8, 61	56	I	S	2B		Liver^k Lung Blood vessels^j	Liver^k Bile duct Urinary bladder^o	Liver^k Bile duct Urinary bladder^p Mammary gland	Bile duct^d Urinary bladder^c	Rabbit: Urinary bladder^o
4-Aminobiphenyl	1, 74	91	S	S	1	Urinary bladder^c	Urinary bladder^{c,w} Liver^k Blood vessels^j	Mammary gland Intestine		Urinary bladder^p	Rabbit: Urinary bladder^{c,o}
Analgesic mixtures containing phenacetin	24, 135	310	S	L	1	Urinary bladder^c Kidney/pelvis^c		Liver^z Kidney/pelvis^x Kidney/cortex^x			
ortho-Anisidine	27, 63	57	I	S	2B		Urinary bladder^w	Urinary bladder^w Kidney/pelvis^w Thyroid^h			
Arsenic and arsenic compounds	23, 39	100	S	L	1	Skin Liver^j Lung Urinary bladder^x	Lung		Lung		
Benzidine	29, 149	123	S	S	1	Urinary bladder^c	Liver^k	Liver^k Bile duct^d Mammary gland Zymbal gland Large intestine	Liver^k Bile duct^d	Urinary bladder^c	
N,N-Bis(2-chloroethyl)-2-naphthylamine (Chlornaphazine)	4, 119	130	S	L	1	Urinary bladder^c	Lung	Connective tissue^u			

Table 3. Some agents (chemicals, mixtures and parasites) producing urinary bladder neoplasms (IARC Monographs, Volumes 1–69)

| Agent | Vol., page | Suppl. 7, page | Evidence of carcinogenicity | | | Target organs | | | | | |
			H	A	Group	Human	Mouse	Rat	Hamster	Dog	Other
Bracken fern	*40, 47*	135		S	2B		Lung Small intestine Haematopoietic system[m]	Small intestine **Urinary bladder**[c] Mammary gland[b]			*Guinea-pig:* Small intestine **Urinary bladder**[c]
4-Chloro-*ortho*-phenylenediamine	27, 81	60	I	S	2B		Liver[k]	**Urinary bladder**[w]			
para-Chloro-*ortho*-toluidine	*48, 123*	60	L	S	2A	**Urinary bladder**[c]	Spleen[j] Connective tissue[j]				
Citrus Red No. 2	*8, 101*	60	I	S	2B		**Urinary bladder**[c,o] Lung Lymphoid system[n]	**Urinary bladder**[o]			
Coal-tar pitches	35, 83	174	S	S	1	**Urinary bladder**[x] Skin Lung	Skin				*Rabbit:* Skin
Coal tars	35, 83	175	S	S	1	Skin Lung **Urinary bladder**[x] Haemato-poietic system[m]	Skin				
para-Cresidine	27, 92	61	I	S	2B		**Urinary bladder**[v,w] Liver[k]	**Urinary bladder**[p] Liver[k] Bile duct[d]			
Cyclophosphamide	26, 165	182	S	S	1	**Urinary bladder**[x] Haemato-poietic system[m]	Lung Mammary gland Lymphoid system[n]	**Urinary bladder**[o, w] Blood vessels[j] Mammary gland Haematopoietic system[m]			

Table 3. Some agents (chemicals, mixtures and parasites) producing urinary bladder neoplasms (IARC Monographs. Volumes 1–69)

Agent	Vol, page	Suppl. 7, page	Evidence of carcinogenicity			Target organs					
			H	A	Group	Human	Mouse	Rat	Hamster	Dog	Other
3,3'-Dichlorobenzidine	29, 239	193	I	S	2B		Liver^z Haematopoietic system^m	Mammary gland Zymbal gland Haematopoietic system^m	**Urinary bladder**^{w}	**Urinary bladder**^{w} Liver	
1,3-Dichloropropene (technical grade, 1% epichlorohydrin)	41, 113	195	I	S	2B		**Urinary bladder**^{w} Lung Forestomach	Liver^z Forestomach			
Diesel engine exhaust	46, 41		L	S	2A	Lung **Urinary bladder**^{c}	Lung Skin	Lung			
3,3'-Dimethoxy-benzidine (ortho-Dianisidine)	4, 41	198	I	S	2B			**Urinary bladder**^{o} Zymbal gland Intestine Skin	Fore-stomach		
para-Dimethylamino-azobenzene	8, 125	62	I	S	2B		Liver Connective tissue	Liver Skin			
Direct Black 38 (technical grade)	29, 295	125	I	S	2A		Liver^k Mammary gland	Liver^k **Urinary bladder**^{c} Large intestine		**Urinary bladder**^{o}	
Disperse Blue 1	48, 139		I	S	2B		Lung Liver^k	**Urinary bladder**^{l,p,v} **			
2-(2-Formyl-hydrazino)-4-(5-nitro-2-furyl)thiazole	7, 151	63	I	S	2B		Forestomach Lung Haematopoietic system^m	Liver^k Mammary gland Kidney/cortex^b Kidney/pelvis^w Intestine	Fore-stomach^o **Urinary bladder**^{w}		

Table 3. Some agents (chemicals, mixtures and parasites) producing urinary bladder neoplasms (IARC Monographs. Volumes 1–69)

Agent	Vol., page	Suppl. 7, page	Evidence of carcinogenicity			Target organs					
			H	A	Group	Human	Mouse	Rat	Hamster	Dog	Other
4,4'-Methylene bis(2-chloroaniline) (MOCA)	57, 271		I	S	2A		Liver[k] Blood vessels[j]	Liver[k] Lung Mammary gland Zymbal gland Blood vessels[j]		Urinary bladder[w]	
N-Methyl-N-nitroso-urea	17, 227	66	I	S	2A		Many sites	Many sites Urinary bladder[o,w]	Many sites	Many sites	
Mineral oils (untreated or mildly treated)	33, 87	252	S	S	1	Skin GI tract Urinary bladder[c]	Skin				
2-Naphthylamine	4, 97	261	S	S	1	Urinary bladder[c]	Liver Lung	Urinary bladder[c]	Urinary bladder[c]	Urinary bladder[c,o]	Monkey: Urinary bladder[w]
Niridazole	13, 123	67	I	S	2B		Forestomach Lung Mammary gland Ovary Urinary bladder[c,w,l]	Urinary bladder[c]	Fore-stomach Urinary bladder[q]		
Nitrilotriacetic acid and its di- and trisodium salts	48, 181		I	S	2B		Kidney[b]	Urinary bladder[v,w] Kidney/cortex[s] Kidney/pelvis[w]			
2-Nitroanisole	65, 369		I	S	2B		Liver[k]	Haemato-poietic system[m] Urinary bladder[w] Kidney/pelvis[w] Large intestine[c]			

Table 3. Some agents (chemicals, mixtures and parasites) producing urinary bladder neoplasms (IARC Monographs. Volumes 1–69)

Agent	Vol., page	Suppl. 7, page	Evidence of carcinogenicity H	A	Group	Target organs Human	Mouse	Rat	Hamster	Dog	Other
N-[4-(5-Nitro-2-furyl)-2-thiazolyl]-acetamide (NFTA)	7, 185	67	I	S	2B		Haemato-poietic system[m] Forestomach	Mammary gland Kidney/-pelvis[w]	Fore-stomach Urinary bladder[w]		Guinea-pig: Liver Bile ducts[d] Urinary bladder[o,v] Rabbit: Urinary bladder[o,w]
N-Nitrosodi-n-butyl-amine	17, 51	67	I	S	2B		Forestomach Oesophagus Urinary bladder[o,v] Lung Liver	Liver Urinary bladder[c,v,w] Lung Oesophagus	Fore-stomach Lung/-trachea Urinary bladder[c,o,v,w] Nasal cavity		
Phenacetin	24, 135	310	L	S	2A	Kidney/pelvis[x] Urinary bladder[x]	Kidney/-cortex[s]	Kidney/cortex[x] Kidney/pelvis[x] Nasal cavity Urinary bladder[w]			
Ponceau 3R	8, 199	70	I	S	2B			Liver[k] Urinary bladder[c]			
Saccharin and sodium saccharin	22, 111	334	I	S	2B		Urinary bladder[c] Thyroid[b]	Urinary bladder[x]			
Schistosoma haematobium	61, 45		S	L	1	Urinary bladder[c,v]					
Sodium-ortho-phenylphenate	30, 330	392	I	S	2B		Liver	Urinary bladder[o,**] Kidney/pelvis[w]			Monkey: Urinary bladder[p]

Table 3. Some agents (chemicals, mixtures and parasites) producing urinary bladder neoplasms (IARC Monographs. Volumes 1–69)

Agent	Vol., page	Suppl. 7, page	Evidence of carcinogenicity			Target organs					
			H	A	Group	Human	Mouse	Rat	Hamster	Dog	Other
Tobacco smoke	38, 37	359	S	S	1	Lung Urinary bladder[c] Kidney/ pelvis[b] Oral cavity Larynx Pancreas	Skin (condensate)	Lung	Larynx		

[a] Adenoma
[b] Adenocarcinoma
[c] Carcinoma
[d] Cholangioma/cholangiocarcinoma
[e] Fibroadenoma
[f] Fibrosarcoma
[g] Follicular-cell adenoma
[h] Follicular-cell adenoma and carcinoma
[i] Follicular-cell carcinoma
[j] Haemangioma or haemangiosarcoma
[k] Hepatoma and/or hepatocellular carcinoma
[l] Leiomyoma/leiomyosarcoma
[m] Leukaemia
[n] Lymphoma
[o] Papilloma
[p] Papilloma and transitional-cell carcinoma
[q] Papilloma, transitional-cell
[r] Renal tubule-cell adenoma
[s] Renal-tubule cell adenoma and carcinoma
[t] Renal-tubule cell carcinoma
[u] Sarcoma
[v] Squamous-cell carcinoma
[w] Transitional-cell carcinoma
[x] Unspecified
[z] Neoplastic nodule/hepato-cellular adenoma
[*] Bladder implantation in pellets
[**] Bladder calculi

Table 4. Some agents (chemicals and mixtures) producing kidney (renal tubule-cell) neoplasms (IARC Monographs. Volumes 1–69)

Agent	Vol., page	Suppl. 7, page	Evidence of carcinogenicity H	A	Group	Human	Mouse	Rat	Hamster	Dog	Other
Aflatoxins Aflatoxin B1	56, 245		S	S	1	Liver[k]	Lung Liver[k]	Liver[k] Bile duct[d] **Kidney[x]**	Bile duct[d]		Monkey: Bile duct[d] Fish: Liver
Aflatoxin G1				S			Liver **Kidney[b]**				Fish: Liver
Analgesic mixtures containing phenacetin	24, 135	310	S	L	1	Urinary bladder[c] Kidney/pelvis[c]		Liver[z] Kidney/pelvis[x] **Kidney/cortex[x]**			
Benzofuran	63, 431		I	S	2B		Liver[a] Forestomach[o,c] Lung	**Kidney[b]**			
Bromodichloromethane	52, 179		I	S	2B		Liver[k] **Kidney[s]**	Liver[z] **Kidney[s]** Large intestine[b]			
Caffeic acid	56, 115		I	S	2B		Forestomach[o,c] **Kidney[b]** Lung	Forestomach[o,c] **Kidney[b]**			
Captafol	53, 353		I	S	2A		Heart[j] Small intestine[b]	**Kidney[s]** Liver[z]			
Chloroform	20, 401	152	I	S	2B		Liver[k] **Kidney[x]**	Liver[z] **Kidney[s]** Thyroid			
Cycasin	10, 121	61	I	S	2B		Liver Lung Lymphoid system[n]	Liver[k] Bile duct **Kidney[b]** Large intestine[b] Nervous system	Bile duct Liver Intestine		Guinea-pig: Liver[k] Bile duct
Daunomycin	10, 145	61	I	S	2B		Connective tissue[u]	Mammary gland[b] **Kidney[s]**			
para-Dichlorobenzene	29, 215	192	I	S	2B		Liver[k]	**Kidney[b]**			

Table 4. (Contd) Some agents (chemicals and mixtures) producing kidney (renal tubule-cell) neoplasms (IARC Monographs. Volumes 1–69)

Agent	Vol., page	Suppl. 7, page	Evidence of carcinogenicity			Target organs					
			H	A	Group	Human	Mouse	Rat	Hamster	Dog	Other
2,4-Dinitrotoluene	65, 309		I	S	2B		**Kidney**[s]	Skin, Mammary gland[e], Liver[k]			
2-(2-Formylhydrazino)-4-(5-nitro-2-furyl)-thiazole	7, 151	63	I	S	2B		Forestomach, Lung, Haemato-poietic system[m]	Liver[k], Mammary gland, **Kidney/cortex**[/b], **Kidney/pelvis**[w], Intestine	Forestomach[o], Urinary bladder[w]		
Gasoline Unleaded	45, 159		I	L	2B		Liver[k]	**Kidney**[s]			
Hexachlorobenzene	20, 155	219	I	S	2B		Liver	Liver[k], Bile duct, **Kidney**[r]	Liver[a,j], Thyroid[a]		
Lead and lead compounds, inorganic; Lead acetate	23, 325	230	I	S	2B		**Kidney**[a,c]	**Kidney**[a,c], Brain			
Lead phosphate								**Kidney**[a,c]			
Lead subacetate							**Kidney**[a,c]	**Kidney**[a,c], Brain			
Methyl mercury compounds	58, 239		I		2B		**Kidney**[a,b]				
Methyl mercury chloride				S			**Kidney**[a,b]				
Nitrilotriacetic acid and its di- and tri-sodium salts	48, 181		I	S	2B		**Kidney**[b], Urinary bladder[w]	**Kidney/cortex**[s], **Kidney/pelvis**[w], Urinary bladder[v,w]			
Nitrobenzene	65, 381		I	S	2B		Lung, Thyroid[g]	Liver[k], **Kidney**[r], Thyroid[h]			

Table 4. (Contd) Some agents (chemicals and mixtures) producing kidney (renal tubule-cell) neoplasms (IARC Monographs. Volumes 1–69)

Agent	Vol., page	Suppl. 7, page	Evidence of carcinogenicity			Target organs					
			H	A	Group	Human	Mouse	Rat	Hamster	Dog	Other
N-Nitroso-diethanolamine	17, 77	67	I	S	2B			Liver[k] **Kidney**[a]	Lung/trachea Nasal cavity[b]		
N-Nitrosodiethylamine	17, 83	67	I	S	2A		Liver[k,j] Oesophagus Forestomach Lung	Liver[k,j] Bile duct[d] Oesophagus **Kidney**[x]	Lung Liver Nasal cavity Oesophagus Forestomach	Nasal cavity	Guinea-pig, rabbit, pig, monkey: Liver[k]
N-Nitrosodimethyl-amine	17, 125	67	I	S	2A		Liver[k,j] Lung **Kidney**[a,c]	Liver[k,j] Bile duct[d] Lung **Kidney**[a,c] Nasal cavity	Liver[k,j] Bile duct[d] Nasal cavity[b]		Guinea-pig, rabbit: Liver[k] Bile duct[a]
N-Nitrosomorpholine	17, 263	68	I	S	2B		Liver[k] Lung	Liver[k,j] Nasal cavity Lung **Kidney**[c] Bile duct[d]	Lung Nasal cavity Oesophagus Forestomach		
Ochratoxin A	56, 489		I	S	2B		Liver[k] **Kidney**[s]	**Kidney**[s]			
Potassium bromate	40, 207	70	I	S	2B			**Kidney**[a,b] Thyroid[x]			
Tetrachloroethylene	63, 159		L	S	2A	Lymphoid system[n] Cervix Oesophagus	Liver[k]	**Kidney**[s] Haemato-poietic system[m]			
Tobacco smoke	38, 37	359	S	S	1	Lung Urinary bladder[x] **Kidney**[b] Oral cavity Larynx Pancreas	Skin (condensate)	Lung	Larynx		

Table 4. (Contd) Some agents (chemicals and mixtures) producing kidney (renal tubule-cell) neoplasms (IARC Monographs. Volumes 1–69)

Agent	Vol., page	Suppl. 7, page	Evidence of carcinogenicity			Target organs					
			H	A	Group	Human	Mouse	Hamster	Rat	Dog	Other
Trichloroethylene	63, 75		L	S	2A	Liver Lymphoid system[n]	Liver[k] Lung Lymphoid system[n]		**Kidney**[s] Testis		
1,2,3-Trichloropropane	63, 223		I	S	2A		Liver[k] Forestomach Oral cavity Uterus		Forestomach Oral cavity Preputial/ clitorial gland Pancreas Mammary gland **Kidney**[t]		
Tris(2,3-dibromo-propyl)phosphate	20, 575	369	I	S	2A		Liver[k] Forestomach Lung **Kidney**[s]		**Kidney**[s]		

[a] Adenoma
[b] Adenocarcinoma
[c] Carcinoma
[d] Cholangioma/cholangiocarcinoma
[e] Fibroadenoma
[f] Fibrosarcoma
[g] Follicular-cell adenoma
[h] Follicular-cell adenoma and carcinoma
[i] Follicular-cell carcinoma
[j] Haemangioma or haemangiosarcoma
[k] Hepatoma and/or hepatocellular carcinoma
[l] Leiomyoma/leiomyosarcoma
[m] Leukaemia
[n] Lymphoma
[o] Papilloma
[p] Papilloma and transitional-cell carcinoma
[q] Papilloma, transitional-cell
[r] Renal tubule-cell adenoma
[s] Renal-tubule cell adenoma and carcinoma
[t] Renal-tubule cell carcinoma
[u] Sarcoma
[v] Squamous-cell carcinoma
[w] Transitional-cell carcinoma
[x] Unspecified
[z] Neoplastic nodule/hepatocellular adenoma

Table 5. Some agents (chemicals and mixtures) producing thyroid follicular-cell neoplasms (*IARC Monographs*. Volumes 1–69)

Agent	Vol., page	Suppl. 7, page	H	A	Group	Human	Mouse	Rat	Hamster	Dog	Other
Acrylamide	60, 389		I	S	2A		Lung Skin (initiator)	Mammary gland Oral cavity Brain Uterus Clitoral gland **Thyroid**[h]			
Amitrole (3-amino-1,2,4-triazole)	41, 293	92	I	S	2B		Liver[k] **Thyroid**[x]	Pituitary gland **Thyroid**[h]			
ortho-Anisidine and its hydrochloride	27, 63	57	I	S	2B		Urinary bladder[w]	Urinary bladder[w] Kidney/pelvis[w] **Thyroid**[h]			
Chlordane and heptachlor	53, 115		I	S	2B		Liver[k]	Liver[z] **Thyroid**[x]			
Chlorendic acid	48, 45		I	S	2B		Liver[k] Lung **Thyroid**[g]	Liver[k] Lung Pancreas (exocrine)			
Chlorinated paraffins (C12, Cl 60%)	48, 55		I	S	2B		Liver[k] Lung **Thyroid**[h]	Liver[k] **Thyroid**[h] Haematopoietic system[m]			
CI Basic Red 9	57, 215		I	S	2B		Liver[k]	Liver[k] Skin Zymbal gland **Thyroid**[h]			
2,4-Diaminoanisole	27, 103	61	I	S	2B		**Thyroid**[h]	**Thyroid**[h] Skin Preputial/clitoral gland Zymbal gland Mammary gland			

Table 5. (Contd) Some agents (chemicals and mixtures) producing thyroid follicular-cell neoplasms (*IARC Monographs*. Volumes 1–69)

Agent	Vol., page	Suppl. 7, page	Evidence of carcinogenicity H	Evidence of carcinogenicity A	Group	Human	Mouse	Rat	Hamster	Dog	Other
4,4'-Diaminodiphenyl ether (4,4'-oxydianiline)	29, 203	61	I	S	2B		Liver[k] Harderian gland Thyroid[g]	Liver[k] Thyroid[h]			
Ethylene thiourea	7, 45	207	I	S	2B		Liver	Thyroid[i]			
Griseofulvin	10, 153	391	I	S	2B		Liver	Thyroid[x]			
HC Blue No. 1	57, 129		I	S	2B		Liver[k] Thyroid[g]	Lung			
4,4'-Methylene-dianiline dihydro-chloride	39, 347	66	I	S	2B		Liver[k] Thyroid[g]	Liver[z] Thyroid[l]			
Methylthiouracil	7, 53	66	I	S	2B		Thyroid[a]	Thyroid[a,c]	Thyroid[a]		
Nitrobenzene	65, 381		I	S	2B		Lung Thyroid[g]	Liver[k] Kidney[f] Thyroid[h]			
Propylthiouracil	7, 67	329	I	S	2B		Thyroid[c] Pituitary gland	Thyroid[a,c]	Thyroid[c]		*Guinea-pig:* Thyroid[a]
Tetrachlorodibenzo-*para*-dioxin	69		L	S	1	Lung All sites	Liver[k] Thyroid[g]	Liver[k] Thyroid[g] Lung Nasal cavity Oral cavity Tongue			

Table 5. (Contd) Some agents (chemicals and mixtures) producing thyroid follicular-cell neoplasms (IARC Monographs. Volumes 1–69)

Agent	Vol., page	Suppl. 7, page	Evidence of carcinogenicity			Target organs					
			H	A	Group	Human	Mouse	Rat	Hamster	Dog	Other
4,4'-Thiodianiline	27, 147	72	I	S	2B		Liver, Thyroid[h]	Liver, Thyroid[i], Zymbal gland, Uterus			
Thiourea	7, 95	72	I	S	2B			Liver, Thyroid[a,c], Zymbal gland			
Toxaphene	20, 327	72	I	S	2B		Liver	Thyroid[h]			

[a] Adenoma
[b] Adenocarcinoma
[c] Carcinoma
[d] Cholangioma/cholangiocarcinoma
[e] Fibroadenoma
[f] Fibrosarcoma
[g] Follicular-cell adenoma
[h] Follicular-cell adenoma and carcinoma
[i] Follicular-cell carcinoma
[j] Haemangioma or haemangiosarcoma
[k] Hepatoma and/or hepatocellular carcinoma
[l] Leiomyoma/leiomyosarcoma
[m] Leukaemia
[n] Lymphoma
[o] Papilloma
[p] Papilloma and transitional-cell carcinoma
[q] Papilloma, transitional-cell
[r] Renal tubule-cell adenoma
[s] Renal-tubule cell adenoma and carcinoma
[t] Renal-tubule cell carcinoma
[u] Sarcoma
[v] Squamous-cell carcinoma
[w] Transitional-cell carcinoma
[x] Unspecified
[z] Neoplastic nodule/hepato-cellular adenoma

oils, and tobacco smoke. For these mixtures there are no bioassay data in which tumours of the urinary bladder occurred in exposed animals of any species. Also, chronic infection with the parasite *Schistosoma haematobium* leads to bladder tumours only in humans and some species of non-human primates, not in rodents (IARC, 1994).

Carcinoma of the urinary bladder was one of the first human cancers to be recognized as having an association with occupational exposure to chemicals (Rehn, 1895), especially chemicals used in dyestuff manufacturing. These were much later shown to be aromatic amines. Rats and mice are not uniformly susceptible to carcinogenesis in the urinary bladder by aromatic amines, however, and much research effort was required to identify the dog (Hueper *et al.*, 1938; Bonser, 1943) and the Syrian hamster (Sellakumar *et al.*, 1969) as surrogate species that more closely resemble humans in their response to bladder carcinogens of the aromatic amine family. This is not necessarily the case for bladder carcinogens of other chemical classes. For analgesic mixtures containing phenacetin, human evidence is supported by bioassay data in rats, although the primary tumour site in both humans and rats is the renal medulla. The remaining eight human bladder carcinogens are individual chemicals or groups of chemicals that vary greatly in the extent to which human and animal target organ sites overlap. For 4-aminobiphenyl, benzidine, cyclophosphamide, 2-naphthylamine, and phenacetin, bladder tumours were identified in one or more experimental animal species. 4-Aminobiphenyl is carcinogenic to the bladder in dogs, rabbits, and mice, also producing tumours in mice at other sites; in rats, tumours were only detected at sites other than the bladder. For benzidine, bladder tumours were found only in the dog; benzidine produced tumours only at sites other than the bladder in mice, rats and hamsters. Cyclophosphamide produced tumours in the bladder and at other sites in rats, but only at other sites in mice. 2-Naphthylamine produced bladder tumours in rats, dogs, monkeys and hamsters, but not mice (in which only liver and lung (newborn) tumours were produced). Phenacetin produced tumours of the bladder and also the kidney in rats, but only in

the renal cortex in mice. For arsenic and arsenic compounds, the anti-tumour drug chlornaphazine (a 2-naphthylamine derivative), and for *para*-chloro-*ortho*-toluidine, all of which are associated with increased risk of bladder cancer in humans, no bladder tumours were detected in the available animal bioassays.

Some of the carcinogens listed in Table 3, for which data in humans are *inadequate* but data in animals are *sufficient*, are associated with the formation of urinary calculi (urolithiasis) in rats under the conditions of bioassays in which bladder tumours occurred. These include the dye Disperse Blue 1 and sodium *ortho*-phenyl phenate[1]. Neither chemical produced bladder tumours or stones in mice, in which species each was carcinogenic only at a site other than the bladder. Melamine[2] (2,4,6-triamino-1,3,5-triazine) (not in Table 3, Group 3) was carcinogenic only to the urinary bladder in rats and produced urinary calculi under conditions where tumours developed, but only a single positive bioassay had been reported when this chemical was evaluated (IARC, 1986a) and evidence for carcinogenicity to animals was considered *inadequate* because of the association of tumours with bladder stones. Saccharin[2] and its salts produced only bladder tumours (and urinary precipitate) in rats; evidence for tumours at another site in mice (thyroid) was based on a single experiment.

Epithelial Neoplasms of the Renal Cortex

Twenty-nine compounds, groups of compounds, or complex mixtures for which there is at least *sufficient* evidence of carcinogenicity in animals are summarized in Table 4. Tumour histology has been footnoted as described in the Monographs. However, adenoma, adenocarcinoma or carcinoma not further specified would refer to tumours of the tubule epithelium. Only one of these, tobacco smoke, is definitely linked to cancer of the renal cortex in humans.

Of these 29 agents, nine are carcinogenic to the renal cortex in both rats and mice: aflatoxins, bromodichloromethane, caffeic acid, chloroform[1], lead compounds, nitrilotriacetic acid and its salts[1], *N*-nitrosodimethylamine, ochratoxin A, and tris-(1,3-dibromopropyl)phosphate. Others: benzofuran,

---

[1] Subsequently re-evaluated in *IARC Monographs* Volume 73 (October, 1998) with no change in overall evaluation.
[2] Subsequently re-evaluated in *IARC Monographs* Volume 73 (October, 1998) with a change in overall evaluation.

captafol, cycasin, daunomycin, *para*-dichloroben-zene[1], 2-(2-formylhydrazino)-4-(5-nitro-2-furyl) thiazole, hexachlorobenzene, nitrobenzene, *N*-nitrosodiethanolamine, *N*-nitrosodiethylamine, *N*-nitrosomorpholine, potassium bromate[1], tetra-chloroethylene, trichloroethylene and 1,2,3-trichloropropane produced tumours of the renal cortex only in rats, indicating that for carcinogenesis at this organ site, the rat is by far the more sensitive species. All these agents except potassium bromate also produced tumours in mice or hamsters or both, but only at sites other than the kidney.

For only one carcinogen in Table 4, methyl mercury chloride, is the kidney the only target organ (in mice only). There are also several compounds for which evidence of carcinogenicity is confined to the kidney, but is considered *limited* in the *IARC Monographs*. Often the evidence was evaluated as *limited* because only a single bioassay had been performed at the time of the evaluation. These include 2-amino-4-nitrophenol (male rats only; IARC, 1993a); chlorothalonil[2] (male and female rats) (IARC, 1983), citrinin (male rats only; females not tested) (IARC, 1986b) and hexachlorobutadiene[1] (male and female rats) (IARC, 1979a); and *d*-limonene[2] (male rats only; IARC, 1993b). Unleaded gasoline, given to rats by inhalation, was carcinogenic only to the kidney and only in males; in mice, it increased the incidence of liver tumours in females only, in which animals a few renal tumours occurred also (IARC, 1989). Hexachloroethane[2] caused a low incidence of kidney tumours in male and female rats, but induced hepatocellular carcinomas in male and female mice (IARC, 1979b).

Oestrogens, whether natural or synthetic and whether steroidal or non-steroidal in structure, are carcinogenic to the kidney in male hamsters, but not in other species. In humans the kidney is not a target organ for medicinal oestrogens, which are carcinogenic to female breast, endometrium and liver under certain conditions of medical use (IARC, 1987), and oestrogens have not been included in Table 4.

Follicular Cell Neoplasms of the Thyroid Gland
Twenty compounds that cause follicular cell neoplasms of the thyroid in rats and/or mice, and occasionally in other species, are summarized in Table 5. None of these is unequivocally associated with thyroid cancer in humans. The only compound for which there is some evidence of carcinogenicity to humans at this site is 2,3,7,8-tetrachloro-dibenzo-*para*-dioxin (TCDD; Group 1), where the most convincing evidence is for all sites combined (IARC, 1997). Elevated mortality (four deaths) from thyroid carcinoma in persons exposed to TCDD has been recorded in one study (Saracci *et al.*, 1991).

For many compounds, elevated thyroid tumour incidence was accompanied by elevated hepatocellular tumour incidence in the same species (see McClain & Rice, this volume), with or without tumours at any other sites. In some cases, liver tumours but no thyroid tumours were reported in one species, and thyroid tumours but no liver tumours in another, but in some of these cases the thyroid gland (especially in mice) was not examined. Thyroid tumours plus tumours in at least one extrahepatic site were observed for many compounds, in at least one test species, usually the rat (e.g., acrylamide, CI Basic Red 9, 2,4-diamino-anisole, TCDD, 4,4'-thiodianiline, and thiourea). Only a few compounds produced tumours only in the thyroid (e.g., methylthiouracil [rat, mouse, hamster], propylthiouracil [rat, hamster, guinea pig], 2,4-diaminoanisole [mouse]) or in the thyroid plus the pituitary but at no other sites (e.g., amitrole [rat], propylthiouracil [mouse]). However, a number of compounds which have undergone only limited testing and are currently in IARC Group 3 (Table 2) have to date produced tumours only in the thyroid. These include sul-famethoxazole and 4,4'-methylene bis(*N,N*-dimethyl)benzenamine in rats (IARC, 1982).

Discussion
In *IARC Monographs* evaluations, mechanistic evidence that neoplasms at any site in rodents might not be predictive of a carcinogenic hazard to humans is only applied to the final overall evaluation, and only to the overall evaluation of agents for which there was *sufficient* evidence in bioassays in animals and *inadequate* evidence in humans. When bioassay data are only available from a single study, or there are other deficiencies in the available published studies that in the opinion of an IARC Working Group provide less than *sufficient*

---

[1] Subsequently re-evaluated in *IARC Monographs* Volume 73 (October, 1998) with no change in overall evaluation.
[2] Subsequently re-evaluated in *IARC Monographs* Volume 73 (October, 1998) with a change in overall evaluation.

evidence of carcinogenicity in animals, such agents would be placed in Group 3 without invoking considerations of carcinogenic mechanism or mode of action (Table 2). Only when there is *sufficient* evidence of carcinogenicity to animals, *inadequate* evidence for cancer in humans, and mechanistic evidence that the tumours seen in exposed animals are not predictive of carcinogenicity to humans, might an agent be downgraded from Group 2B to Group 3. In the IARC classification scheme, it is not possible for any agent that causes tumours in animals by any mechanism or mode of action to be classified as *probably not carcinogenic to humans* (Group 4).

References

Bonser, G.M. (1943) Epithelial tumours of the bladder in dogs induced by pure β-naphthylamine. *J. Path. Bact.*, 55, 1–6

Hueper, W.C., Wiley, F.H. & Wolfe, H.D. (1938) Experimental production of bladder tumors in dogs by administration of beta-naphthylamine. *J. industr. Hyg.*, 20, 46–84

IARC (1979a) *IARC Monographs on the Evaluation of the Carcinogenic Risk of Chemicals to Humans, Volume 20: Some Halogenated Hydrocarbons.* IARC, Lyon, pp. 179–193

IARC (1979b) *IARC Monographs on the Evaluation of the Carcinogenic Risk of Chemicals to Humans, Volume 20: Some Halogenated Hydrocarbons.* IARC, Lyon, pp. 467–476

IARC (1982) *IARC Monographs on the Evaluation of the Carcinogenic Risk of Chemicals to Humans, Volume 27: Some Aromatic Amines, Anthraquinones and Nitroso Compounds, and Inorganic Fluorides Used in Drinking Water and Dental Preparations.* IARC, Lyon, pp. 119–126

IARC (1983) *IARC Monographs on the Evaluation of the Carcinogenic Risk of Chemicals to Humans, Volume 30: Miscellaneous Pesticides.* IARC, Lyon, pp. 319–328

IARC (1986a) *IARC Monographs on the Evaluation of the Carcinogenic Risk of Chemicals to Humans, Volume 39: Some Chemicals used in Plastics and Elastomers.* IARC, Lyon, pp. 333–346

IARC (1986b) *IARC Monographs on the Evaluation of the Carcinogenic Risk of Chemicals to Humans, Volume 40: Some Naturally Occurring and Synthetic Food Components, Furocoumarins and Ultraviolet Radiation.* IARC, Lyon, pp. 67–82

IARC (1987) *IARC Monographs on the Evaluation of Carcinogenic Risks to Humans, Supplement 7: Overall Evaluations of Carcinogenicity, an Updating of IARC Monographs Volumes 1 to 42.* IARC, Lyon

IARC (1989) *IARC Monographs on the Evaluation of Carcinogenic Risks to Humans, Volume 45: Occupational Exposures in Petroleum Refining; Crude Oil and Major Petroleum Fuels.* IARC, Lyon, pp. 159–201

IARC (1992) *IARC Monographs on the Evaluation of Carcinogenic Risks to Humans, Volume 54: Occupational Exposures to Mists and Vapours from Strong Inorganic Acids; and other Industrial Chemicals.* IARC, Lyon, pp.13–32

IARC (1993a) *IARC Monographs on the Evaluation of Carcinogenic Risks to Humans, Volume 57: Occupational Exposures of Hairdressers and Barbers and Personal Use of Hair Colourants; Some Hair Dyes, Cosmetic Colourants, Industrial Dyestuffs and Aromatic Amines.* IARC, Lyon, pp. 167–176

IARC (1993b) *IARC Monographs on the Evaluation of Carcinogenic Risks to Humans, Volume 56: Some Naturally Occurring Substances: Food Items and Constituents, Heterocyclic Aromatic Amines and Mycotoxins.* IARC, Lyon, pp. 135–162

IARC (1994) *IARC Monographs on the Evaluation of Carcinogenic Risks to Humans, Volume 61: Schistosomes, Liver Flukes, and Helicobacter pylori.* IARC, Lyon, pp. 45–119

IARC (1997) *IARC Monographs on the Evaluation of Carcinogenic Risks to Humans, Volume 69: Polychlorinated Dibenzo-para-dioxins and Polychlorinated Dibenzofurans.* IARC, Lyon

Rehn, L. (1895) Urinary bladder tumours in Fuschin workers. *Arch. Klin. Chir.*, 50, 588–600 (In German)

Saracci, R., Kogevinas, M., Bertazzi, P.A., Bueno de Mesquita, B.H., Coggon, D., Green, L.M., Kauppinen, T., L'Abbé, K.A., Littorin, M., Lynge, E., Mathews, J.D., Neuberger, M., Osman, J., Pearce, N. & Winkelman, R. (1991) Cancer mortality in workers exposed to chlorophenoxy herbicides and chlorophenols. *Lancet*, 338, 1027-1032

Sellakumar, A.R., Montesano, R. & Saffiotti, U. (1969) Aromatic amines carcinogenicity in hamsters. *Proc. Amer. Assoc. Cancer Res.*, 10, 78

Corresponding author:

Julian D. Wilbourn

Unit of Carcinogen Identification and Evaluation
International Agency for Research on Cancer
150 cours Albert Thomas
69372 Lyon Cedex 08, France

Species Differences in Thyroid, Kidney and Urinary Bladder Carcinogenesis
C.C. Capen, E. Dybing, J.M. Rice and J.D. Wilbourn, eds
IARC Scientific Publications No. 147
International Agency for Research on Cancer, Lyon, 1999

Appendix 2

Chemicals associated with tumours of the kidney, urinary bladder and thyroid gland in laboratory rodents from 2000 US National Toxicology Program/National Cancer Institute bioassays for carcinogenicity

James Huff

Introduction

Since the late 1960s, the US National Cancer Institute (NCI) and since 1978, the US National Toxicology Program (NTP) have studied and evaluated the potential carcinogenicity of nearly 500 chemicals. Most of these were tested in both genders of two species of rodents, typically Fischer 344 inbred rats (and earlier, on occasion, Osborne-Mendel rats) and (C57BL/6 x C3H/HeN MTV-)F_1 (B6C3F$_1$) hybrid mice. Thus, nearly 2000 individual sex-species bioassays have been accomplished in these last three decades since publication of the first NCI Bioassay Technical Report in 1976.

Long-term (usually two-year) carcinogenesis bioassays continue to be the most appropriate and predictive model for identifying those chemicals with the most likelihood to cause cancer in humans (Montesano et al., 1986; Huff et al., 1991a; IARC, 1997; Huff, 1999). In several instances, chemicals were first shown to be carcinogenic in laboratory animals before evidence of cancer was observed in humans (Tomatis, 1979; Huff, 1993; IARC, 1997). Results from long term experiments in animals should continue to be used judiciously to protect public health, to reduce and prevent cancer risks from these agents, and to establish standards of exposures (Fung et al., 1995). Further, chemical carcinogenesis results can be used to identify and set reasonable priorities for chemicals that should be investigated epi-demiologically (Huff et al., 1991a).

Presented in this paper are lists of chemicals shown by the NCI or the NTP to cause tumours of the kidney, urinary bladder, or/and thyroid gland in rats and/or mice. Examples are given of chemicals that induce tumours in two or more of these target organs, as well as some interesting chemical structure correlations. Chemical carcinogenesis target sites in rodents other than these three have been published (Huff et al., 1991b), and are available on-line: http://ntp-server.niehs.nih.gov/-htdocs/Sites/Site_Cnt.html.

Materials and methods

The NTP collection of carcinogenesis results contains detailed information on nearly 500 chemicals tested since the early 1970s, involving nearly 2000 gender-specific bioassays. For almost all chemical agents tested, four unique groups of animals were used: male rats, female rats, male mice, female mice. Each grouping consists of 50–60 animals in each of 2–3 exposure groups and a control or unexposed group. Carcinogenic activity was evaluated separately for each gender-specific grouping. Proposed results and conclusions are presented to and peer-reviewed by independent experts in carcinogenesis and related fields in public meetings. Final data, results, evaluations, and conclusions are prepared as detailed technical reports, and these are made publicly available (Huff et al., 1988; Huff, 1998, 1999).

Within the overall NTP tumour data base, organ-specific effects have been recorded and are available for tabulation and comparisons (Huff *et al.*, 1991b). For this paper, the three target organs selected by the International Agency for Research on Cancer as the subject of a Workshop on carcinogenesis mechanisms in November 1997 form the basis of this compilation: kidney, urinary bladder, thyroid gland.

For a further listing of chemicals that may affect these organs, see also the paper taken from the IARC Monographs (Wilbourn *et al.*, this volume), and other chemical carcinogenesis data collections; these include PHS 149 series (National Cancer Institute, 1999), California EPA Proposition 65 [internet on-line: http://www. calepa.cahwnet.-gov/oehha/docs/9-96lstb.htm], and Gold and Zeiger (1997). Also available on-line are NTP files of long-term bioassay testing results [http://ntp-server.niehs.nih.gov/htdocs/pub.html] and the NTP Reports on Carcinogens [http://ntp-server.niehs.nih.gov/Main_Pages/NTP_ARC_PG.ht ml].

Results

The numbers of chemicals associated with site-specific neoplasia for the 36 organs and systems routinely evaluated histopathologically are given in Table 1. An abbreviated rank-ordered listing is given in Table 2. Kidney ranks second to liver, thyroid gland ranks seventh between mammary gland and adrenal glands, and urinary bladder ranks 11th between Zymbal gland and intestine. Regarding incidences of human cancers in these organs in the United States (Ries *et al.*, 1997; American Cancer Society, 1998), urinary bladder resides in fourth place for men and eighth for women, kidney ranks eighth for men and 13th for women, and thyroid gland tumours are 18th for men and 12th for women.

For the three target organs emphasized in this paper, using the pathology data on the 500 chemicals tested, the rat kidney appears to be the most responsive, with the male rat predominating. Similar results have been obtained for the urinary bladder, but here the responsiveness seems comparable for both male and female rats. For the thyroid gland, rats again show more positive responses than mice, yet mice do respond more often for this organ site than for kidneys and urinary bladder. Each gender within a species is

approximately equal in numbers of positive responses.

Some have reported correlations among certain chemical-associated organs in rodents. Haseman and Lockhart (1993) reported that certain high incidence tumour combinations do occur: rat liver and rat Zymbal gland, mouse lung and rat/mouse mammary glands, and mouse lung and mouse forestomach. However, the relevance of these empirical observations for the most part allows little insight into rodent carcinogenesis or into human relevance and extrapolation. In fact, however, correspondence between various tumour sites is a less common finding among animals exposed to chemicals. For instance, for the three target sites highlighted in this paper, only one combination is statistically associated: liver and thyroid gland; these rarely occur in the same sex-species group, and even more uncommonly in the same animal. The meaning of this observational combination remains obscure (see McClain & Rice, this volume).

The data selected for Tables 3–5 include: the NCI or NTP Technical Report Numbers; the common chemical names; positive (+), negative (-) or equivocal mutagenicity results in *Salmonella typhimurium* (Ames assay), routes of exposure used for the long-term bioassays; levels of evidence of carcinogenicity for each sex-species group (with parentheses indicating a carcinogenic response in the particular organ of concern); carcinogenic responses that may be related to chemical exposure; and whether tumours were also induced at sites other than the subject organ (yes) or in the subject organ only (no). Results for each of the three organs are listed alphabetically in Tables 3–5, and are summarized below in separate commentaries.

Kidney

For the kidney, 64 chemicals induced tumours in one or more of the four gender-species experimental groups (Table 3). Most chemically induced tumours of the kidney were renal tubule cell types, with four chemicals causing transitional cell tumours only and seven causing both neoplasms.

For 11 of the 64 chemicals, carcinogenic effects were observed only in the kidney, for nine of the 11, the effect was observed only in a single gender-species group (three of these were equivocal

Table 1. Numbers of chemicals associated with site-specific neoplasms from nearly 2000 long-term carcinogenesis bioassays

Organ/tissue site	Ranking	Male rats POS[a]	Male rats EE[a]	Female rats POS	Female rats EE	Male mice POS	Male mice EE	Female mice POS	Female mice EE	Totals POS	Totals EE	POS/EE[a]
Adrenal gland	8	11	11	8	8	6	3	4	1	20	17	37
Bone	29	1	2	0	0	0	0	0	0	1	2	3
Brain	23	2	7	2	4	2	1	1	0	3	9	12
Circulatory system	14	4	0	2	1	8	4	9	2	13	5	18
Clitorial gland	19	0	0	13	2	0	0	0	0	13	2	15
Epididymis	33	0	0	0	0	0	1	0	0	0	1	1
Oesphagus	28	3	0	3	0	0	1	0	1	3	1	4
Forestomach	5	19	4	13	5	20	5	21	8	30	12	42
Forestomach/stomach	34	0	1	0	0	0	0	0	0	0	1	1
Glandular stomach	32	0	0	0	2	0	0	0	0	0	2	2
Harderian gland	18	0	0	0	0	10	3	11	2	12	4	16
Heart	27	0	0	0	0	4	0	4	0	4	0	4
Haematopoietic system	4	14	8	12	8	11	6	16	4	34	22	56
Intestines	12	12	3	9	2	1	3	1	0	14	6	20
Kidney	2	41	11	17	4	9	6	1	2	50	14	64
Liver	1	44	10	39	4	76	20	99	10	132	24	156
Lung	3	11	6	12	3	29	6	32	5	46	10	56
Mammary gland	6	4	0	27	7	0	0	11	1	33	7	40
Mesothelium [ac/tv][b]	22	9	3	2	1	1	0	1	0	9	3	12
Nasal cavity	24	9	2	8	1	3	0	3	1	10	1	11
Oral cavity	20	12	1	12	1	0	1	1	0	14	0	14
Ovary	25	0	0	0	0	0	0	10	0	10	0	10
Pancreas	17	8	8	2	2	0	0	0	0	9	8	17
Parathyroid gland	35	0	1	0	0	0	0	0	0	0	1	1
Pituitary gland	26	0	1	1	2	2	0	3	0	4	3	7
Preputial gland	15	8	5	0	0	4	1	0	0	12	6	18
Seminal vesicle	30	1	0	0	0	1	0	0	0	2	0	2
Skin	9	16	5	8	1	4	3	4	1	18	8	26
Spleen	21	8	2	3	1	1	0	2	0	10	2	12
Subcutaneous tissue	16	7	3	3	2	0	4	4	2	10	8	18
Thyroid gland	7	16	8	15	5	8	6	10	2	25	14	39
Ureter	31	2	0	1	0	0	0	0	0	2	0	2
Urinary bladder	11	14	1	13	4	2	1	3	0	19	4	23
Uterus/cervix	13	0	0	9	0	0	0	8	1	17	1	18
Zymbal gland	10	19	3	17	1	1	2	2	2	21	4	25

[a] POS, positive findings, EE, equivocal evidence, POS/EE, positive findings or equivocal evidence
[b] ac/tv, abdominal cavity/tunica vaginalis
Rankings were determined using the POS/EE column totals data. With ties, the site with the most POS was given the higher ranking; e.g.., circulatory system [rank 14], preputial gland [15], and subcutaneous tissue [16] had the same number of POS/EE, but circulatory system following by preputial gland had more POS responses.
Responses by sex and species:
Totals represents the numbers of individual chemicals that caused positive responses [POS], equivocal responses [EE], and combined totals [POS/EE] for each particular organ/system.
The sum of the POS or EE numbers from all of the sex/species columns for an organ site most often is greater than the number in the totals columns, because a given chemical may have caused tumours in more than one sex-species group, but would only be counted once as either a POS or an EE substance.
Testis not listed as no NCI or NTP chemical has caused tumours in this organ.

Table 2. Rank order of chemically induced site-specific neoplasms from nearly 2000 long-term NCI/NTP carcinogenesis bioassays[a]

1.	Liver	19.	Clitoral gland
2.	Kidney	20.	Oral cavity
3.	Lung	21.	Spleen
4.	Haematopoietic system	22.	Mesothelium
5.	Forestomach	23.	Brain
6.	Mammary gland	24.	Nasal cavity
7.	Thyroid gland	25.	Ovary
8.	Adrenal gland	26.	Pituitary gland
9.	Skin	27.	Heart
10.	Zymbal gland	28.	Oesophagus
11.	Urinary bladder	29.	Bone
12.	Intestines	30.	Seminal vesicle
13.	Uterus/cervix	31.	Ureter
14.	Circulatory system	32.	Glandular stomach
15.	Preputial gland	33.	Epididymis
16.	Subcutaneous tissue	34.	Forestomach/stomach
17.	Pancreas	35.	Parathyroid gland
18.	Harderian gland	36.	Testes[b]

[a] See details in Table 1.
[b] Listed even though no chemical has been associated with tumours in this organ.

responses). In no case did a chemical induce tumours of the kidney in all four gender-species groups. Several chemicals caused tumours of the kidney in three of the four groups: bromodichloromethane, chloroprene, nitrilotriacetic acid (NTA), tris(2,3-dibromopropyl)phosphate; for one more the findings were equivocal in one of the three positive groups: ortho-nitroanisole and tris(2-chloroethyl)phosphate. For these five chemicals, none were mutagenic for *Salmonella*. Considering all 59 chemicals tested for mutagenic activity (5 have not been), 19 (32%) induced mutations in *Salmonella*, whereas 40 did not. What this means mechanistically is uncertain, because one would have to evaluate the full scope of genotoxic activity.

Overall, 50 chemicals were positive or equivocal in male rats, 19 in female rats, 15 in male mice, and only three in female mice (with two of the latter being equivocal). Thus, for the kidney, the female B6C3F$_1$ mouse is the least sensitive of the species and strains used for carcinogenicity testing

by the NTP, with only a single chemical of the nearly 500 tested being unequivocally positive for the female mouse kidney: NTA. Perhaps much of this gender and species/strain difference – at least for male and female Fischer 344 rats – might decrease if study duration were lengthened to 30 or more months, since female rats seem to develop tumours at this organ site much later than do male rats of this strain.

Consistently, male rats exhibit a higher background incidence of tumours of the kidney at 24 months than do female rats: 1.0% versus 0.11%. This difference extends to step- or multiple sections as well: 4.6% in males versus 0.75% in females (Eustis *et al.*, 1994). In one limited life-span study of 529 male and 529 female Fischer 344 rats, renal tubule cell tumour rates went from 0.34% in males at 24 months to 0.57% at 140–146 weeks (1.7-fold increase); for females the percentages were 0.17% and 0.95% (5.6 fold increase) (Solleveld *et al.*, 1984). More work and some life time chemical exposure studies need to be accomplished to solidify these findings.

Urinary bladder

For the urinary bladder, 23 chemicals induced tumours in one or more of the four gender-species experimental groups (Table 4). Five chemicals caused tumours only of the urinary bladder: *meta*-cresidine and *N*-nitrosodiphenylamine were positive in both sexes of rats; two were single sex-species carcinogens, one in male rats (melamine) and one in female rats (*para*-benzoquinone dioxime); with another that was positive in male rats yielding equivocal evidence in female rats (4-amino-2-nitrophenol).

Most chemicals caused transitional cell tumours, with both transitional and squamous cell types induced by three chemicals. CI Disperse blue 1, an anthraquinone, was associated with tumours of three cellular types: transitional, squamous, and smooth muscle (mesenchymal). In this case the situation was somewhat confusing because about one-half the animals had bladder stones (National Toxicology Program, 1986); further, one other anthraquinone likewise caused tumours of the urinary bladder in both male and female rats. Squamous cell tumours are thought to arise from transitional epithelial cells (Jokinen, 1990).

Table 3. Chemicals Associated with Site-Specific Tumour Induction in Kidney [Renal tubule cell, RTC, tumours unless otherwise noted]

Technical Report No.	Chemical name	Salmonella[a]	Route	MR	FR	MM	FM	Other tumour sites
383	1-Amino-2,4-dibromoanthraquinone	+	Feed	[P]	P	N	P	Yes
111	1-Amino-2-methylanthraquinone	+	Feed	[P]	P	N	P	Yes
339	2-Amino-4-nitrophenol	+	Gavage	[SE]	NE	NE	NE	No
089	o-Anisidine hydrochloride [T cell][c]	nd	Feed	[P]	P	P	P	Yes
067	Aspirin,Phenacetin,Caffeine[T & RTC]	nd	Feed	N	[E]	N	N	Yes
469	3'-Azido-3'-deoxythymidine	+	Gavage	nd	nd	[EE]	CE	Yes
370	Benzofuran	–	Gavage	NE	[SE]	CE	CE	Yes
424	o-Benzyl-p-chlorophenol [T & RTC]	–	Gavage	NE	[EE]	[SE]	NE	No
452	2,2-Bis[bromomethyl]-1,3-propanediol*	–,+	Feed	CE	CE	[CE]	CE	Yes
321	Bromodichloromethane	–	Gavage	[CE]	[CE]	[CE]	CE	Yes
434	1,3-Butadiene*	+	Inhal	nd	nd	[CE]	CE	Yes
436	tert-Butyl alcohol	–	Water	[SE]	NE	EE	SE	Yes
308	Chlorinated paraffins: C12, 60% Cl	–	Gavage	[CE]	CE	CE	CE	Yes
000	Chloroform	–	Gavage	[P]	N	P	P	Yes
467	Chloroprene	–	Inhal	[CE]	[CE]	[CE]	CE	Yes
041	Chlorothalonil	–	Feed	[P]	[P]	N	N	No
335	C.I. Acid Orange 3 [T cell]	+	Gavage	NE	[CE]	NE	NE	No
430	C.I. Direct Blue 218*	–	Feed	SE	NE	CE	CE	Yes
407	C.I. Pigment Red 3	+	Feed	SE	SE	[SE]	NE	Yes
411	C.I. Pigment Red 23	+	Feed	[EE]	NE	NE	NE	No
196	Cinnamyl anthranilate	–	Feed	[P]	N	P	P	Yes
422	Coumarin	+	Gavage	[SE]	[EE]	SE	CE	Yes
463	D & C Yellow No. 11	?,+W	Feed	[SE]	SE	nd	nd	Yes
401	2,4-Diaminophenol dihydrochloride	+	Gavage	NE	NE	[SE]	NE	No
400	2,3-Dibromo-1-propanol	+	Dermal	[CE]	[CE]	CE	CE	Yes
319	1,4-Dichlorobenzene[p-dichlorobenzene]	–	Gavage	[CE]	NE	CE	CE	Yes
423	3,4-Dihydrocoumarin [T & RTC]	–	Gavage	[SE]	NE	NE	SE	Yes
456	1,2-Dihydro-2,2,4-trimethylquinoline	–	Dermal	[SE]	NE	NE	NE	Yes
323	Dimethyl methylphosphonate [T & RTC]	–	Gavage	[SE]	NE	IS	NE	Yes
466	Ethylbenzene	–	Inhal	[CE]	[SE]	SE	SE	Yes
382	Furfural*	?,–	Gavage	SE	NE	CE	SE	Yes
356	Furosemide	–	Feed	[EE]	NE	NE	SE	Yes
252	Geranyl acetate*	–	Gavage	N	N	N	N	Yes
361& 068	Hexachloroethane	–	Gavage	[CE]	NE	P	P	Yes
366	Hydroquinone	–	Gavage	[SE]	SE	NE	SE	Yes
291	Isophorone	–	Gavage	[SE]	NE	EE	NE	Yes
347	d-Limonene	–	Gavage	[CE]	NE	NE	NE	No
408	Mercuric chloride	–	Gavage	SE	EE	[EE]	NE	Yes
359	8-Methoxypsoralen	+	Gavage	[CE]	NE	nd	nd	Yes
369	α–Methylbenzyl alcohol	–	Gavage	[SE]	NE	NE	NE	No
348	Methyldopa sesquihydrate	nd	Feed	NE	NE	[EE]	NE	No
313	Mirex [T cell]	–	Feed	[CE]	CE	nd	nd	Yes
266	Monuron	–	Feed	[CE]	NE	NE	NE	Yes

Table 3. (Contd) Chemicals associated with site-specific tumour induction in kidney [renal tubule cell, RTC, tumours unless otherwise noted

Technical Report No.	Chemical name	Salmonella	Route	Levels of Evidence of Carcinogenicity MR	FR	MM	FM	Other tumour sites
006	Nitrilotriacetic acid	–	Feed	[P]	P	[P]	[P]	Yes
006	NTA Trisodium[d] [T & RTC]	–	Feed	[P]	[P]	N	N	Yes
416	o-Nitroanisole [T & RTC]	+	Feed	[CE]	[CE]	CE	SE	Yes
341	Nitrofurantoin	+	Feed	[SE]	NE	NE	CE	Yes
358	Ochratoxin A	–	Gavage	[CE]	[CE]	nd	nd	Yes
468 & 443	Oxazepam	–	Feed	[EE]	NE	C	CE	Yes
232	Pentachloroethane	–	Gavage	[E]	N	P	P	Yes
465	Phenolphthalein	?,-	Feed	[CE]	SE	CE	CE	Yes
367	Phenylbutazone[e] [T & RTC]	–	Gavage	[EE]	[SE]	SE	NE	Yes
333	N-Phenyl-2-Naphthylamine	–	Feed	NE	NE	N	[EE]	No
476	Primidone [Primaclone]	+	Feed	[EE]	NE	CE	CE	Yes
409	Quercetin	+	Feed	[SE]	NE	nd	nd	No
457	Salicylazosulfapyridine [T cell]	–	Gavage	SE	[SE]	CE	C	Yes
311	Tetrachloroethylene	–	Inhal	[CE]	SE	CE	CE	Yes
450	Tetrafluoroethylene	nd	Inhal	[CE]	[CE]	CE	CE	Yes
475	Tetrahydrofuran	–	Inhal	[SE]	NE	NE	C	Yes
243	Trichloroethylene [& TR 002 & 273]	–	Gavage	[SE]	[SE]	CE	CE	Yes
384	1,2,3-Trichloropropane	+	Gavage	[CE]	CE	CE	CE	Yes
449	Triethanolamine*	–	Dermal	[EE]	NE	EE	SE	Yes
391	Tris[2-chloroethyl] phosphate	–	Gavage	[CE]	[CE]	[EE]	EE	Yes
076	Tris[2,3-dibromopropyl] phosphate	nd	Feed	[P]	[P]	[P]	P	Yes

Number of chemicals causing tumours in **KIDNEY** = 64

[a] Salmonella results: + = Positive; +W = Weakly Positive; ? = Inconclusive; - = Negative

[b] [ ] = animal group in which tumours of the kidney were observed. MR, male rat; FR, female rat; MM, male mouse; FM, female mouse

CE = Clear evidence of carcinogenicity; P = Evidence of carcinogenicity; SE = Some evidence of carcinogenicity; EE or E = Equivocal evidence of carcinogenicity; NE or N = No Evidence of carcinogenicity; IS = Inadequate study; nd = no NCI or NTP data

[c] T=Transitional cell; RTC = Renal tubule cell

[d] Monohydrate; two studies done on this salt form, with data combined.

[e] Transitional cell tumours are causative in female rats, while renal tubule cell tumours may be related

Note: for tables 3–5, the different abbreviations for levels of evidence of carcinogenicity reflect simply designation changes over time; that is, P became CE and SE; E became EE; N became NE.

* Possible association is one sex of one species

Table 4. Chemicals associated with site-specific tumour induction in urinary bladder
[transitional cell tumours unless otherwise noted]

Technical report no.	Chemical name	Salmonella[a]	Route	Levels of Evidence of Carcinogenicity[b] MR	FR	MM	FM	Other tumour sites
234	Allyl isothiocyanate	+W,-	Gavage	[P]	E	N	N	Yes
383	1-Amino-2,4-dibromoanthraquinone	+	Feed	[CE]	[CE]	CE	CE	Yes
094	4-Amino-2-nitrophenol	+	Feed	[P]	[E]	N	N	No
216	11-Aminoundecanoic acid	–	Feed	[P]	N	E	N	Yes
089	o-Anisidine hydrochloride	nd	Feed	[P]	[P]	[P]	[P]	Yes
067	Aspirin, Phenacetin, and Caffeine	nd	Feed	N	[E]	N	N	Yes
179	p-Benzoquinone dioxime	+	Feed	N	[P]	N	N	No
452	2,2-Bis[Bromomethyl]-1,3-propanediol	–,+	Feed	[CE]	CE	CE	CE	Yes
458 & 213	Butyl benzyl phthalate	–	Feed	SE	[EE]	NE	NE	Yes
063	4-Chloro-o-phenylenediamine	+	Feed	[P]	[P]	P	P	Yes
467	Chloroprene **	–	Inhal	CE	CE	CE	CE	Yes
299	C.I. Disperse Blue 1 [T,SqC & L] [c]	+	Feed	[CE]	[CE]	EE	NE	Yes
105	m-Cresidine	+	Gavage	[P]	[P]	IS	N	No
142	p-Cresidine [T,SqC]	+	Feed	[P]	[P]	[P]	[P]	Yes
269	1,3-Dichloropropene [Telone II]	+	Gavage	CE	SE	IS	[CE]	Yes
374	Glycidol*	+	Gavage	CE	CE	CE	CE	Yes
245	Melamine	–	Feed	[P]	N	N	N	No
006	Nitrilotriacetic acid [NTA]	–	Feed	P	[P]	P	P	Yes
006	Nitrilotriacetic acid trisodium[d]	–	Feed	P	[P]	N	N	Yes
416	o-Nitroanisole [T,SqC]	+	Feed	[CE]	[CE]	CE	SE	Yes
164	N-Nitrosodiphenylamine	–	Feed	[P]	[P]	N	N	No
457	Salicylazosulfapyridine	–	Gavage	[SE]	[SE]	CE	CE	Yes
153	o-Toluidine hydrochloride	–,+	Feed	P	[P]	P	P	Yes

Number of chemicals causing tumours in **URINARY BLADDER** = 23

[a] Salmonella results: + = Positive; +W = Weakly Positive; ? = Inconclusive; - = Negative

[b] [ ] = animal group in which tumours of the urinary bladder were observed.

CE = Clear evidence of carcinogenicity; P = Evidence of carcinogenicity; SE = Some evidence of carcinogenicity; EE or E = Equivocal evidence of carcinogenicity; NE or N = No Evidence of carcinogenicity; IS = Inadequate experiment; nd = no NCI or NTP data

[c] T=transitional cell; SqC=Squamous cell; L=leiomyoma or leiomyosarcoma

[d] = Monohydrate

* Possible association in one sex of one species

** Possible association in both sexes of one species

Two chemicals caused tumours of the urinary bladder in each of the four groups: *ortho*-anisidine hydrochloride and *para*-cresidine (isomeric *meta*-cresidine was positive in male and female rats). Fifteen induced tumours of the urinary bladder in male rats, 17 in female rats, three in male mice, and three in female mice. As with the lack of chemically caused kidney tumours in female mice, both male and female B6C3F$_1$ mice seem considerably less sensitive than are rats to chemical induction of urinary bladder tumours. Thirteen of the 24 chemicals induced mutations in *Salmonella*. There do not appear to be any significant differences between 104 week and 140–146 week studies in background tumour incidences of the urinary bladder in male and female rats (Solleveld *et al.*, 1984).

Thyroid gland

For thyroid gland, 39 chemicals induced tumours in one or more of the four gender-species experimental groups (Table 5). All but seven chemicals caused follicular cell tumours only; four of these caused C cell tumours, and the other three caused both C cell and follicular cell tumours. Of these 39, seven chemicals induced only tumours of the thyroid gland, with four of these having only equivocal evidence of carcinogenicity; for two of these there were marginal responses in both sexes of one species. Thus, for practical purposes, only three chemicals of the nearly 500 tested induced only thyroid gland tumours: 3-amino-4-ethoxy-acetanilide, *N,N*'-diethylthiourea, and trimethyl-thiourea.

Four chemicals caused tumours of the thyroid gland in each of the tested experimental groups: 2,4-diaminoanisole sulfate, ethylene thiourea (ETU), 4,4'-methylenedianiline dihydrochloride, and 4,4'-thiodianiline. One other chemical – 4,4'-oxydianiline – caused thyroid gland tumours in three of the four groups. Moreover, three of the positive chemicals were anilines and three others were thiourea derivatives.

Regarding gender or species specificity, 24 chemicals were associated with thyroid tumours in male rats, 20 in female rats, 14 in male mice, and 12 in female mice. This represents a more balanced sensitivity than was seen for the kidney or for the urinary bladder. For both C cell and follicular cell tumours in control rats, the incidences increased

considerably between 104 weeks and 140–146 weeks (Solleveld *et al.*, 1984). Twenty of the 39 chemicals were mutagenic to *Salmonella*.

Comparative target sites

Considering the three tumour-organ sites collectively, rats appear to be more responsive than mice to chemicals inducing tumours at these sites. This is especially true for kidneys and urinary bladder.

In this data set of chemicals, several cause tumours in two or three of these selected target sites (Table 6). *ortho*-Anisidine hydrochloride not only causes tumours of the urinary bladder in each of the four sex-species groups but also causes tumours of the kidney and thyroid gland in male rats. Chloroprene represents the one chemical that causes tumours at each of the three sites in both sexes of rats, and kidney tumours in male mice as well. Still others have some interesting carcinogenic features (Table 7). For example, salicylazo-sulfapyridine is a goitrogen that does not induce tumours of the thyroid gland, yet does cause tumours of the kidney and urinary bladder (National Toxicology Program, 1997).

Tumour rates in control animals

Background, naturally occurring, or 'spontaneous' tumour rates for these three target sites are low, compared to other more common spontaneous tumours in laboratory animals (Table 8) (Haseman *et al.*, 1990; Haseman & Elwell, 1996). One exception to these low control rates is C cell tumours of the thyroid gland in Fischer 344 rats.

Of course different species, strains, and genders often vary with respect to tumour incidence at a given organ site. As examples, C57BL/6 mice have a much lower liver tumour rate than do C3H mice, female Sprague-Dawley rats have considerably more mammary tumours than do female Fischer 344 rats, and Fischer 344 rats have a high rate of leukaemias and tumours of the testis. In fact, contra-intuitively perhaps, organ systems with very high control rates of tumours rarely if ever are associated with carcinogenic effects. Interstitial cell tumours of the testis in male Fischer rats, for instance, have never been evaluated by NTP as being a carcinogenic response to a chemical.

Therefore, one needs to know some historical context of background tumour rates before

Table 5. Chemicals associated with site-specific tumour induction in thyroid gland
[follicular cell tumours unless noted otherwise]

Technical report no.	Chemical name	Salmonella[a]	Route	MR	FR	MM	FM	Other tumour sites
				Levels of Evidence of Carcinogenicity[b]				
021	Aldrin	–	Feed	[E]	[E]	P	N	Yes
112	3-Amino-4-ethoxyacetanilide	+	Feed	N	N	[P]	N	No
089	o-Anisidine hydrochloride	nd	Feed	[P]	P	P	P	Yes
069	Azinphosmethyl	+W,+	Feed	[E]	N	N	N	Yes
452	2,2-Bis[bromomethyl]-1,3-propanediol	–,+	Feed	[CE]	[CE]	CE	C	Yes
436	tert-Butyl alcohol	–	Water	SE	NE	[EE]	[SE]	Yes
308	Chlorinated paraffins: C12, 60% Cl	–	Gavage	CE	[CE]	CE	[CE]	Yes
467	Chloroprene	–	Inhal	[CE]	[CE]	CE	CE	Yes
285	C.I. Basic Red 9 monohydrochloride	+	Feed	[CE]	[CE]	CE	CE	Yes
407	C.I. Pigment Red 3	+	Feed	SE	SE	[SE]	NE	Yes
309	Decabromodiphenyl oxide	–	Feed	SE	SE	[EE]	NE	Yes
084	2,4-Diaminoanisole sulfate [C & F cell][c]	+	Feed	[P]	[P]	[P]	[P]	Yes
149	N,N'-Diethylthiourea	–	Feed	[P]	[P]	N	N	No
388	Ethylene thiourea [ETU]	–,+W	Feed	[CE]	[CE]	[CE]	[CE]	Yes
374	Glycidol	+	Gavage	[CE]	[CE]	CE	CE	Yes
271	HC Blue 1*	+	Feed	EE	SE	E	E	Yes
009	Heptachlor	–	Feed	N	[E]	P	P	Yes
340	Iodinated glycerol	+	Gavage	[SE]	NE	NE	E	Yes
448	Isobutyl nitrite*	+	Inhal	CE	CE	SE	SE	Yes
331	Malonaldehyde, sodium salt	–	Gavage	[CE]	[CE]	NE	NE	Yes
428	Manganese sulfate monohydrate	–	Feed	NE	NE	[EE]	[EE]	No
408	Mercuric chloride*	–	Gavage	SE	EE	EE	NE	Yes
186	4,4'-Methylenebis[N,N-dimethyl]-benzenamine	+	Feed	[P]	[P]	E	P	Yes
248	4,4'-MethylenedianilineDiHCl[C & F cell]	+	Water	[P]	[P]	[P]	[P]	Yes
143	1,5-Naphthalenediamine [C & F cell]	+	Feed	N	P	[P]	[P]	Yes
443 & 468	Oxazepam	–	Feed	EE	NE	CE	[CE]	Yes
205	4,4'-Oxydianiline	+	Feed	[P]	[P]	P	[P]	Yes
016	Phosphamidon [C cell]	+	Feed	E	[E]	N	N	Yes
476	Primidone [Primaclone]	+	Feed	[EE]	NE	[CE]	CE	Yes
231	Stannous chloride [C cell]	–	Feed	[E]	N	N	N	No
209	2,3,7,8-Tetrachlorodibenzo-p-Dioxin	–	Gavage	[P]	P	P	[P]	Yes
131	Tetrachlorodiphenylethane [TDE]	–	Feed	[E]	N	N	N	No
033	Tetrachlorvinphos [C cell]	–	Feed	N	[P]	P	P	Yes
446	1-Trans-Delta-9-Tetrahydrocannabinol	–	Gavage	NE	NE	[EE]	[EE]	No
047	4,4'-Thiodianiline	+	Feed	[P]	[P]	[P]	[P]	Yes
037	Toxaphene	+	Feed	[E]	[E]	P	P	Yes
129	Trimethylthiourea	–	Feed	N	[P]	N	N	No
391	Tris[2-chloroethyl] phosphate*	–	Gavage	CE	CE	EE	EE	Yes
238	Ziram [C cell]	+	Feed	[P]	N	N	E	Yes

Number of chemicals causing tumours in **THYROID GLAND** = 39

[a] Salmonella results: + = Positive; +W = Weakly Positive; ? = Inconclusive; - = Negative
[b] [ ] = Animal group in which tumours of the thyroid glands were observed. CE = Clear evidence of carcinogenicity; P = Evidence of carcinogenicity; SE = Some evidence of carcinogenicity; EE or E = Equivocal evidence of carcinogenicity; NE or N = No Evidence of carcinogenicity; IS = Inadequate experiment; nd = no NCI or NTP data.
[c] [C cell]=chemical causes C cell tumours of the thyroid gland; F = Follicular cell
* Possible association in one sex of one species

Table 6. Chemicals causing tumours at two or three of the selected organs: kidney, urinary bladder, thyroid gland			
Chemical	**Kidney**	**Urinary bladder**	**Thyroid gland**
o-Anisidine HCl	Male rat	Male rat, female rat, Male mice, female mice	Male rat
2,2-bis [Bromomethyl]-1,3-propanediol	Male rat [?] Male mice	Male rat	Male rat Female rat
tert-Butyl alcohol	Male rat		Male mice [?] Female mice
Chlorinated paraffins: C12,60%Cl	Male rat		Female rat, Female mice
Chloroprene	Male rat, Female rat, Male mice	Male rat [?], Female rat [?]	Male rat Female rat
C.I.Pigment red 3	Male mice		Male mice
Glycidol		Male mice [?]	Male rat Female rat
Mercuric chloride	Male mice [E]		Male rat [?]
NTA	Male rat Male mice Female mice	Female rat	
NTA trisodium monohydrate	Male rat Female rat	Female rat	
o-Nitroanisole	Male rat Female rat	Male rat Female rat	
Oxazepam	Male rat [E]		Female mice
Salicylazosulfapyridine	Female rat	Male rat Female rat	
Tris[2-chloroethyl]phosphate	Male rat Female rat Male mice [E]		Male rat [?] Female rat [?]

[?], may have been related to chemical; [E], equivocal evidence of carcinogenicity

attempting to compare across species, strains, or genders – including humans. A further caution is selection of appropriate species and strains and genders when planning and designing long term carcinogenesis experiments, especially if one has information from previous long-term experiments, shorter toxicity studies, or structure-effect correlations regarding likely target organs. For instance, B6C3F$_1$ mice appear to be a relatively insensitive model to study chemicals thought likely to cause kidney or urinary bladder tumours. Similarly, as other examples, one would be ill-advised to use the Fischer 344 rat to study a potential leukaemogen or a likely testicular tumourigen, or to use female Fischer rats to identify a possible carcinogen for the pituitary gland or mammary gland because of the high background rates of these tumours in this particular strain.

Table 7. Interesting chemical grouping observations regarding chemicals causing tumours at these selected sites: kidney, urinary bladder, thyroid gland

Chemical	Observations
1-Amino-2,4-dibromoanthraquinone	**Kidney** and **urinary bladder**, male and female rats
1-Amino-2-methylanthraquinone	**Kidney**, male rat
1,4,5,8-Tetraamino-anthraquinone [CI Disperse Blue 1]	**Urinary bladder**, male and female rats
*2-Amino-4-nitrophenol	**Kidney**, male rat
*4-Amino-2-nitrophenol	**Urinary bladder**, male rat; equivocal female rat
o-Anisidine HCl	**Kidney**, male rat; **urinary bladder,** male and female rats and mice; thyroid gland, male rat
o-Toluidine HCl	**Urinary bladder**, female rat
Aspirin, phenacetin, and caffeine	**Kidney** and **urinary bladder**, equivocal female rat
Phenacetin	**Kidney** and **urinary bladder**, humans and animals
1,3-Butadiene	**Kidney**, female mice,
Chloroprene	**Kidney**, male and female rats, male mice; **urinary bladder**, male [?] and female [?] rats; thyroid gland, male and female rats
Isoprene	**Kidney**, male rats
*m-Cresidine	**Urinary bladder**, male and female rats
p-Cresidine	**Urinary bladder**, both sexes of rats and mice
2-Naphthylamine	**Urinary bladder**, several species including humans
*N-Phenyl-2-naphthylamine	**Kidney**, equivocal in male mice; metabolized to 2-naphthylamine
Salicylazosulfapyridine	**Kidney**, male rats; **urinary bladder**, male and female rats; goitrogen causing no tumours of thyroid glands
Tetrachloroethylene	**Kidney**, male rats
Tetrafluoroethylene	**Kidney**, male and female rats

*Chemicals causing tumours only at this site.

Discussion and conclusions

Organ site specificity is a relatively common outcome of carcinogenicity testing (Haseman et al., 1986; Huff et al., 1991b). That is, many chemicals frequently induce cancers in only one, two, or three organ-systems, and in some cases these organs are rodent-specific with no exact counterpart in humans. Conversely, in many other cases, chemicals affect carcinogenesis in multiple organs, in both genders, of multiple strains and of multiple species.

Target site concordance between laboratory animals and humans does occur with significant frequency. Wilbourn et al. (1986) and others (Tomatis et al., 1989; Huff, 1994a, 1998, 1999) have shown remarkable tissue or organ concordance of carcinogenicity between those agents causing cancer in humans and that have been tested adequately in laboratory animals.

Correspondence between various tumour sites is not a common finding among animals exposed to chemicals; for instance, for the three target sites

Table 8. Background tumour rates for Fischer 344 rats and B6C3F₁ mice			
Male rat	Female rat	Male mice	Female mice
Kidney transitional cell tumours			
2/1352 [0.14%]	1/1348 [0.07%]	1/1351 [0.07%]	0/1349
range = 0–2%	0–2%	0–2%	0%
Kidney tubule cell tumours			
13/1352 [0.14%]	1/1348 [0.07%]	3/1351 [0.07%]	4/1349 [0.03%]
range = 0–6%	0–2%	0–2%	0–2%
Thyroid gland C cell tumours			
195/1347 [14.5%]	182/1347 [13.5%]	2/1343 [0.15%]	0/1340
range = 4–35%	4–24%	0–2%	0%
Thyroid gland follicular cell tumours			
28/11347 [2.08%]	12/1347 [0.89%]	26/1343 [0.15%]	26/1340 [1.94%]
range = 0–8%	0–6%	0–6%	0–8%
Urinary bladder squamous cell tumours			
0/1337	0/1332	0/1325	0/1325
Urinary bladder transitional cell tumours			
4/1337 [0.30%]	4/1332 [0.30%]	1/1325 [0.08%]	0/1325
range = 0–2%	0–2%	0–2%	0%

highlighted in this paper, only one combination is statistically associated: liver and thyroid gland; these rarely occur in the same sex-species group, and even more uncommonly in the same animal. Other organ combinations do occur with a statistical association, however: rat liver and rat Zymbal gland, mouse lung and rat/mouse mammary glands, and mouse lung and mouse forestomach, as examples (Haseman & Lockhart, 1993). These may be valuable when doing necropsy and histopathology because if one observes a grossly visible liver tumour in rats, then one could look more closely at Zymbal glands; likewise, if a liver tumour in mice is found, then step sections of the thyroid glands could be done. Whether this observational knowledge may lead to other insights remains to be discerned.

Other than ionizing radiation and perhaps dioxins (Huff, 1994b; Huff et al., 1994), no other chemicals or occupational exposure circumstances are yet known that induce cancer of the thyroid gland in humans. Further, urinary bladder carcinogens appear to be more common in humans than those inducing tumours of the kidney, although kidney tumours often go undiagnosed or undiscovered (Barrett & Huff, 1991; Huff, 1992). In addition, several other agents are suspected of causing cancer of the urinary bladder in humans, including chlorinated drinking water (Morris, 1995), or kidney cancers, including occupational exposures to trichloroethylene (Henschler et al., 1995; Vamvakas et al., 1998) and to gasoline (Lynge et al.,1997).

Thus, in few instances are there compelling findings to support the notion that species-specific carcinogenic effects occur. Arsenic, for example, has been long cited as an example of an exposure circumstance causing cancer in humans (including cancer of kidney and urinary bladder), and yet has not been shown convincingly to cause cancer in laboratory animals (IARC, 1987). At the same time, one must realize that arsenic has yet to be studied adequately in laboratory animals, and to make a final "exception" conclusion is premature (Chan & Huff, 1997; Huff et al., 1998). Benzene carcinogenicity was another long believed exception to the human-animal paradigm until appropriate and adequate tests were done, showing carcinogenicity in animals in multiple sites, species, strains, and genders carcinogenicity in animals (Huff et al., 1989; Maltoni et al., 1989). Perhaps arsenic will prove to be similar.

More difficult to prove are "species-specific effects" in animals with little or no human data for comparison. In some cases, human data have accrued, dispelling long histories of discounting the initial animal results. Relevant examples include 1,3-butadiene (see Huff et al., 1985 for the first animal data; see Matanoski et al., 1990 for the first human evidence); dioxins (see Kociba et al., 1978 for the animal findings; IARC, 1997 for human data; Huff et al., 1994; Huff, 1994b); vinyl chloride (Viola et al., 1971 and Maltoni & Lefemine, 1974 for first animal data; Creech & Johnson, 1974 for first human data).

Other instances of discovering carcinogenicity in animals and only subsequently in humans (Tomatis, 1979; Huff, 1993; Vainio et al., 1995; IARC, 1997) should give us pause when attempting, by using posed mechanisms or theoretical rodent tumour specificity, to declare any agent that is clearly carcinogenic to animals as being irrelevant to humans. The IARC November 1997 Workshop (this volume) is a tentative beginning of how one might approach these difficult scientific and public health situations.

Acknowledgments

For their useful and constructive comments and suggestions, I thank Joseph Haseman, William Jirles, Ghanta Rao and Jackie Stillwell

References

American Cancer Society (1998) *Cancer Facts and Figures – 1998*. American Cancer society, Atlanta

Barrett, J.C. & Huff, J.E. (1991) Cellular and molecular mechanisms of chemically induced renal carcinogenesis. Chapter 45: 287–306. In: *Nephrotoxicity. Mechanisms,*

Early Diagnosis & Therapeutic Management. Bach P.H., Gregg, J., Wiks, M.F. & Delacruz, L. (eds.) Marcel Dekker, Inc., New York. (Reprinted as revised and updated: Renal Failure 13: 211–225, 1991)

Chan, P. & Huff, J.E. (1997) Arsenic carcinogenesis in animals and in humans: mechanistic, experimental, and epidemiological evidence. *Environ. Carcinog. Ecotox. Rev.,* C15[2], 83–122

Creech, J.L. & Johnson, M.N. (1974) Angiosarcoma of the liver in the manufacture of polyvinyl chloride. *J. Occup. Med.,* **16**, 150–151

Eustis, S.L., Hailey, J.R., Boorman, G.A. & Haseman, J.K. (1994) Utility of multiple-section sampling in the histological evaluation of the kidney for carcinogenicity studies. *Toxicol. Pathol.,* **22**, 457–472

Fung, V.A., Barrett, J.C. & Huff, J.E. (1995) The carcinogenesis bioassay in perspective: application in identifying human cancer hazards. *Environ. Health Perspect.,* **103**, 680–683

Gold, L.S. & Zeiger, E. (eds) (1997) Handbook of Carcinogenic Potency and Genotoxicity Databases. CRC Press, Boca Raton, FL

Haseman, J.K. & Lockhart, A.-M. (1993) Correlations between chemically related site-specific carcinogenic effects in long-term studies in rats & mice. *Environ. Health Perspect.,* **102**, 50–454

Haseman, J.K. & Elwell, M.R. (1996) Evaluation of false positive and false negative outcomes in NTP long-term rodent carcinogenicity studies. *Risk Anal.,* **16**, 813–820

Haseman, J.K., Tharrington, E.C., Huff, J.E. & McConnell, E.E. (1986) Comparison of site-specific and overall tumor incidence analyses for 81 recent National Toxicology Program carcinogenicity studies. *Regul. Toxicol. Pharmacol.,* **6**, 155–170

Haseman, J.K., Eustis, S.L. & Arnold, J. (1990) Tumor incidences in Fischer 344 rats: NTP historical data. In: Boorman, G.A., Eustis, S.L., Elwell, M.R., Montgomery, C.A., MacKensie, W.F. (eds). Pathology of the Fischer Rat. Academic Press, New York. pp. 555–564

Henschler, D., Vamvakas, S., Lammert, M., Dekant, W., Kraus, B., Thomas, B. & Ulm, K.(1995) Increased incidence of renal cell tumors in a cohort of cardboard workers exposed to trichloroethylene. *Arch. Toxicol.,* **69**, 291–299

Huff, J.E. (1992) Chemical toxicity and chemical carcinogenesis. Is there a causal connection? A comparative morphological evaluation of 1500 experiments. In: Vainio, H., Magee, P., McGregor, D. & McMichael, A. (eds). *Mechanisms of Carcinogenesis in Risk Identification.* IARC Sci. Pub. 116: 437-475. International Agency for Research on Cancer, Lyon, France

Huff, J.E. (1993) Chemicals and cancer in humans: first evidence in experimental animals. *Environ. Health Perspect.*, **100**, 201–210

Huff, J.E. (1994a) Chemicals causally associated with cancers in humans and in laboratory animals: A perfect concordance. In: Waalkes, M.P. & Ward, J.M. (eds). *Carcinogenesis*. Raven Press, New York, pp. 25–37

Huff, J.E. (1994b) Dioxins and mammalian carcinogenesis. In: Schecter, A. (ed.) *Dioxins and Health*. Plenum Press, New York, pp. 389–407

Huff, J.E. (1998) Carcinogenesis results in animals predict cancer risks to humans. In: Wallace, R.B. [ed], *Maxcy-Rosenau-Last's Public Health & Preventive Medicine*. 14th Ed. Appleton & Lange, Norwalk, CT, pp. 543–550; 567–569

Huff, J.E. (1999) Value, validity, and historical development of carcinogenesis studies for predicting and confirming carcinogenic risks to humans. In: Kitchin, K.T., ed., *Testing, Predicting, and Interpreting Chemical Carcinogenicity*, Marcel Dekker, pp. 21–123

Huff, J.E., Melnick, R.L., Solleveld, H.A., Haseman, J.K., Powers, M. & Miller, R.A. (1985) Multiple organ carcinogenicity of 1,3-butadiene in B6C3F1 mice after 60 weeks of inhalation exposure. *Science*, **227**, 548–549

Huff, J.E., McConnell, E.E., Haseman, J.K., Boorman, G.A., Eustis, S.L., Schwetz, B.A., Rao, G.N., Jameson, C.W., Hart, L.G. & Rall, D.P. (1988) Carcinogenesis studies: Results from 398 experiments on 104 chemicals from the U.S. National Toxicology Program. *Ann. N.Y. Acad. Sci.*, **534**, 1–30

Huff, J.E., Haseman, J.K., DeMarini, D.M., Eustis, S.L., Maronpot, R.R., Peters, A.C., Persing, R.L., Chrisp, C.E. & Jacobs, A.C. (1989) Multiple-site carcinogenicity of benzene in Fischer rats and B6C3F1 mice. *Environ. Health Perspect.*, **82**, 125–163

Huff, J.E., Haseman, J.K. & Rall, D.P. (1991a) Scientific concepts, value, and significance of chemical carcinogenesis studies. *Ann. Rev. Pharmacol. Toxicol.*, **31**, 621–652

Huff, J.E., Cirvello, J., Haseman, J.K. & Bucher, J.R. (1991b) Chemicals associated with site-specific neoplasia in 1394 long-term carcinogenesis experiments in laboratory rodents. *Environ. Health Perspect.*, **93**, 247–271

Huff, J.E., Lucier, G. & Tritscher, A. (1994) Carcinogenicity of TCDD: experimental, mechanistic, and epidemiologic evidence. *Ann. Rev. Pharmacol. Toxicol.*, **34**, 343–372

Huff, J.E., Chan, P. & Waalkes, M. (1998) Arsenic carcinogenicity testing. *Environ. Health Perspect.* [letter] **106**, A170

IARC (1987) *IARC Monographs on the Evaluation of Carcinogenic Risks to Humans, Supplement 7. Overall Evaluation of Carcinogenicity: An Updating of IARC Monographs, Volumes 1 to 42.* IARC, Lyon, pp. 100–106

IARC (1997) *Polychlorinated dibenzo-para-dioxins and polychlorinated dibenzofurans. IARC Monographs on the Evaluation on the Evaluation of Carcinogenic Risks to Humans.* Volume 65. IARC, Lyon, pp. 33–636

Jokinen MP (1990) Urinary bladder, ureter, and urethra. In: Boorman, G.A., Eustis, S.L., Elwell, M.R., Montgomery, C.A., MacKenzie, W.F., eds, *Pathology of the Fischer Rat. Reference and Atlas*, Academic Press, New York, pp. 105–126

Kociba, R.J., Keyes, D.G., Beyer, J.E., Carreon, R.M., Wade, C.E., Dittenber, D.A., Kalnins, R.P., Frauson, L.E., Park, C.N., Barnard, S.D., Hummel, R.A. & Humiston, C.G. (1978) Results of a two-year chronic toxicity and oncogenicity study of 2,3,7,8-tetrachlorodibenzo-p-dioxin in rats. *Toxicol. Appl. Pharmacol.*, **46**, 279–303

Lynge, E., Andersen, A., Nilsson, R., Barlow, L., Pukkala E., Nordlinder, R., Boffetta, P., Grandjean, P., Heikkila, P., & Horte, L.G. (1997) Risk of cancer and exposure of gasoline vapors. *Am. J. Epidemiol.*, **145**, 449–458

Maltoni, C. & Lefemine, G. (1974) Carcinogenicity bioassays on vinyl chloride. I. Research plan and early results. *Environ. Res.*, **6**, 340–351

Maltoni, C., Cilberti, A., Cotti, G., Conti, B. & Belpoggi, F. (1989) Benzene, an experimental multipotential carcinogen: results of long-term bioassays performed at the Bologna Institute of Oncology. *Environ. Health Perspect.*, **82**, 109–124

Matanoski, G.M., Santos-Burgoa, C. & Schwartz, L. (1990) Mortality of a cohort of workers in the styrene-butadiene polymer manufacturing industry (1943-1982). *Environ. Health Perspect.*, **86**, 107–117

Montesano, R., Bartsch, H., Vainio, H., Wilbourn, J. & Yamasaki, H. (eds) (1986) Long-term and Short-term Assays for Carcinogens. A critical appraisal. IARC Scientic Publication No. 83. International Agency for Research on Cancer. Lyon, France

Morris, R.D. (1995) Drinking water and cancer. *Environ. Health Perspect.*, **103**, [Suppl 8]: 225–231

National Cancer Institute (1999) Survey of Compounds Which Have Been Tested for Carcinogenic Activity. U.S. Public Health Service Publication No. 149, 1951–1999. National Cancer Institute, Bethesda, MD

National Toxicology Program (1986) Toxicology and carcinogenesis studies of CI Disperse Blue 1 [CAS No 2475-45-8] in F344/N rats and B6C3F1 mice (feed studies). NTP Tech Rept Ser No 289. National Toxicology Program, Research Triangle Park, NC

National Toxicology Program (1997) Toxicology and carcinogenesis studies of Salicylazosulfapyridine [CAS No 599-79-1] in F344/N rats and B6C3F1 mice (gavage studies). NTP Tech Rept Ser No 457. National Toxicology Program, Research Triangle Park, NC

Ries, L.A.G., Kosary, C.L., Hankey, B.F., Miller, B.A., Harras, A. & Edwards, B.K. (eds) (1997) SEER Cancer Statistics Review, 1973-1994. NIH Pub No 97-2789. National Cancer Institute, Bethesda, MD

Solleveld, H.A., Haseman, J.K. & McConnell, E.E. (1984) Natural history of body weight gain, survival, and neoplasia in the F344 rat. *J. Natl Cancer Inst.*, **72**, 929–940

Tomatis, L. (1979) The predictive value of rodent carcinogenicity tests in the evaluation of human risks. *Ann. Rev. Pharmacol. Toxicol.*, **19**, 511–530

Tomatis, L., Aitio, A., Wilbourn, J. & Shuker, L. (1989) Human carcinogens so far identified. *Jpn J. Cancer Res.*, **80**, 795–807

Vainio, H., Wilbourn, J., Sasco, A.J., Partensky, C., Gaudin, N., Heseltine, E. & Eragne, I. (1995) Identification of human carcinogenic risk in IARC Monographs. *Bull. Cancer,* **82**, 339–348 (in French)

Vamvakas, S., Bruning, T., Thomasson, B., Lammert, M., Baumuller, A., Bolt, H.M., Dekant, W., Birner, G., Henschler, D. & Ulm, K. (1998) Renal cell cancer correlated with occupational exposure to trichloroethlene. *J. Cancer Res. Clin. Oncol.*, **124**, 374–382

Viola, P.L., Bigotti, A. & Caputo, A. (1971) Oncogenic response of rat skin, lungs, and bone to vinyl chloride. *Cancer Res.*, 31, 516–522

Wilbourn, J., Haroun, L., Heseltine, E., Kaldor, J., Partensky, C. & Vainio, H. (1986) Response of experimental animals to human carcinogens: an analysis based upon the IARC Monographs Programme. *Carcinogenesis,* 7, 1853–1863

Corresponding author

James Huff
National Institute of Environmental Health Sciences,
PO Box 12233
Research Triangle Park
NC 27709, USA